# Violence
## IN
# Families

## Assessing Prevention and Treatment Programs

Rosemary Chalk and Patricia A. King, Editors

Committee on the Assessment of Family Violence Interventions
Board on Children, Youth, and Families

Commission on Behavioral and Social Sciences and Education
National Research Council
and
Institute of Medicine

NATIONAL ACADEMY PRESS
Washington, D.C. 1998

NOTICE: The project that is the subject of this report was approved by the Governing Board of the National Research Council, whose members are drawn from the councils of the National Academy of Sciences, the National Academy of Engineering, and the Institute of Medicine. The members of the committee responsible for the report were chosen for their special competences and with regard for appropriate balance.

This report has been reviewed by a group other than the authors according to procedures approved by a Report Review Committee consisting of members of the National Academy of Sciences, the National Academy of Engineering, and the Institute of Medicine.

This study was supported by the Carnegie Corporation of New York under contract number B5936, the U.S. Department of Health and Human Services under contract number HPU 940003, and the U.S. Department of Justice under contract 95-1J-CX-0001. Any opinions, findings, conclusions, or recommendations expressed in this publication are those of the author(s) and do not necessarily reflect the view of the organizations or agencies that provided support for this project.

### Library of Congress Cataloging-in-Publication Data

Violence in families : assessing prevention and treatment programs /
Rosemary Chalk and Patricia A. King, editors ; Committee on the
Assessment of Family Violence Interventions, Board on Children,
Youth, and Families, National Research Council and Institute of
Medicine.
p. cm.
Includes bibliographical references (p. ) and index.
ISBN 0-309-05496-6 (cloth)
1. Family violence—United States—Prevention—Evaluation.
2. Crisis intervention (Psychiatry)—United States—Evaluation.
3. Evaluation research (Social action programs)—United States.
I. Chalk, Rosemary A. II. King, Patricia A., 1942-  . III. Board on
Children, Youth, and Families (U.S.). Committee on the Assessment
of Family Violence Interventions.
HV6626.2.V56 1998
362.82'927'0973—dc21                                     97-45375

## COMMITTEE ON THE ASSESSMENT OF
## FAMILY VIOLENCE INTERVENTIONS

PATRICIA A. KING (*Chair*), Georgetown University Law Center
JACQUELYN C. CAMPBELL, Johns Hopkins University School of Nursing
DAVID S. CORDRAY, Vanderbilt Institute for Public Policy Studies
DIANA J. ENGLISH, Office of Children's Administration Research,
    Department of Social and Health Services, State of Washington
JEFFREY A. FAGAN, School of Public Health, Columbia University
RICHARD J. GELLES, Family Violence Research Program, University of
    Rhode Island
JOEL B. GREENHOUSE, Department of Statistics, Carnegie Mellon University
THE HONORABLE SCOTT HARSHBARGER, Office of the Attorney
    General, Commonwealth of Massachusetts
DARNELL F. HAWKINS, Departments of African-American Studies and
    Sociology, University of Illinois, Chicago
THE HONORABLE CINDY LEDERMAN, Eleventh Judicial Circuit of
    Florida, Miami
ELIZABETH McLOUGHLIN, San Francisco Injury Center, San Francisco
    General Hospital
ELI NEWBERGER, Family Development Program, Children's Hospital,
    Boston
JOY D. OSOFSKY, Department of Pediatrics and Psychiatry, Louisiana State
    University Medical Center
HELEN RODRIGUEZ-TRIAS, Pediatrician/Consultant in Health
    Programming, Brookdale, California
SUSAN SCHECHTER, School of Social Work, University of Iowa
MICHAEL E. SMITH, School of Law, University of Wisconsin, Madison
BILL WALSH, Investigations Unit, Youth and Family Crimes Bureau, Dallas
    Police Department
CAROLE L. WARSHAW, Cook County Hospital, Chicago
ROSALIE WOLF, Institute on Aging, The Medical Center of Central
    Massachusetts, Worcester

JACK P. SHONKOFF (*Liaison*), Board on Children, Youth, and Families
CATHY SPATZ WIDOM (*Liaison*), Committee on Law and Justice,
    Commission on Behavioral and Social Sciences and Education

ROSEMARY CHALK, *Study Director*
NANCY CROWELL, *Staff Officer*
KATHERINE DARKE, *Research Assistant*
SEBLE MENKIR, *Research Assistant* (through August 1995)
CINDY PRINCE, *Project Assistant*
NIANI SUTARDJO, *Project Assistant* (through August 1996)

# Contents

# Tables and Figures

## TABLES

## FIGURES

The National Academy of Sciences is a private, nonprofit, self-perpetuating society of distinguished scholars engaged in scientific and engineering research, dedicated to the furtherance of science and technology and to their use for the general welfare. Upon the authority of the charter granted to it by the Congress in 1863, the Academy has a mandate that requires it to advise the federal government on scientific and technical matters. Dr. Bruce M. Alberts is president of the National Academy of Sciences.

The National Academy of Engineering was established in 1964, under the charter of the National Academy of Sciences, as a parallel organization of outstanding engineers. It is autonomous in its administration and in the selection of its members, sharing with the National Academy of Sciences the responsibility for advising the federal government. The National Academy of Engineering also sponsors engineering programs aimed at meeting national needs, encourages education and research, and recognizes the superior achievements of engineers. Dr. William A. Wulf is president of the National Academy of Engineering.

The Institute of Medicine was established in 1970 by the National Academy of Sciences to secure the services of eminent members of appropriate professions in the examination of policy matters pertaining to the health of the public. The Institute acts under the responsibility given to the National Academy of Sciences by its congressional charter to be an adviser to the federal government and, upon its own initiative, to identify issues of medical care, research, and education. Dr. Kenneth I. Shine is president of the Institute of Medicine.

The National Research Council was organized by the National Academy of Sciences in 1916 to associate the broad community of science and technology with the Academy's purposes of furthering knowledge and advising the federal government. Functioning in accordance with general policies determined by the Academy, the Council has become the principal operating agency of both the National Academy of Sciences and the National Academy of Engineering in providing services to the government, the public, and the scientific and engineering communities. The Council is administered jointly by both Academies and the Institute of Medicine. Dr. Bruce M. Alberts and Dr. William A. Wulf are chairman and vice chairman, respectively, of the National Research Council.

# Preface

In May 1993, a group of 35 research scholars, state and federal officials, and representatives from law enforcement, social services, and health care systems met at the Wingspread Conference Center in Racine, Wisconsin. The purpose of this meeting was to examine whether it would be feasible to synthesize the body of research knowledge that had emerged in the past few decades regarding the development, implementation, and effectiveness of interventions designed to treat and prevent family violence. The participants agreed that efforts are needed to bridge the gap that now exists between research resources and policy needs in addressing the problem of family violence, and that one way to address this gap is to synthesize the rigorous evaluations of public-sector programs designed to treat or reduce incidents of child and spousal abuse and abuse of the elderly. They emphasized that, although no single strategy for prevention or treatment has yet proven to be effective in the research literature, the existing evaluations of relevant program interventions should be identified and analyzed to disseminate important lessons learned from past efforts to reduce family violence.

In response to the guidance of the Wingspread meeting participants, the Board on Children, Youth, and Families of the Commission on Behavioral and Social Sciences and Education (CBASSE) of the National Research Council (NRC) and the Institute of Medicine (IOM) established a Committee on the Assessment of Family Violence Interventions in August 1994. Funding was provided by several agencies within the U.S. Department of Health and Human Services (DHHS) and the U.S. Department of Justice (DOJ). The sponsoring agencies within DHHS include the Centers for Disease Control and Prevention, the Administration for Children and Families, the Office of Maternal and Child

Health, the National Institute of Mental Health, and the Substance Abuse and Mental Health Services Administration. The National Institute of Justice was the DOJ sponsor. Funding was also provided by the Carnegie Corporation of New York. The Office of Health Promotion and Disease Prevention within DHHS served a valuable administrative role in coordinating the DHHS agency contributions for this project.

This study is the latest in a series of reports by the NRC that examine the emerging social science research base on violence and families. It builds on five earlier NRC publications related to this topic.

*Understanding and Preventing Violence—Volume 1* (National Academy Press, 1993). This report is a comprehensive review of America's experience of violence, taking an interdisciplinary approach to examining the causes and consequences of interpersonal violence. The report includes a chapter on violence in families that describes the array of family violence interventions, research findings about police interventions and battered women's shelters, and the difficulties of evaluating and comparing interventions in this area.

*Understanding and Preventing Violence—Volume 3: Social Influences* (National Academy Press, 1994). This volume includes four background papers that review research on violent victimization; violence between spouses and intimates; gender and interpersonal violence; and the role of alcohol and psychoactive drugs in violent events. The paper on spousal and intimate violence by Jeffrey Fagan and Angela Browne examines the state of empirical and theoretical knowledge on violence between adult partners and presents a social epidemiology of intimate violence, characteristics of victims and assailants, and an assessment of risk markers for marital violence.

*Understanding Child Abuse and Neglect* (National Academy Press, 1993). This report presents a research agenda for studies of child maltreatment. It reviews the state of research on different forms of child maltreatment, including physical and sexual abuse, emotional maltreatment, and neglect. The research agenda emphasizes the importance of studies that address the nature and scope of child maltreatment, its causes and consequences, the assessment of prevention and treatment interventions, and the need for a science policy to guide the development of research in this field.

*Violence and the American Family* (National Academy Press, 1994). This workshop report presents a summary of the Wingspread meeting that called for the development of an in-depth analysis of the state of knowledge regarding family violence interventions.

*Understanding Violence Against Women* (National Academy Press, 1996). The result of a study requested by Congress in the 1994 Omnibus Crime Prevention Act, this report presents an agenda for research on intimate partner violence and sexual assault. The study identifies gaps in the knowledge base in this area and recommends a strategy for building comprehensive and interdisciplinary studies that can examine the causes and consequences, nature and scope, and prevention and intervention for violence against women.

These NRC reports provide important insights into what is known about interventions in the field of family violence. But their assessment of rigorous evaluation studies of treatment and prevention programs is limited. In this study, our committee sought to extract knowledge from research concerning the evaluations of family violence interventions as well as insights reported in other assessments of selected interventions. The committee met six times over a 24-month period to identify major conceptual themes and to review the relevant knowledge base in formulating its conclusions and recommendations. This synthesis of research and program evaluation knowledge was augmented by expert opinion through two workshops, commissioned papers, consultant reports, and five site visits designed to draw on the experiences and insights of service providers in the health, social service, and legal communities. The study also included a review of the methodological issues associated with research in areas characterized by weak conceptual clarity and immature measurement (Institute of Medicine, 1994).

The committee benefited from an inter-agency working group organized to help guide the early stages of development and the dissemination of this study and to share agency research resources. Program officers from the sponsoring agencies also participated in the committee workshops. We are grateful to each of these officials for their thoughtful contributions over the course of the study: Bernard Auchter and Christy Visher from the National Institute of Justice; Ashley Files, Matthew Guidry, and James Harrell from the Office of Health Promotion and Disease Prevention; Lynn Short from the Centers for Disease Control and Prevention; Frank Sullivan from the Substance Abuse and Mental Health Services Administration; Audrey Yowell from the Office of Maternal and Child Health; Malcolm Gordon from the National Institute of Mental Health; William Riley from the Administration for Children and Families; and Michael Levine from the Carnegie Corporation of New York.

The committee's study identification and data collection effort required an extensive staff effort; these studies appeared in dozens of journals and had not been previously assembled into a research database. Study director Rosemary Chalk and research assistants Katherine Darke and Seble Menkir, in consultation with committee member David Cordray, identified search strategies and citation indexes to gather the appropriate studies. The results of their effort are presented in Tables 3-1 and 3-2. Katherine Darke provided an important contribution in the preparation of the individual research review tables that are included in Chapters 4 through 6.

The committee held two workshops in Washington, D.C. to inform its deliberations. The first workshop was designed to elicit expertise and perspective from service providers associated with treatment and prevention interventions in child maltreatment, domestic violence, and elder abuse. Background papers prepared by the workshop participants were published in an interim report by the committee (*Service Provider Perspectives on Family Violence Interventions,* 1995). The participants observed that much of the information regarding family violence programs does not appear in the research literature, and that reforms in community-based interventions have not been studied in a systematic manner.

The second workshop focused on evaluation methods and research designs associated with the assessment of family violence interventions. The participants included researchers who had studied selected interventions in health care, social services, and law enforcement settings. They reviewed specific methodological challenges and creative strategies that have been used in the selection and retention of research subjects, the ethical and legal concerns associated with research in this field, and the quality of data that is associated with administrative records in public agencies.

The site visits were coordinated by Katherine Darke, who contacted local organizations and developed comprehensive itineraries for committee members and staff in each of the five cities that served as the subjects of these meetings (Boston, Dallas, New York City, Miami, and Seattle). A detailed listing of these organizations is included in Appendix A.

Several consultants provided background information that was very helpful to the committee's work. Jodi Short and Joseph Youngblood contributed materials on the nature and scope of family violence and federal intervention programs (Chapter 2). Anne Flitcraft, Patti Culross, Patricia Mrazek, and Michelle Forcier prepared background materials on health care interventions for domestic violence (Chapter 6). Terry Fulmer and Georgia Anetzberger prepared a research review on elder abuse interventions that informed several chapters. The material in Chapter 3 that pertains to client referrals, screening, and baseline assessment benefited from a publication prepared by Georgine Pion and David Cordray (Cordray and Pion, 1993). Chapter 5 benefited from contributions by Diane Juliar and Juliana Blome and a research paper on legal interventions for family violence developed by Alissa Pollitz Worden. The committee is grateful to all these contributors.

The committee also benefited from the tremendous support of the staff of the Board on Children, Youth, and Families and the Institute of Medicine: Cynthia Abel, Nancy Crowell, Katherine Darke, Seble Menkir, Faith Mitchell, Deborah Phillips, and Michael Stoto contributed careful readings, draft chapters, and literature searches that identified relevant materials throughout the development of the project. Lauren R. Meader, Julie Walko, and Susan M. Fourt of the National Research Council Library provided invaluable assistance in identifying and collecting research materials. Special thanks are due to senior project assistants Niani Sutardjo and Cindy Prince who provided administrative support during the study, including the organization of meetings, workshops, and the preparation of several drafts of the report. Project assistants Karen Autrey and Roger Butts helped to prepare the final draft for publication. Communications director Anne

Bridgman was particularly helpful in the final stages of preparing the report and planning its dissemination. We also thank our editors Rona Briere and Christine McShane, whose efforts contributed significantly to the organization and presentation of the panel's views. Most of all, thanks and acknowledgment of extraordinary effort are due to the members of the committee and our study director Rosemary Chalk.

> Patricia A. King, *Chair*
> Committee on the Assessment of
> Family Violence Interventions

# Violence

## IN

# Families

## Assessing Prevention and Treatment Programs

# Executive Summary

In the past three decades, family violence—which includes child maltreatment, domestic violence, and elder abuse—has emerged as a major social, health, and law enforcement issue. In addition to child and adult homicides, family violence contributes to a broad array of fatal and nonfatal injuries and medical and psychiatric disorders each year. In addition, family violence has been associated with numerous social problems, including teenage pregnancy, runaway and homeless youth, alcoholism and substance abuse, and crime and delinquency. The association of family violence victimization with such an extensive range of health, mental health, and behavioral dysfunctions suggests that interventions that can lead to the reduction or prevention of family violence would contribute to the resolution of these other problems as well.

The rate of family violence victimization in the U.S. population is widely regarded as a serious problem that affects large numbers of children and adults, but there are currently no generally agreed-on national statistics that measure the experience with family violence across the life span. Varying estimates of the scope of the different forms of family violence exist that draw on self-report surveys, crime reports, and child protective services records. Recent government surveys indicate that almost 3 million children in the United States are annually reported to child protective services agencies as alleged victims of maltreatment (including neglect, physical abuse, sexual abuse, and emotional maltreatment), and at least one-third of these cases are confirmed. National crime victimization surveys indicate that the rate of reported violent attacks by family members was 9.3 per 1,000 in 1992-1993. Other self-report surveys have indicated annual rates of domestic violence that range from 12 per 1,000 (for acts of marital rape) to 116

*1*

per 1,000 (for any act of violence). There are no self-report surveys of elder abuse, and the surveys of elder abuse reporting and recognition are incomplete.

The U.S. General Accounting Office has estimated that treatment services for child maltreatment alone (such as child protective services, child mental health services, and court expenses) cost in the range of $500 million annually. Preliminary estimates of the costs of direct services and enforcement efforts aimed at family violence in Canada range between $1.5 and $4.2 billion. These estimates are generally regarded as conservative, since family violence may be a hidden but contributing factor to injuries, disorders, and crimes for which services or enforcement efforts are provided.

The urgency and magnitude of the problem of family violence have caused policy makers, service providers, and advocates to take action in the absence of scientific knowledge that could inform policy and practice. The rush to *do something* has resulted in a broad array of community agency services, law enforcement approaches, and health care practices—a wealth of program experimentation that is extensive but uncoordinated. Most interventions have their origins in local and national advocacy efforts, and as such they have remained largely undocumented and unanalyzed in the research literature. Programs are often put into place without collecting baseline information about existing services or client characteristics, testing preliminary designs, or specifying—let alone measuring—the outcomes that the interventions are expected to achieve.

Existing interventions include child and adult protective services, battered women's shelters, special police and prosecution units focused on child maltreatment and domestic violence, victim advocates in health and law enforcement agencies, fatality review teams, guidelines and treatment protocols for health care providers, family support services (including home visitation and intensive family preservation services), and child advocacy centers. They can be arrayed conceptually along a continuum of strategies that include prevention, identification, protection, treatment, enforcement, punishment, and deterrence. Many services have been put into place with limited resources. The extent to which interventions have been implemented as designed is seldom documented, and often they are not fully implemented because of budget shortages in local agencies.

For the research community, service providers, program sponsors, and policymakers, the challenge is to determine if and where the research evidence is sufficient to guide a critical examination of selected components of family violence interventions. This examination is complicated by the fragmentation and uneven distribution of the research and program literature. Service providers and researchers who focus on one type of family violence or one institutional setting (social services, law enforcement, or health care) are often unfamiliar with key interventions and research evaluations in other areas. Yet there are multiple interventions focused directly or indirectly on family violence alongside each other in most communities, raising important but unexamined questions about interactive and synergistic effects.

Services are separated by the institutional settings and community jurisdictions in which they are located. Family violence interventions may focus on victims, offenders, service providers, witnesses, families, or communities. Interventions are generally specific to a certain type of maltreatment. Although many different agencies play important roles in seeking to prevent, identify, treat, or punish family violence, their efforts are largely uncoordinated. As a result, they lack shared strategies and common frameworks that could guide efforts to identify common goals, create common measures of service performance, pool resources when appropriate, and guide the implementation and development of selected interventions.

## THE ROLE OF SCIENCE IN THE
## ASSESSMENT OF INTERVENTIONS

In reviewing the research literature on evaluations of family violence interventions, the Committee on the Assessment of Family Violence Interventions identified 114 evaluation studies conducted in the period 1980-1996 that have sufficient scientific strength to provide inferences about the effects of specific interventions in the area of child maltreatment, domestic violence, and elder abuse. Because the committee was charged with focusing on questions about the effectiveness of interventions (rather than, for example, questions about the severity of the problem of family violence or the process of implementing interventions), we identified a core group of studies for review that included a control or comparison group (rather than simply conducting pre- and postintervention studies on the clients of a specific treatment or prevention program). Hundreds of other descriptive research studies or process evaluations have been published that provide other insights into the characteristics of an intervention and its clientele, but they do not have sufficient rigor to examine the impact or the relative effectiveness of the intervention compared with other treatment or prevention efforts.

In most cases, the set of 114 studies that forms the evidentiary base for this report also used reliable research instrumentation to measure the impact of the intervention itself on child or adult cognitive skills, attitudes, behavior, and physical and mental health as well as the impact on rates of family violence reports. However, it is important to note that comparison groups can be severely distorted by selection bias, differential attrition, and failure to consider critical unmeasured differences among groups—factors that have plagued the literature in the family violence area. In addition, the number of participants in these individual evaluation studies is often very small, which reduces their strength in examining the overall effectiveness of the intervention in addressing family violence. What can be said about the relative effectiveness of specific innovative interventions is also limited by the absence of reliable research information about the nature, quality, and impact of existing community services.

A critical review of this core group of studies illuminates both the quality of

TABLE S-1  Total Number of Quasi-Experimental
Evaluations of Family Violence Interventions by Service
Sector, 1980-1996

|  | Type of Family Violence | | |
| --- | --- | --- | --- |
| Service Sector | Child Maltreatment | Domestic Violence | Elder Abuse |
| Social service | 50 | 7 | 2 |
| Legal | 4 | 19 | 0 |
| Health care | 24 | 8 | 0 |

SOURCE: Committee on the Assessment of Family Violence Interventions,
National Research Council and Institute of Medicine, 1998.

the family violence evaluation research and the developmental history of this
field. Almost half of the studies identified (50 of 114 studies) involve evaluations
of social service interventions for child maltreatment (see Table S-1). The majority of evaluations of domestic violence interventions (19 of 34 studies) focus on
law enforcement strategies. Rigorous evaluations for elder abuse interventions in
any institutional setting are almost nonexistent. Evaluations of any type of family violence intervention in health care settings (with the exception of home
visitation programs) are comparatively rare.

In some areas, nevertheless, the body of research is sufficient to inform
policy choices, program development, evaluation research, data collection, and
theory building; the committee's conclusions and policy recommendations about
these interventions are highlighted below. In other areas, although the research
base is not yet mature enough to guide policy and program development, in the
committee's judgment some interventions are ready for rigorous evaluation studies. For this second tier of interventions, the committee makes recommendations
for future evaluation studies, also presented below. The committee has also
identified a set of four topics for basic research that reflect current insights into
the nature of family violence and trends in family violence interventions.

## CONCLUSIONS

The committee's conclusions are derived from our analysis of the research
literature as well as discussions with service providers:

• Findings from small-scale studies are often adopted into policy and professional practice without sufficient independent replication or reflection on their
possible shortcomings;
• Identification and treatment interventions predominate over preventive

strategies in all areas of family violence, reflecting a current emphasis on after-the-fact interventions rather than proactive approaches in the design of interventions;

- Interventions exist in an uncoordinated system of services whose effects interact on the problem of family violence in a way that presents a major challenge to their evaluation;

- Secondary prevention efforts have emerged in some areas (such as home visitation services and child witness to violence interventions) that show some promise of impact on the problem of family violence by concentrating services on targeted populations at risk;

- An increasing emphasis on the need for integration of services is stimulating interest in comprehensive and cross-problem approaches that can address family violence in the context of other problem behaviors; and

- The duration and intensity of the mental health and social support services needed to influence behaviors that result from or contribute to family violence may be greater than initially estimated.

## RECOMMENDATIONS FOR CURRENT POLICIES AND PRACTICES

It is premature to offer policy recommendations for most family violence interventions in the absence of a research base that consists of well-designed evaluations. However, the committee has identified two areas (home visitation and intensive family preservation services) in which a rigorous set of studies offers important guidance to policy makers and service providers. In four other areas—reporting practices, batterer treatment programs, record keeping, and collaborative law enforcement strategies—the committee has drawn on its judgment and deliberations to encourage policy makers and service providers to take actions that are consistent with the state of the current research base.

**Recommendation 1: The committee recommends that states initiate evaluations of their current reporting laws addressing family violence to examine whether and how early case detection leads to improved outcomes for the victims or families and promote changes based on sound research. In particular, the committee recommends that states refrain from enacting mandatory reporting laws for domestic violence until such systems have been tested and evaluated by research.**

In reviewing the research base associated with the relationship between reporting systems and the treatment and prevention of family violence, we observed that no existing evaluation studies can demonstrate the value of mandatory reporting systems compared with voluntary reporting procedures in addressing child maltreatment or domestic violence. For elder abuse, studies suggest that a high level of public and professional awareness and the availability of comprehensive services to identify, treat, and prevent violence are preferable to reporting requirements in improving rates of case detection.

The absence of a research base to support mandatory reporting systems raises questions as to whether they should be recommended for all areas of family violence. The committee therefore suggests that it is important for the states to proceed cautiously at this time and to delay adopting a mandatory reporting system in the area of domestic violence until the positive and negative impacts of such a system have been rigorously examined in states in which domestic violence reports are now required by law. In the committee's view, mandatory reporting systems have some disadvantages in cases involving domestic violence, especially if the victim objects to such reports, if comprehensive community protections and services are not available, and if the victim is able to gain access to therapeutic treatment or support services in the absence of a reporting system.

**Recommendation 2: In the absence of research that demonstrates that a specific model of treatment can reduce violent behavior for many domestic violence offenders, courts need to put in place early warning systems to detect failure to comply with or complete treatment and signs of new abuse or retaliation against victims, as well as to address unintended or inadvertent results that may arise from the referral to or experience with treatment.**

Court mandates for treatment are becoming increasingly widespread in the area of domestic violence, but the effectiveness of batterer treatment has not been examined in rigorous scientific studies. The research base does not yet suggest a specific treatment model that is appropriate for most batterers. Batterer treatment programs may be helpful for some offenders but require stronger mechanisms to enforce referrals, to establish penalties for failure to comply with program requirements, to identify and develop program components that can address the needs of different types of batterers, and to consider the unintended or inadvertent results that may be a consequence of the treatment program, such as the possible desensitizing effects of an offender's recognition that other individuals are batterers or exposure to experiences with diverse forms of violent or coercive behavior.

**Recommendation 3: The committee recommends that health care and social service providers develop safeguards to strengthen their documentation of abuse and histories of family violence in both individual and group records, regardless of whether the abuse is reported to authorities.**

Such documentation should be designed to record voluntary disclosures by both victims and offenders and to enhance early and coordinated interventions that can provide a therapeutic response to experiences with abuse or neglect. Safeguards are required, however, to ensure that such documentation does not lead to victim stigmatization, encourage discriminatory practices, or violate assurances of privacy and confidentiality.

**Recommendation 4: Collaborative strategies among caseworkers, police, prosecutors, and judges are recommended as law enforcement interventions that have the potential to improve the batterer's compliance with treatment as well as the certainty of the use of sanctions in addressing domestic violence.**

In the committee's view, collaborative law enforcement strategies that create a web of social control for offenders are worth testing to determine if such efforts can achieve a significant deterrent effect in addressing domestic violence. Collaborative strategies include such efforts as victim support and offender tracking systems that are designed to increase the likelihood that domestic violence cases will be prosecuted when an arrest has been made, that sanctions and treatment services will be imposed when evidence exists to confirm the charges brought against the offender, and that penalties will be invoked for failure to comply with treatment conditions. Creating the deterrent effect, however, requires extensive coordination and reciprocity among diverse sectors of the law enforcement and social services community that may be difficult to implement and evaluate.

Early efforts to control domestic violence through deterrence relied on single strategies (such as the use of arrest) that have now been studied. Although the arrest studies provide empirical support for the use of deterrence in dealing with specific groups of batterers, the differing effects of arrest for employed/unemployed and married/unmarried individuals call into question the reliance of law enforcement officers on arrest as the sole or central component of their response to domestic violence incidents in communities where domestic violence cases are not routinely prosecuted, where sanctions are not imposed by the courts, or where victim support programs are not readily available. What remains to be determined is whether collaborative approaches have the ability to establish deterrence for larger numbers or different types of batterers and how the costs and benefits of increased agency coordination compare with those that could be achieved by a single law enforcement strategy (such as arrest) in dealing with different populations of offenders and victims.

**Recommendation 5: As part of a comprehensive prevention strategy for child maltreatment, the committee recommends that home visitation programs should be particularly encouraged for first-time parents living in social settings with high rates of child maltreatment reports.**

Evaluation studies are needed to determine the factors that may influence the effectiveness of home visitation programs, including (1) the conditions under which home visitation services are provided as part of a continuum of family support programs, (2) the types of parenting behaviors that are most and least amenable to change as a result of home visitation, (3) the duration and intensity of services (including amounts and types of training for home visitors) that are necessary to achieve positive outcomes for high-risk families, (4) the experience of fathers in general and of families in diverse ethnic communities in particular with home visitation interventions, and (5) the need for follow-up services once the period of home visitation has ended.

**Recommendation 6: Intensive family preservation services represent an important part of the continuum of family support services, but they should not be required in every situation in which a child is recommended for out-of-home placement.**

Research findings suggest that intensive family preservation services do not show an ability to resolve underlying family dysfunction or to improve child well-being or family functioning in most families.  However, methodological shortcomings in these studies suggest that measures of child health, safety, and well-being often are not included in evaluations of intensive family preservation services, so it is difficult to determine their impact on children's outcomes as well as placement rates and levels of family functioning.  It is particularly important to include evidence of recurrence of abuse of the child or other family members. Intensive family preservation services may provide important benefits to the child, family, and community in the form of emergency assistance, improved family functioning, better housing and environmental conditions, and increased collaboration among discrete service systems.  These services may also result in child endangerment, however, when a child remains in family environments that threaten the health or physical safety of the child or other family members.

## RESEARCH RECOMMENDATIONS

Determining which interventions should be selected for rigorous and in-depth evaluations in the future will acquire increased importance as the array of family violence interventions expands in social services, law, and health care settings.  For this reason, clear criteria and guiding principles are necessary to guide sponsoring agencies in their efforts to determine which types of interventions are suitable for evaluation research.  Recognizing that all promising interventions cannot be evaluated, public and private agencies need to consider how to invest research resources in areas that show programmatic potential as well as an adequate research foundation.  To assist in this evaluation selection process, the committee developed the following guiding principles:

1. An intervention should be mature enough to warrant evaluation.
2. An intervention should be different enough from existing services that its critical components can be evaluated.
3. Service providers should be willing to collaborate with the researchers and appropriate data should be accessible in the service records.
4. Satisfactory measures should exist to assess service processes and client outcomes.

5. Adequate time and resources should be available to conduct a quality assessment.

With these principles in mind, the committee has identified a set of interventions that are the focus of current policy attention and service innovation efforts but have not received significant attention from research. In the committee's judgment, each of these nine interventions has reached a level of maturation and preliminary description in the research literature to justify their selection as strong candidates for future evaluation studies: (1) family violence training for health and social service providers and law enforcement officials; (2) universal screening for family violence victims in health care and child welfare settings; (3) comprehensive community initiatives; (4) shelter programs and other domestic violence services; (5) protective orders; (6) child fatality review panels; (7) mental health and counselling services for child maltreatment and domestic violence; (8) child witness to violence prevention and treatment programs; and (9) elder abuse services.

The committee identified four research topics that require further development to inform policy and practice. These topics raise fundamental questions about the approaches that should be used in designing treatment, prevention, and deterrence strategies:

- Cross-problem research (such as the relationship between substance abuse and family violence);
- Studies of family dynamics and processes that interact with family violence;
- Cost analysis and service system studies that describe the existing set and distribution of services focused on different forms of family violence;
- Social setting issues that warrant study because of their implications for the design of treatment, support, prevention, and deterrence strategies.

## CHALLENGES TO EFFECTIVE EVALUATIONS

In recommending this research agenda, the committee recognizes that such research is complicated by a number of factors. Service providers and researchers are realizing that family violence is an interactive, dynamic, and complex problem that requires approaches across multiple levels of analysis (individual, family, community) and multiple service systems. The presence or absence of policies and programs in one domain may directly affect the implementation and outcomes of service strategies in another. Services also interact with the characteristics of the client: some people need more support or stronger sanctions, depending on their histories and life circumstances; others need only a limited amount of assistance, treatment, or sanction to improve.

The lack of collaboration between researchers and service providers has impeded the development of appropriate measures and study designs in assessing the effectiveness of programs. It has also discouraged research on the design and implementation of service interventions and the multiple pathways to services that address the causes and consequences of family violence.

To improve evaluations of family violence interventions and to provide a research base that can inform policy and practice, major challenges must be addressed. These challenges include issues of study design and methodology, as well as logistical concerns, that must be resolved in order to conduct rigorous research in open service systems in which many factors are not under the control of the research investigator. Meeting these challenges will require collaborative partnerships among researchers, service providers, and policy makers to generate approaches and data sources that are useful to all. The establishment and documentation of a series of consensus conferences on relevant outcomes, and appropriate measurement tools, will strengthen and enhance evaluations of family violence interventions and lead to improvements in the design of programs, interventions, and strategies.

The development of the next generation of evaluation studies will benefit from the building blocks of knowledge that have been put into place over the past 15 years. This research base, and the convergence of the field around such issues as the recognition of the interactive nature of the service system in different institutional settings, the existence of multiple subgroups of offenders, the need for research experimentation to guide treatment and prevention efforts, and the use of multiple measures of program outcomes suggest that a richer and deeper understanding of family violence interventions lies within reach in the decade ahead.

# 1

# Introduction

The need for evidence of the effectiveness of family violence interventions arises every day in a variety of settings: in courtroom deliberations, in which judges must decide appropriate punishment and treatment for offenders; in child protection investigations, in which caseworkers must consider what services to recommend for their clients; and in clinical settings, in which health professionals are expected to develop an appropriate response in examining suspicious injuries of adult and child patients. Indicators of program effectiveness are the focus of attention when program and service budgets are under review, in public hearings in which victims and advocates seek legislation to strengthen existing services or to develop new ones, and in media reports that compare the merits of customary practice with innovative approaches to addressing child maltreatment, domestic violence, and elder abuse.

Scientific research has not been able to provide clear guidance in determining the comparative effectiveness of specific efforts. Much of the literature simply describes individual programs rather than rigorously evaluating their outcomes. And most evaluations of family violence interventions simply describe the intervention that was provided (without providing much detail about the implementation process), estimate the number of clients served over selected time periods, review the types and costs of the services provided, or examine specific skills or knowledge obtained as the result of a training program. These types of studies are commonly referred to as process evaluations, because they focus on the processes of the intervention rather than its results.

An emphasis on theory and outcomes has been missing in evaluations of family violence interventions: What behaviors was the intervention seeking to influence, and how do they relate to the overall problem of child maltreatment, domestic violence, or elder abuse? Did the child, adult, or family actually improve as a result of the program and, if so, how was this measured? Did the community experience a lower rate of family violence following the intervention? Did changes in skills or knowledge result in modifications in behavior among offenders or lead to new services in communities that reduced the violence and provided more safety or improved health? And are the results of a single program or comprehensive community intervention transferable to a larger and more diverse population of clients and multiple communities?

Both public and private agencies now seek to move beyond anecdotal reports in a search for data that can guide policy and program decisions. Yet service providers, public officials, clients, and researchers themselves are frustrated by the difficulties of measuring and assessing the impacts of treatment and prevention programs. The enormous complexity of the phenomena, the comparatively short history with service interventions, the shifting legal and social doctrines that shape public policy, the interactive nature of the problems and the services themselves, and the demographic transformations affecting American families and communities present tremendous challenges to the use of science in this field. The urgency and magnitude of these problems and the scale of resources that our society invests in treatment and prevention efforts demand better results.

## SCOPE OF THE PROBLEM

Family violence victimization in the general population is widely regarded as a serious problem that affects large numbers of children and adults across the life span. Estimates of the scope of the problem vary according to the source of the information that provides the basis of the estimate and the definitions used in describing the nature of the problem. But although the exact dimensions of child maltreatment, domestic violence, and elder abuse are frequently disputed, conservative estimates suggest that these problems affect millions of children, women, and men in the United States. In 1996, a government survey (NIS-3) reported that 2.8 million cases of child maltreatment were known to local child protection agencies or community sources (including teachers, health care professionals, and other service providers) in 1993, when the data were collected (National Center on Child Abuse and Neglect, 1996b). This estimate indicates a rate of 41.9 children per 1,000, or 1 in 24 in the U.S. child population (National Center on Child Abuse and Neglect, 1996b:3-17).

No government survey has yet been published that estimates the national incidence of domestic violence in the United States. The National Crime Victimization Survey, which collects data about incidents reported as crimes, has reported that the annual rate of physical attacks by family members for women was 9.3 per 1,000 in 1992-1993 (Bachman and Saltzman, 1995). Population-based surveys suggest that the rate of adult violence involving family members may be much higher—the National Family Violence Surveys (Straus and Gelles, 1990), for example, have reported an annual rate of 116 per 1,000 women for a violent act by an intimate partner and 34 per 1,000 for "severe violence" by an intimate partner.

The rate of child deaths attributed to abuse and neglect remained relatively stable (around 2,000 per year) from 1979 through 1988 (McClain et al., 1993). Of the 4,869 female homicide victims reported in 1993, 31 percent (1,531) were killed by intimate partners (husbands, ex-husbands, or boyfriends) (Federal Bureau of Investigation, 1993). No reliable statistics are kept for rates of elder abuse or deaths attributed to the maltreatment of older persons. There are no self-report surveys of elder abuse, and the surveys of elder abuse reporting and recognition are incomplete.

## FRAGMENTATION OF THE FIELD

The study of family violence consists of many separate areas of research focused on the study of child maltreatment, domestic violence, and elder abuse (Ohlin and Tonry, 1989). Each area has its own terminology, theories, experts, funding sources, data collection efforts, research instruments, and scholarly journals. Those who study domestic violence have rarely communicated with, or even read the works of, those who study child abuse. This specialization and fragmentation, combined with a lack of methodological rigor, have contributed to a research literature that has been characterized as "extensive but not definitive" (Ohlin and Tonry, 1989:5).

The absence of unifying theories, common measures, and datasets has discouraged efforts to draw inferences between studies of family violence and studies of other forms of criminal and violent behavior. Little is known, for example, about the pathways or nature of the relationship between childhood experiences with violence in the home and juvenile delinquency or adult criminal behavior, even though research has suggested that children who experience maltreatment have an increased risk both of arrest as a juvenile or adult and of committing a violent crime (Widom, 1992). Similarly, much uncertainty exists about the extent to which men who batter their intimate partners engage in other forms of violent or criminal behavior. The organization of research in this field, within both academic centers and federal research bureaucracies, often isolates different forms of family violence research and discourages efforts to integrate research on violence within the family and research on violence within the community.

The fragmentation that characterizes the research field also exists in the service delivery system. As a result of history and social forces, the law enforcement, social services, and health care efforts that are focused on different aspects of family violence must address diverse policy objectives. These goals include the punishment and rehabilitation of offenders, the protection of victims and communities, the reduction of unnecessary costs, a respect for due process and fairness (often difficult to achieve when conflicting testimony exists or physical evidence is not available), concern for the rights and developmental needs of children and vulnerable adults, the mitigation of the adverse effects of experiences with violence, and the prevention of new incidents of violence in the home. Such services are subject to enormous social and political influences in the wake of sensational cases. The result is a patchwork of separate efforts that operate in a semiautonomous manner, although the presence or absence of one component may have direct implications for another. The basic dimensions of this loosely coupled system of treatment, prevention, and control interventions have remained ambiguous and unexamined in the research literature, and little is known about their basic character, operation, or impact.

Treatment and prevention programs are fragmented by the focus of the interventions: some efforts are designed to respond to the needs of the victims; others deal exclusively with the offenders. Some programs focus on children, others on adults. Some programs seek to serve individuals; others emphasize the importance of serving their clients in the context of their relationships as parent, child, intimate partners, or members of a family unit.

Service providers and researchers are realizing that family violence is an interactive and dynamic problem that requires approaches across multiple levels of analysis and multiple service systems (National Research Council, 1993b, 1996). This realization has profound consequences for the development of the next generation of treatment and prevention programs as well as the design of studies of their effectiveness. The emergence of a public health response and comprehensive community initiatives focused on family violence has stimulated interest in examining collaborative approaches to multiple problems within a family. These multiple problems may exist entirely within the context of family violence (such as the impact of witnessing spousal violence on the developmental outcomes of children) or they may co-exist within a family with a broad range of behaviors (such as poverty, family violence, and alcoholism or substance abuse). Artificial barriers between separate programs and institutional services still remain, but in some regions they are yielding to more integrated and inclusive approaches that focus on the need to support individuals, families, and communities as they seek to reduce the incidence of violent behavior in families. Evaluation of these comprehensive community efforts is in its infancy, challenged by the complexities noted below as well as the difficulties of evaluating programs that are not yet fully developed.

## CHALLENGES TO EFFECTIVE EVALUATIONS

The evaluation research literature has provided limited guidance in the design of treatment and prevention interventions for family violence. Significant methodological and logistical problems include difficulties in constructing and gaining access to appropriate sample sizes, limited availability of comparison and control groups, weak research measures and survey instruments, short time intervals for follow-up studies, and high attrition rates in both the interventions themselves and the evaluation studies. Some interventions that are in widespread practice have *never* been evaluated (such as the use of mandatory reporting procedures for child maltreatment cases), whereas extensive attention has focused on a few interventions in specialized settings (such as arrest policies for domestic violence, the use of home visitation services as a preventive intervention for child maltreatment, and intensive family preservation services that seek to provide family support services in crisis-oriented setting).

This imbalance between the need for knowledge in areas that are hard to measure and the availability of knowledge in discrete areas of policy and practice creates two major quandaries that this report seeks to address: (1) how to review the implications of current research findings in a form that can be useful for researchers, service providers, and policy makers in various institutional settings who are concerned with discrete and multiple aspects of family violence, (2) how to determine which interventions should be strong candidates for the next generation of evaluation studies. The problem of selecting interventions for evaluation will acquire increased significance as larger numbers of agencies in social services, law enforcement, and health care seek to address the complex dimensions of the problem of family violence within the loosely coupled but interactive system of services that has emerged at the national and local level.

In addition to the generic challenges to effective evaluations, studies in this specific area are complicated by a number of factors:

• Most family violence interventions have resulted from advocacy efforts in communities that focus on the specific needs of children, women, and the elderly. Many evaluations focus on a single program rather than an overall intervention or service strategy.

• Many interventions are not fully implemented, and the status of their implementation is often missing in evaluation reports.

• The urgent emphasis on meeting the needs of victims and taking action against offenders has caused services to be developed in the absence of a knowledge base about the causes and consequences of family violence. As a result, the theoretical frameworks that guide specific interventions are often not explicit and may vary among individual programs. In addition, limited attention has been paid, in either the research literature or the design of interventions, to the impact of unsubstantiated reports of family violence on the affected parties.

• Measures of the nature and scope of family violence often come from court or administrative records rather than health records or the observation of families and couples themselves. Administrative records often include biases that distort the ability of researchers to identify key trends or risk and protective factors that may influence patterns of aggression and the outcomes of interventions.

• When evaluations are closely coupled with program development, the research base may not have an opportunity or sufficient resources to develop an array of studies that can build on the strengths of qualitative and quantitative research. The programmatic emphasis on examining the results of an intervention within a short time period can inhibit efforts to learn more about the basic nature of the services that were provided and the characteristics of clients who did or did not respond to them.

• Researchers are often prevented by resource constraints as well as the nature of service systems from designing experimental studies that make use of an appropriate control group in comparing the relative effects of a selected program. Controlled studies are especially difficult to develop when services are limited by budgetary restrictions, access to services is determined by multiple agencies within a community, and service providers are not accustomed to working with researchers. Controlled studies are also not feasible in circumstances in which random assignments cannot be made for ethical or legal reasons, such as felony violence.

• Even when it is possible to conduct rigorous evaluations, program advocates have sometimes resisted scientific study because of concerns that the research will interfere with the basic service mission of the program, that the researchers do not have the capacity to measure significant interactions, or that negative findings may weaken support for existing services. Researchers, as well, have sometimes displayed a lack of appreciation for the complexities of dealing with the problems of family violence and underserved populations, focusing on factors that are relatively easy to measure, such as attendance rates or length of service, rather than addressing more difficult issues, such as the capacity to change one's own or another's behavior or consideration of the presence of multiple stressors and interactive processes that may be significant in examining the impact of policy and programs.

• The lack of opportunities for collaboration between researchers and service providers has impeded the development of appropriate measures and study designs in assessing the impact of programs. It has also discouraged research on the design and implementation of service interventions and the multiple pathways to services that address the causes and consequences of family violence.

These complications have hindered the development of a useful body of scientific knowledge about the impact of family violence interventions. In the absence of such knowledge, program decisions are influenced by anecdotal reports, marketing or lobbying efforts, and the fiscal realities of budgetary politics. Proponents of law enforcement programs may argue that stiffer penalties and mandatory sentences for offenders are effective in reducing the incidence of domestic violence and child maltreatment, but such claims lack empirical evidence. Similarly, advocates for women and children may argue that public funds should be spent on social service and public health programs designed to meet the needs of victims of abuse and neglect, but such claims lack valid indicators of effectiveness.

## CHARGE TO THE COMMITTEE

The Committee on the Assessment of Family Violence Interventions was convened by the National Research Council to undertake five primary tasks:

1. Document the impact of family violence on public- and private-sector services in the United States, especially in the area of spousal abuse. This analysis should include an assessment of what is known about the scope and cost of service interventions, the adequacy and validity of current reporting and detection data that are used to estimate the incidence and prevalence of selected types of family violence, and areas of bias in the current reporting system that may exaggerate or underestimate estimates of service intervention costs.

2. Synthesize the relevant research literature and develop a conceptual framework for clarifying what is known about relationships among the risk and protective factors associated with family violence. This framework should make distinctions between areas in which evidence of harm is clear in the interaction of certain risk and protective factors and areas in which knowledge is limited or uncertain.

3. Characterize what is known about both prevention efforts and specific interventions in dealing with family violence, including an assessment of what has been learned about the strengths and limitations of each approach and factors to consider in designing program evaluations.

4. Highlight successful components and, to the extent possible, identify "best practice" models of specific intervention programs for different forms of family violence. This task includes the examination of policy and program elements and service delivery system features that appear to contribute to or inhibit the development of effective program responses to family violence.

5. Develop criteria and principles that can guide the development of future evaluations of family violence interventions, especially the identification of outcomes and methodological issues that are essential to rigorous evaluation efforts.

Early in the course of our deliberations, the committee recognized that the research literature associated with evaluations of family violence interventions was relatively immature and scattered across a wide range of research fields. Judging that the absence of an integrative review of this literature has discouraged efforts to understand the nature, objectives, and outcomes of interventions, the committee sought to develop a report that would describe the ways in which interventions and service strategies interact with families and communities. Although some types of interventions have been in place for decades (for example, child protective services), they have not been subjected to rigorous evaluations to examine their impact on offenders and victims. Experience with other types of interventions is relatively new; many interventions now in place for domestic violence, for example, are not yet fully implemented and have not yet been evaluated. The committee therefore directed its efforts toward reviewing the knowledge base associated with the array of interventions currently in place, identifying the evaluation studies that met minimal standards of scientific quality, highlighting the major challenges to evaluations of these interventions, and examining how problems such as weak design and limited study samples could be resolved in developing the next generation of evaluation studies.

In developing the criteria and principles to guide future evaluations, the committee was not asked to address the nature of public policy, funding, and other critical factors that could influence whether or not these principles and criteria are actually used. Clearly, there is a need for further consideration of the potential roles of public agencies, both federal and state, and private foundations in improving the quality of both quantitative and qualitative evaluations for family violence interventions. The types of collaborations that might foster progress in examining the impact of the wide range of services already in place in this field also deserves attention. The committee does address the need for improved partnerships among research, practice, and policy in this report, but specific questions pertaining to the adequacy of funding for research, infrastructure, and implementation were beyond the scope of our study.

## STUDY APPROACH

### Definition of Family Violence

The term *family violence* is applied to a broad range of acts whose presence or absence results in harm to individuals who share parent-child or adult intimate relationships. These relationships are often long-term and generally involve aspects of financial or physical interdependence.[1] The definition of family violence adopted by this committee is based on one developed by the Committee on Family Violence convened by the National Institute of Mental Health (1992:6):

---

[1]Emery (1989) has reviewed the frustrations associated with efforts to come up with precise definitions of family violence, especially in the context of child maltreatment. He concludes that professionals who are responsible for intervention should be encouraged "to use definitions of and responses to family violence that match those used for assaults between strangers" (p. 321), implementing the recommendations of the 1984 Attorney General's Task Force on Family Violence.

The report of the NRC Panel on Research on Child Abuse and Neglect (National Research Council, 1993a) includes an entire chapter on definitional issues in child abuse research. Both Emery (1989) and the NRC committee criticized the research community for the absence of a standardized definition of child maltreatment for research studies. A similar lack of consensus exists on definitional issues in domestic violence (see e.g., Gelles and Straus, 1988; Fagan and Browne, 1994) and in elder abuse (Pillemer and Suitor, 1988).

Family violence includes child and adult abuse that occurs between family members or adult intimate partners. For children, this includes acts by others that are physically and emotionally harmful or that carry the potential to cause physical harm. Abuse of children may include sexual exploitation or molestation, threats to kill or abandon, or a lack of the emotional or physical support necessary for normal development. For adults, family or intimate violence may include acts that are physically and emotionally harmful or that carry the potential to cause physical harm. Abuse of adult partners may include sexual coercion or assaults, physical intimidation, threats to kill or to harm, restraint of normal activities or freedom, and denial of access to resources.

Despite progress in identifying the characteristics of family violence, serious problems remain in defining the severity of the injury or threat, the amount of harm, and the extent of the consequences associated with its occurrence (Ohlin and Tonry, 1989). The question of what constitutes a family relationship is also complicated by the diversity of intimate or dependent caregiving relationships in home environments. Furthermore, uncertainty remains about the strength of the relationship among the different forms of family violence. Definitional issues are discussed further in Chapter 2.

This report examines opportunities for interactions among child maltreatment, domestic violence, and elder abuse in terms of both research and service. These relationships are important because the forms of family violence may share common risk factors or may represent a developmental continuum, such as the case of an abused child who becomes either a batterer or a victim of domestic violence. They are also important because opportunities may exist in the service delivery system to combine or integrate services and to reinforce individual program goals by adopting common strategies. The report does not address the issues of sibling violence or violence among same sex intimate adults, primarily because research in these fields is less well developed and the committee did not identify evaluations of interventions for these forms of family violence that met the selection criteria for the study.

Although the report often emphasizes the interactions among different forms of family violence, it is important to maintain diverse approaches in examining the array of programs, services, and interventions. In some situations, the origins of domestic violence may have stronger theoretical links to other forms of violence against women, such as rape and sexual harassment, than to other forms of family violence. Similarly, some forms of child maltreatment may have stronger theoretical links to interpersonal violence, such as pedophilia, assault, and homicide, than to other forms of family violence. The complexity of the field is daunting to scientific study; theory building remains in an early stage of development.

## Levels of Attention

In formulating its approach, the committee developed distinctions among strategies, interventions, and programs. Although these terms are often used interchangeably in discussions of program effectiveness, they are not synonymous. By *strategies*, the committee refers to a general course of treatment, control, or prevention that is designed to achieve a broad social goal, such as the prevention of family violence, the identification and protection of victims, and the punishment or deterrence of offenders.

The term *interventions* refers to the array of services and policies used to implement strategies at the individual, family, and community levels. Examples of interventions include parenting education programs for child maltreatment cases, treatment services for batterers, and universal screening for pregnant women to enhance the access to services of victims of domestic violence. Interventions include not only organized services but also legal, judicial, and regulatory policies and procedures, such as protective orders and mandatory reporting systems, some of which have been evaluated in the research literature.

*Programs* are community-specific examples of particular interventions. Batterer treatment interventions, for example, may be voluntary or mandatory, depending on the setting and context of a particular program. Some interventions consist solely of a single community's program; other interventions may be composed of several programs that share a common theoretical framework but rely on different approaches in achieving their goals. These program variations often are regarded as the same intervention. The home visitation intervention, for example, consists of several models, some of which rely on public health nurses who establish contact with mothers during their pregnancy and provide frequent visits after birth; others rely on paraprofessionals who meet with the mother after her discharge from a hospital. The home visitation intervention is part of a broader child abuse prevention strategy designed to detect risk factors for child maltreatment and to strengthen parenting skills through public health and family support services.

This report focuses primarily on interventions rather than individual programs or broad strategies. Specific program examples are used when they illustrate community efforts to implement a particular intervention or when they have served as the subject of an evaluation study. Table 1-1 identifies the specific family violence interventions that are reviewed in this report. Each intervention is numbered by chapter and by type of violence (A-child, B-domestic, C-elderly). Thus, for example, intervention 4A-1 is the first child abuse intervention discussed in Chapter 4. Figure 1-1 illustrates how the interventions reviewed in this report can be arrayed in terms of the general strategies of identification, prevention, protection, treatment, legal separation, and deterrence.

## Approach to the Evidence

The committee has identified interventions that have been evaluated in the literature, as well as key interventions worthy of study because of their perceived value to victims and communities in responding to family violence. Some evaluations that did not meet the committee's criteria for inclusion nonetheless are discussed in the report because they offer insights concerning outcome measurement and program implementation.

The literature review covers scientific journals, federal research reports, national research databases, state agency reports, and foundation studies. In our search we identified and reviewed over 2,000 studies to determine if they included evaluations that relied on a scientific design that included the use of a control or comparison group. The use of a control group is critical to good evaluation research, because it allows the researcher to compare the relative effects of the intervention under study to what might be expected in its absence (Metcalf and Thornton, 1992). In selecting evaluation studies for detailed analysis, the committee relied on the following criteria:

- The evaluation involved a program intervention that was designed to treat or prevent some aspect of child maltreatment, domestic violence, or elder abuse;
- The evaluation was conducted between 1980 and 1996 (this time period was selected to provide a contemporary history of the evaluation research literature while maintaining manageable limits on the scope of the evidence considered by the committee);
- The evaluation used an experimental or quasi-experimental design and included measurement tools and outcomes related to family violence; and
- The evaluation included a comparison group as part of the study design.

A total of 114 evaluation studies were identified that met this standard (see Table 1-2). Most of the studies reviewed by the committee have been published in the peer-reviewed literature, although some state agency reports, foundation reports, and studies in progress are included in the research base for this report. In addition, the committee relied on 35 research review papers that include detailed analyses of independent research studies, even though the individual studies within each review paper may not be consistent with the selection criteria outlined above.

The committee initiated its search with a review of the relevant on-line databases that include evaluation studies of family violence interventions.[2] We

---

[2]Research efforts focused on searches of 18 relevant electronic databases, including the National Criminal Justice Reference Section, the National Child Abuse and Neglect Data System, Medline, the Legal Resource Index, the Criminal Justice Periodical Index, ERIC, Social SciSearch,

*continued on page 28*

TABLE 1-1   Array of Interventions by Type of Family Violence and Institutional Setting

| Institutional Setting | Child Abuse | Domestic Abuse | Elder Abuse |
|---|---|---|---|
| Social service | 4A-1. Parenting practices and family support services | 4B-1. Shelters for battered women | 4C-1. Adult protective services |
| | 4A-2. School-based sexual abuse prevention | 4B-2. Peer support groups for battered women | 4C-2. Training for caregivers |
| | 4A-3. Child protective services investigation and casework | 4B-3. Advocacy services for battered women | 4C-3. Advocacy services to prevent elder abuse |
| | 4A-4. Intensive family preservation services | 4B-4. Domestic violence prevention programs | |
| | 4A-5. Child placement services | | |
| | 4A-6. Individualized service programs | | |
| Law enforcement | 5A-1. Mandatory reporting requirements | 5B-1. Reporting requirements | 5C-1. Reporting requirements |
| | 5A-2. Child placement by the courts | 5B-2. Protective orders | 5C-2. Protective orders |
| | 5A-3. Court-mandated treatment for child abuse offenders | 5B-3. Arrest procedures | 5C-3. Education and legal counseling |
| | 5A-4. Treatment for sexual abuse offenders | 5B-4. Court-mandated treatment for domestic violence offenders | 5C-4. Guardians and conservators |
| | | 5B-5. Criminal prosecution | 5C-5. Arrest, prosecution, and other litigation |

| | | |
|---|---|---|
| | 5A-5. Criminal prosecution of child abuse offenders | 5B-6. Specialized courts |
| | | 5B-7. Systemic approaches |
| | 5A-6. Improving child witnessing | 5B-8. Training for criminal justice personnel |
| | 5A-7. Evidentiary reforms | |
| | 5A-8. Procedural reforms | |
| Health care | 6A-1. Identification and screening | 6B-1. Domestic violence screening, identification, and medical care responses | 6C-1. Identification and screening |
| | 6A-2. Mental health services for child victims of physical abuse and neglect | 6B-2. Mental health services for domestic violence victims | 6C-2. Hospital multidisciplinary teams |
| | 6A-3. Mental health services for child victims of sexual abuse | | 6C-3. Hospital-based support groups |
| | 6A-4. Mental health services for children who witness domestic violence | | |
| | 6A-5. Mental health services for adult survivors of child abuse | | |
| | 6A-6. Home visitation and family support programs | | |

SOURCE: Committee on the Assessment of Family Violence Interventions, National Research Council and Institute of Medicine, 1998.

24

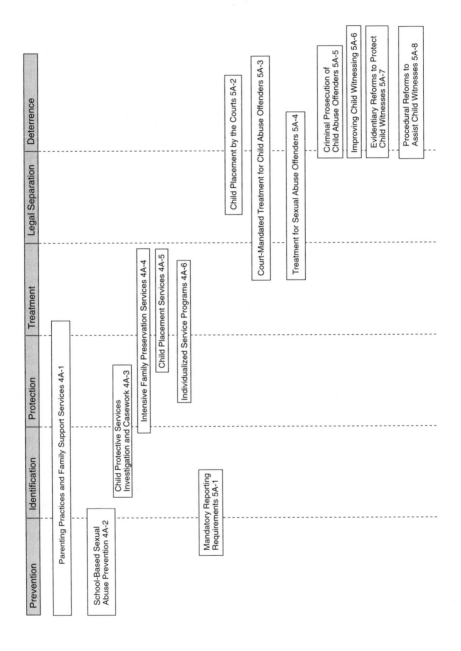

Prevention | Identification | Protection | Treatment | Legal Separation | Deterrence

Parenting Practices and Family Support Services 4A-1

School-Based Sexual Abuse Prevention 4A-2

Child Protective Services Investigation and Casework 4A-3

Intensive Family Preservation Services 4A-4

Child Placement Services 4A-5

Individualized Service Programs 4A-6

Mandatory Reporting Requirements 5A-1

Child Placement by the Courts 5A-2

Court-Mandated Treatment for Child Abuse Offenders 5A-3

Treatment for Sexual Abuse Offenders 5A-4

Criminal Prosecution of Child Abuse Offenders 5A-5

Improving Child Witnessing 5A-6

Evidentiary Reforms to Protect Child Witnesses 5A-7

Procedural Reforms to Assist Child Witnesses 5A-8

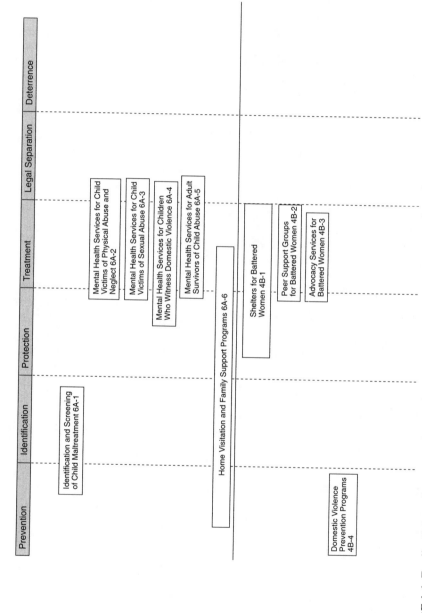

FIGURE 1-1 Family violence interventions by type of strategy. (*Continued on next page.*)

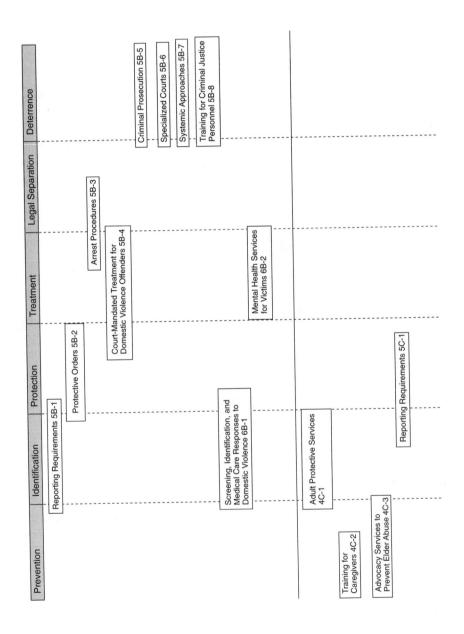

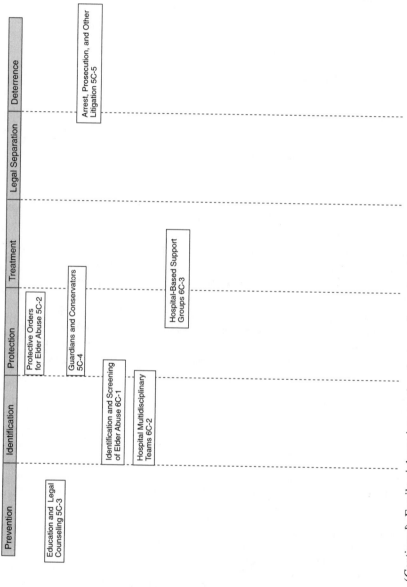

FIGURE 1-1 (*Continued*) Family violence interventions by type of strategy. SOURCE: Committee on the Assessment of Family Violence Interventions, National Research Council and Institute of Medicine, 1998.

TABLE 1-2  Total Number of Quasi-Experimental
Evaluations of Family Violence Interventions by Service
Sector, 1980-1996

| Service Sector | Type of Family Violence | | |
|---|---|---|---|
| | Child Maltreatment | Domestic Violence | Elder Abuse |
| Social service | 50 | 7 | 2 |
| Legal | 4 | 19 | 0 |
| Health care | 24 | 8 | 0 |

SOURCE: Committee on the Assessment of Family Violence Interventions,
National Research Council and Institute of Medicine, 1998.

also contacted several public and private national clearinghouses, which aided in identifying unpublished materials that were included in the literature review. In addition, we learned of a small number of evaluation studies that meet our criteria but have recently been completed or exist only as state agency reports and have not been included in the literature or national clearinghouse collections.

It is important to note that the range of evaluation studies presented in this report does not reflect the current range of treatment and prevention interventions. The research literature is primarily focused on small or innovative programs that provide an opportunity for research study. Science-based evaluations are rarely conducted on major existing interventions, such as foster care, domestic violence shelters, adult protective services, health care provider training programs, and court procedures, because research samples and appropriate measures are not available to assess the intervention, the intervention was already in place prior to the development of evaluation methods, the organizational setting is not

---

PsychINFO, Dissertation Abstracts Online, A-V Online, PAIS Online, IAC Business A.R.T.S., U.S. Political Science Documents, British Education Index, AgeLine, Religion Index, and Public Opinion Online. Boolean search terms were employed to identify evaluation studies (descriptive, quasi-experimental, and causal) of family violence interventions.

The committee also contacted several public and private national clearinghouses to determine if their collections included evaluation studies that might not be identified in the electronic database searches. The relevant clearinghouses included the National Center on Child Abuse and Neglect (NCCAN) (Fairfax, Virginia); the Family Violence and Sexual Assault Institute (Tyler, Texas); the National Clearinghouse for the Defense of Battered Women (Philadelphia); the National Resource Center on Domestic Violence (Harrisburg, Pennsylvania), and the Family Violence Prevention Fund (San Francisco).

These sources aided in identifying unpublished materials that were included in the literature review. The NCCAN clearinghouse provided a CD-ROM of its resources and customized searches of additional databases in its collection.

conducive to evaluation, or policy and program sponsors are not prepared to provide funds to examine the impact of the intervention.

As noted later in this report, rigorous evaluations are focused primarily on social service interventions in the area of child maltreatment and legal interventions for domestic violence. Experimental evaluations of interventions for elder abuse are almost nonexistent.

## Organization of the Report

The report begins by examining what is known about the scope of family violence, risk factors, the nature and scope of interventions, and their impact and costs (Chapter 2). Next we examine the state of the art of evaluations, identify obstacles to evaluations in this field, and explore potential improvements to the use of qualitative and quantitative information (Chapter 3). Chapter 3 also highlights the importance of structuring partnerships between researchers and service providers so that relevant expertise can be applied to study designs, the selection of outcomes of interest, and the use of appropriate measures.

Chapters 4, 5, and 6 provide a comprehensive review and assessment of existing interventions in the areas of child maltreatment, domestic violence, and elder abuse. These chapters characterize the state of evaluation research and summarize what is known about treatment and preventive interventions in social service, law enforcement, and health care sectors, respectively. Interagency family violence interventions and comprehensive services or community change interventions are discussed in Chapter 7. These four chapters aim to capture the insights of the research base as well as those of service providers—a perspective generally not found in the scholarly literature.

Chapter 8 discusses a number of cross-cutting issues that arose in our assessment of treatment and prevention interventions. Chapter 9 presents the committee's recommendations.

## THE COMMITTEE'S PERSPECTIVE

The committee considered several different conceptual schemes in considering how to organize the material reviewed in this report. We could have presented this material in terms of the life spans of victims and offenders: child, adult, and elder. We could have sought to distinguish between victims and perpetrators and between treatment, prevention, and enforcement interventions by focusing chapters on each approach. However, we decided that an approach that divides the targets of the interventions would perpetuate the fragmentation that has characterized this area of research, policy, and practice.

The committee decided that the intended audience of this report, which includes researchers, service providers, and policy makers from distinct institutional settings, would be best served by a synthesis of research that brings the relevant knowledge to bear on specific services and policies within their own organizational service system. At this stage in the development of family violence interventions, the institutional settings of the interventions exercise a major influence on their objectives, resources, and method of implementation.

This choice of a categorical structure for the report, however, was disturbing to several committee members, who would prefer to see a more holistic approach that builds on the needs of children, adults, and the elderly. In our analysis of cross-cutting themes in Chapter 8, we highlight key issues that cut across these institutional sectors. We also highlight, in Chapter 7, examples of interventions that experiment with comprehensive community approaches and that seek to replace bureaucratic structures with service systems focused on the developmental and multiple needs of clients and communities rather than the convenience of the service provider. These approaches, while not yet evaluated, represent an important dimension in the design of family violence interventions that requires further examination.

In the decades ahead, research will provide more powerful insights that can lead to improved services, policy, and practice. But the integration of research knowledge and the development of interventions will require consistent and explicit attention to the ways in which the domains of science, law, health care, and social services interact. The absence or presence of interventions in one setting— such as shelters for battered women—may directly influence the operation and effectiveness of services in another domain—such as arrest policies for batterers. This interactive process is often missed in current assessments of family violence interventions, although it is often intrinsic to the experience of service providers.

The interactions among service systems add a new level of complexity to the design of both interventions and evaluations. Addressing this complexity will require collaborative partnerships between researchers and service providers to develop approaches that are consistent with the needs of the scientific process, that can be implemented in large systems of ongoing services as well as smaller innovative programs, and that can provide guidance in determining what works, for whom, and under what conditions. An integrated research foundation, the development of reliable measures and large datasets, careful descriptions of the goals of an intervention and the characteristics of clients, and documentation of the services that were actually provided all provide important opportunities for such partnerships. Through such efforts, the institutions and agencies that have supported the development of the interventions themselves can acquire the capacity to look closely at what they have achieved and to translate this knowledge into improved efforts to address the problem of family violence.

# 2

# Family Violence and
# Family Violence Interventions

In the 1960s, physical child abuse and child neglect were recognized as significant problems that required identification and intervention. In the 1970s, similar attention was called to domestic violence. In the 1980s, child sexual abuse and elder abuse gained attention. Each type of family violence developed its own set of definitions, research, and interventions. In recent years, researchers have begun to examine family violence across the life span, seeking commonalities among various forms of child maltreatment, domestic violence, and elder abuse (Barnett et al., 1997). Although the very nature of family relationships makes it reasonable to look for common risk and protective factors and interactions among the forms of family violence, debate continues about what determines the appropriate unit of analysis: the individuals who perpetrate or are victims of violent behavior, the family, the community, or broader social-cultural norms.

How the nature of family violence is conceptualized has important implications for the ways in which interventions are structured and outcomes are measured in evaluating them. This chapter examines similarities and differences in research on child maltreatment, domestic violence, and elder abuse in definitions, measurement, risk factors, and interventions. Each area has developed its own approach to the problems under study, resulting in tremendous variation in theoretical frameworks, research instrumentation, scholarly journals, and funding sources. Although studies of the field of family violence are now emerging, research in this area has traditionally been fragmented into separate areas of inquiry.

## DEFINITIONAL ISSUES

How family violence is measured and studied and who is identified to receive interventions depend on its definition. The multiple dimensions of family violence make definition tasks both difficult and controversial, and definitions have evolved somewhat differently for child maltreatment, domestic violence, and elder abuse. Although precise definitions are required for research and data collection, the situational context of many cases of family violence often challenges efforts to establish consistent criteria that can govern case reporting and selection decisions. The types of cases deemed appropriate for intervention may differ by service sector as well as within service settings. Despite these differences, common concerns have emerged that influence efforts to define family violence: a trend toward broadening the set of behaviors that are viewed as abuse or neglect, the role of cultural norms, the role of intentionality, the balance of power in the offender-victim relationship, and the influence of service-sector resources on definitions.

### Broadening of Definitions

Early definitions of child maltreatment were narrowly focused on issues of physical harm and endangerment. They were often based on a medical diagnostic approach, emphasizing the more serious forms of physical abuse and neglect that can result in physical injury and poor health. More recent definitions focus on the impact of maltreatment on development, expanding the category of abuse and neglect to include actions viewed as harmful to children, such as emotional abuse or educational or medical neglect, even though they are not necessarily associated with immediate physical injury. The negative impacts of exposure to domestic violence on children have recently been recognized. Some perpetrators of domestic violence have been charged not only with assault of their wives, but also reported as child abusers for exposing their children to their violent behavior. The National Center on Child Abuse and Neglect (1988) recognizes six major types of child maltreatment: physical abuse, sexual abuse, emotional abuse, physical neglect, educational neglect, and emotional neglect.

Similarly, initial definitions of domestic violence focused on acts of physical violence directed toward women by their spouses or partners (Gelles and Straus, 1974; Martin, 1976). Survey research found women also committed acts of physical violence against their husbands, suggesting that the initial definition might be too restrictive (Straus et al., 1980; Gelles, 1987; Gelles and Straus, 1988; Straus and Gelles, 1986). Further research broadened the definition to include sexual violence, marital rape, and acts of emotional or psychological abuse. Feminist scholars conceptualize domestic violence as coercive control of women by their partners (Yllo, 1993); the coercion can be physical, emotional, or sexual.

The recognition of elder abuse through adult protective services has led to definitions similar to those of child maltreatment. Elder abuse is generally defined to include physical and sexual violence, psychological abuse, and neglect. However, elder abuse definitions frequently go beyond those of child maltreatment to include financial abuse or exploitation. Elder abuse may also be a continuation of domestic violence in the relationship, in which case the issue of coercive control is pertinent.

Definitions of family violence have also broadened with respect to who is considered family. For domestic violence, the trend is to include all intimate relationships, such as cohabiting couples, same-sex couples, and ex-spouses, as well as currently married couples. Dating couples and ex-boyfriends/girlfriends may also be included. For child maltreatment, a distinction is made between abuse and neglect; the definition of neglect is generally limited to acts by a child's parents or legal caregiver. For child physical and sexual abuse, no consensus exists as to how broadly the set of potential abusers should be defined (National Research Council, 1993a), although, in the context of family violence, strangers are not included. For elder abuse, family members as well as legal or informal caregivers can be involved, and self-neglect has sometimes been counted in elder abuse data. In addition, violence between siblings and violence by children directed at their parents may be included in family violence.

The broadening of definitions of the various forms of family violence has been criticized by some on the grounds that it leads to a diffusion of effort within service agencies that have limited resources. Others have noted, however, that because emotional abuse and emotional neglect are often associated with other forms of maltreatment, the broader definitions create opportunities for early interventions that may be successful in preventing more serious and lethal forms of violence.

How broadly or narrowly family violence is defined has an obvious impact on its prevalence. Wyatt and Peters (1986) demonstrated empirically the impact of variations in definitions of sexual abuse on the estimated prevalence rates reported in a number of studies. Table 2-1 presents the rates of violence from various studies broken down by physical violence, sexual abuse, emotional abuse, and neglect. Physical violence is the most commonly measured form of maltreatment of adults and is second only to neglect in the maltreatment of children. Although clinical reports suggest that emotional abuse (such as yelling, criticism, ridicule, and threats) may be pervasive and central components of family violence, no rigorous measures currently exist to assess the extent of this type of behavior.

## The Role of Culture

Definitions of family violence vary not only over time, but also across cultures. Behavior that may be considered the norm by some groups may be consid-

TABLE 2-1  Past Year Rates of Family Violence (per 1,000 persons)

| Study and Author | Sample Size | All Maltreatment | All Physical Violence |
|---|---|---|---|
| Children | | | |
| NIS-3 (National Center on Child Abuse and Neglect, 1996a) | | 41.6 (reported) | 9.2 |
| NCANDS (National Center on Child Abuse and Neglect, 1996b) | | 43 (reported) | 3.4 |
| National Committee to Prevent Child Abuse (1996) | | 47 (reported) 16 (substantiated) | — |
| 1985 National Family Violence Survey (Straus and Gelles, 1988) | 3,232 | — | 498 |
| Finkelhor et al. (1990) | | | |
| Females | 1,374 | — | — |
| Males | 1,252 | — | — |
| Siblings | | | |
| 1975 National Family Violence Survey (Straus et al., 1980) | | — | 800 |
| Adult Women | | | |
| 1985 National Family Violence Survey (Straus and Gelles, 1988) | 6,002 | — | 116 |
| National Crime Victimization Survey (Bachman and Saltzman, 1995) | ~50,000 | — | 9.3 |
| Adult Men | | | |
| 1985 National Family Violence Survey (Straus and Gelles, 1988) | 6,002 | — | 124 |
| National Crime Victimization Survey (Bachman and Saltzman, 1995) | ~50,000 | — | 1.4 |
| Elderly Adults | | | |
| Pillemer and Finkelhor (1988) | 2,020 | 32 | 20 |

NOTE:  Dash indicates absence of data.
  [a]Prevalence rates of sexual abuse before age 18.
  [b]Ten or fewer sample cases.

SOURCE:  Committee on the Assessment of Family Violence Interventions, National Research Council and Institute of Medicine, 1998.

| Severe Physical Violence | Sexual Abuse or Marital Rape | Emotional or Psychological Abuse | Neglect | Fatal Abuse |
|---|---|---|---|---|
| — | 4.4 | 7.9 | 20.1 | |
| — | 2 | <0.1 | 6 | — |
| — | — | — | — | 0.0019 |
| 23 | — | 63.4 | — | — |
| — | 270[a] | — | — | — |
| — | 160[a] | — | — | — |
| 530 | — | — | — | — |
| 34 | 12 | 74 | — | — |
| — | 1 | — | — | — |
| 48 | not asked | 74.8 | — | — |
| — | —[b] | — | — | — |
| — | — | 11 | 4 | — |

ered abusive by others. Debate continues over the extent to which definitions of family violence can accommodate cultural variability without promoting different thresholds for intervention on the basis of race, ethnicity, or socioeconomic status. Agreement across cultural groups may be easy to reach on severe forms of family violence, such as beating a family member to death. Less severe behaviors are more subject to cultural differences. For example, a number of child advocates, researchers, and some parent groups believe that corporal punishment is abusive and harmful to children and should be illegal (Straus, 1994). In contrast, many working-class parents believe in strict child discipline practices and favor its use. Role expectations derived from traditional family relationships (which commonly viewed children and wives as property of the head of the household) can also contribute to conflict and violence when major changes occur in the status of women and children within a society. Pervasive gender inequality may be embedded in cultural norms and may influence patterns and rates of victimization.

As U.S. society becomes more diverse, cultural practices such as "coining" (a curing ritual that involves the forceful pressing of coins on a child's body, resulting in bruises) among Vietnamese populations and female genital mutilation among some African and Middle Eastern populations will increasingly be the focus of debate. Although such practices may meet criteria for abuse in the United States, it is important to understand their social and cultural contexts, at least in the perceptions of the families involved, in order to influence behavioral changes.

American society lacks a clear definition of caregiver responsibility for elders comparable to parental responsibilities for children, and conflicts may arise in certain cultures, classes, and social groups as to what types of arrangements constitute maltreatment. Recently, some researchers have questioned the legal and clinical definitions of elder abuse, suggesting that it is the older person's perception of a particular behavior, influenced by culture and tradition, that should be the salient factor in identification and intervention (Gebotys et al., 1992; Hudson, 1994).

## The Role of Intentionality

Although some definitions of family violence require that acts be intentional (see, e.g., Gelles and Straus, 1979; National Research Council, 1993b), recent trends in research definitions have been to focus on acts that are harmful or potentially harmful rather than on intent (Zuravin, 1991). Although intent is often difficult to determine, it is often important in determining the type of intervention necessary when decisions are made to investigate a family.

Neglect of children and the elderly may result from ignorance or lack of resources rather than malevolence. Parental knowledge of children's developmental abilities (especially feeding and toilet training), parental abilities to supervise young children, and parental expectations regarding the needs and behavior of young children have been identified as key areas in which significant variation exists within neighborhoods and between social classes and cultures. These discrepancies may be particularly difficult to resolve in identifying cases of maltreatment that occur in settings characterized by extreme poverty, substance abuse, community violence, and transience (including immigration and homelessness).

Elder abuse may also be unintentional because of the caregiver/perpetrator's ignorance of the needs of the elderly or because of his or her own infirmity. The lack of a clear definition of caregiver responsibility for elders also makes determining intentional withholding of care difficult. Whether behavior is labeled as abusive or neglectful may depend on its frequency, duration, intensity, severity, and consequences.

## Dependence and Power

Running through discussions of child maltreatment, domestic violence, and elder abuse is the idea of unequal power in the relationship between abuser and victim. In all three domains, abusers may use violence to control the victim. It is expected that children are dependent and that parents have more power than their children and will exert control over them. However, if the parent abdicates responsibility for caring for the child, neglect can occur. If the parent uses excessive physical force in exerting control, abuse can occur. For the incapacitated elderly, it is also expected that they are dependent on family or a caregiver; the typical elder abuse victim was thought to be frail and dependent. Although some research has found that elder abuse may be more likely when an adult child remains financially dependent on his or her parent rather than when the elderly parent has become dependent (Pillemer and Suitor, 1992), the adult child may still have power over the elderly parent by virtue of size, strength, and mobility.

The feminist analysis of domestic violence posits that physical violence is but one tactic used by abusers to exert control over their partners. In this paradigm, physical violence, emotional abuse, sexual violence, social isolation, and withholding of financial resources all serve to undermine a woman's autonomy and limit her power in the relationship. Feminist theory focused on gender inequalities offers a framework for a broad set of interventions designed to expose the pattern of male dominance and control in violent relationships and the ways in which society tolerates and legitimizes social inequalities that can contribute to entrapment.

## Influence of the Service Sector on Definitions

There is an interplay between the conceptualization of the types of family violence and the service sector in which interventions take place. For example, the identification of the "battered child syndrome" in the health care system at first focused the definitions of child maltreatment on physical injury (Kempe et al., 1962). As the legal and social service systems became involved and the emphasis in services became that of protecting the child, acts that threatened the child's well-being became a relevant factor in defining maltreatment; the definitions were subsequently broadened to include emotional abuse, sexual abuse, and neglect (National Research Council, 1993a). It is important to note that legal definitions encompass stringent standards in each category of abuse focused on thresholds for legal intervention that may not be useful in other service systems.

Similarly, the emphasis in domestic violence was first on physical injury. Even the term "battered wife" echoed the earlier use of "battered child," and much attention was focused and continues to be focused on the identification and documentation of physical injury in medical settings. Also for domestic violence, an emphasis on physical injury carried over to early legal interventions. For example, evidence of physical injury was often deemed necessary before an arrest was made. As a result of research studies and programs to change community attitudes toward the needs of battered women, definitions broadened beyond physical injury to include sexual and emotional abuse and threats of harm. Recent legislation now recognizes the stalking of estranged or former partners as domestic violence.

The recognition of elder abuse grew out of adult protective services—that is, services for adults who, for whatever reason, are unable to care for themselves. The similarity to child protective services heavily influenced definitions of elder abuse. It has been suggested that there has been an overreliance on the child abuse model. Recent findings suggest that domestic violence may be a more useful framework for study and intervention, since the individuals involved are legally independent adults. To some health researchers, however, the family violence paradigm is also not suitable. They recommend that elder abuse be considered from the perspective of "inadequate care," since it is easier to measure unmet needs than inappropriate behavior (Fulmer and O'Malley, 1987).

## MEASUREMENT ISSUES

Even if there were consensus on definitions, estimates of the scope of family violence would vary because of the different methods used to measure its incidence and prevalence. Detailed discussions of measuring the scope of family violence are available elsewhere (National Research Council, 1993a,b; 1996). Data on family violence are available from clinical data, administrative data, and social surveys. Each type of data has its own strengths and weaknesses and is useful for different purposes.

Clinical studies, carried out by psychiatrists, psychologists, and counselors, continue to be a frequent source of data on family violence. This is primarily due to the fact that these investigators have the most direct access to cases of family violence. The clinical or agency setting (including hospital emergency departments and battered women's shelters) provides access to extensive in-depth information about particular cases of violence. Studies of violence toward women have relied heavily on samples of women who seek help at battered women's shelters (Dobash and Dobash, 1979; Giles-Sims, 1983; Pagelow, 1984). Such samples are important because they are often the only way of obtaining detailed data on severely battered women. Such data are also necessary to study the impact of intervention programs. However, because they are based on small, nonrepresentative samples, such data cannot be used to estimate the incidence and prevalence of domestic violence.

Administrative data collected from official sources, such as child protective services, police departments, and adult protective services, provide the bulk of the information from which estimates of the incidence and prevalence of family violence are made. There are a number of factors that influence how well these data accurately reflect true incidence and prevalence. First, the quality and amount of these data vary by type of violence. All states now mandate reporting of child maltreatment and most states mandate reporting of elder abuse, although the definitions of reportable abuse differ from state to state. Even with mandatory reporting laws, it is widely acknowledged that abuse is underreported (e.g., Kalichman, 1993; Widom, 1988). One study found that only 44 percent of cases known to community professionals were officially known to child protective services agencies (Sedlak, 1991). This discrepancy may be based on the unwillingness of professionals to report, contradictory community standards regarding maltreatment definitions, or screening practices in child protective services agencies (Downing et al., 1990; Zellman, 1992). Furthermore, the number of substantiated cases may vary with the amount of resources devoted to case investigation. There is no administrative data source for domestic violence that is comparable to the state child and elder abuse datasets, and surveillance efforts are often challenged by concerns about victim safety and confidentiality.

Second, segments of the population at risk are subject to different levels of surveillance. Families who, because of their demographic characteristics (e.g., poverty, unemployment, single parenthood), have more frequent contact with public-sector services (e.g., welfare, housing) are more often exposed to mandated reporters and get closer scrutiny. Consequently, children who are poor or members of minority groups are more likely to be identified as maltreated than are more affluent white children (Newberger et al., 1977).

To remedy underreporting, national incidence studies of child maltreatment include official reports supplemented by surveys of other professionals about suspected cases of child abuse that have not been reported. The most recent National Incidence Study of Child Abuse and Neglect (NIS-3) found 2.8 million cases of child maltreatment (National Center on Child Abuse and Neglect, 1996b), a significant increase over the 1.4 million cases known by the agencies surveyed in 1986 (Sedlak, 1991). An unknown part of this increase may be due to broader definitions and broader sampling frames in the survey sample. Based on the NIS methodology, the National Center on Elder Abuse has launched a similar incident study of elder abuse, scheduled to be completed in 1997 (National Center on Elder Abuse and Neglect, 1995).

Researchers often turn to survey research to overcome the problems associated with administrative data. Surveys often find higher rates of violence than do administrative data; however, surveys have their own drawbacks. They are constrained by the low base rate of most forms of abuse and violence in families, as well as the sensitive and taboo nature of the topic. Some investigators cope with the problem of the low base rate by employing purposive or nonrepresentative sampling techniques to identify cases. Another approach has been to use large groups of available subjects. For example, investigators of courtship violence have made extensive use of survey research techniques using college students as subjects (Henton et al., 1983; Laner, 1989a,b; Makepeace, 1981, 1983). Other sources of bias in social survey data on family violence include inaccurate recall, differential interpretation of questions, and intended and unintended response error (Weis, 1989).

Survey results may also vary by question wording and context. For example, when the National Crime Victimization Survey revised its questionnaire to stress, among other things, that they wanted to know about incidents involving relatives and family members as well as acts committed by strangers, the reported violent attacks by family members nearly doubled from 5.4 per 1,000 for women in 1987-1991 to 9.3 per 1,000 in 1992-1993 (Bachman and Saltzman, 1995). This change most likely reflects the change in the survey and not a sudden increase in the rate of violence against women (National Research Council, 1996). The rates for domestic violence are lower than the rates found in other surveys that did not rely solely on crime reports. The 1985 National Family Violence Survey found much higher rates of domestic violence: 116 per 1,000 women reported experiencing violence during the past year; 34 per 1,000 women reported severe violence; and 12 per 1,000 reported marital rape (Straus and Gelles, 1988). In the 1993 Commonwealth Fund Survey of Women's Health, 70 per 1,000 women reported physical violence by an intimate partner.

The source of data has an impact not only on measures of incidence and prevalence of family violence, but also on what factors and variables are identified as risk and protective factors. In an analysis based on clinical data or official report data, risk and protective factors are confounded with factors such as labeling bias and agency or clinical setting catchment area. Researchers have long noted that certain individuals and families are more likely to be correctly and incorrectly labeled as offenders or victims of family violence (Gelles, 1975; Newberger et al., 1977; Hampton and Newberger, 1985). Social survey data are not immune to confounding problems either, as social or demographic factors may be related to willingness to participate in a self-report survey and a tendency toward providing socially desirable responses.

## RISK FACTORS

Researchers have looked, unsuccessfully for the most part, for traits that predispose children or adults to being victims of family violence. Much of the early retrospective research lacked comparison groups and confounded traits that preceded abuse with those that resulted from it. Research next focused on the traits of perpetrators. Although there appears to be a relatively high incidence of psychological and emotional problems among perpetrators of family violence, no characteristic profile of a child abuser, batterer, or elder abuser has emerged. It appears that no single factor can explain family violence. Rather it seems most likely that the complex interaction of personal history, personality traits, and demographic factors with social and environmental influences leads to violence in the family. Understanding better the particular factors that are relevant in a given family, and the sequence in which they emerge, may be important for choosing the most appropriate intervention.

In the sections that follow we review the most widely discussed risk factors in the study of family violence and, when appropriate, identify for which forms of violence and which types of relationships the factors are relevant. To overcome the limitations of studies of single factors, interactive models of risk and protective factors may further understanding of the etiology of family violence (Belsky, 1980; Garbarino, 1987; Lutzker et al., 1984; Malamuth et al., 1993). However, the complexity of analysis associated with these models and the difficulty of distinguishing causal effects from observational data have inhibited their testing and application (National Research Council, 1993b). Hence, research often focuses on risk factors that appear to be subject to change as a result of intervention or that are helpful in identifying at-risk populations. In research on domestic violence, several reviews of case-comparison studies have noted that potential risk markers are highly correlated with each other (e.g., family socioeconomic status and husband's occupational status, witnessing and experiencing violence as a child). This conceptual and statistical redundancy requires careful attention to disentangle risk factors that are directly related to the use of violence from other confounding factors (Hotaling and Sugarman, 1990).

### Risk Factors for Perpetrators

### Age

One of the most consistent risk factors for perpetration is age. As in violence between nonintimates, family violence is most likely to be perpetrated by those between ages 18 and 30. For child abuse, the age of the mother at the birth of the abused child has been found to be related to rates of physical abuse, with younger mothers exhibiting higher rates of abuse (Kinard and Klerman, 1980; Connelly and Straus, 1992). An analysis of data from the 1985 National Family Violence

Survey found young men significantly more likely to abuse their spouses (Fagan and Browne, 1994). Over 20 percent of men between ages 18 and 25 and 16.9 percent of men between ages 26 and 35 committed at least one act of domestic violence in the past year. Violence was reported by 7.2 percent of men ages 36 to 50 and 4.5 percent of those over 50. Youth has not been found to be a risk factor for elder abuse perpetration, although the rate of elder abuse is lower than the rate of other forms of family violence.

## Gender

Men are the most likely offenders in acts of intimate as well as nonintimate violence. However, the differences in the rates of offending between men and women are much smaller for family violence than for violence outside the home. Men and women have comparable rates of child homicide. Although women have been regarded as more likely to be offenders when the child victim is young (under 3 years of age) because of their traditional roles as primary caregivers for infants and toddlers, recent research suggests that extremely stressed or enraged male adults (including birth fathers, stepfathers, and boyfriends) are more often the cause of physical abuse fatalities involving an infant or small child (Levine et al., 1994; U.S. Advisory Board on Child Abuse and Neglect, 1995). In cases of child deaths from neglect, including bathtub drownings, fires started by unsupervised children, dehydration, and starvation, mothers are most often held responsible (Margolin, 1990; U.S. Advisory Board on Child Abuse and Neglect, 1995).

The extent of male victimization is controversial in the field of family violence (Dobash et al., 1992). The earliest studies of spousal violence reported violence by women toward their husbands (see, e.g., Gelles and Straus, 1974). The two National Family Violence Surveys also found a higher than expected incidence of violence toward men—the rate of violence was the same or even higher than that reported toward women (Straus et al., 1980; Straus and Gelles, 1986). In addition, women initiated violence about as often as men did (Straus, 1993). However, the researchers qualified their findings by noting that much of the female violence appeared to be in self-defense and that women, because of their size and strength, appeared to inflict less injury than male attackers. In contrast to the National Family Violence Surveys, the National Crime Victimization Survey found women reporting much higher rates of victimization by partners or ex-partners than men reported. In 1992-1993, the average rate of physical and sexual violence by an intimate was 9.4 per 1,000 for women, but only 1.4 per 1,000 for men (Bachman and Saltzman, 1995). These differences may be accounted for by the fact that the National Crime Victimization Surveys included only victimization serious enough to be considered a crime by the respondents.

Rates of disclosure of experience with violent incidents are thought to be susceptible to several factors, including the wording of the questions, the context in which questions are asked about sexual or intimate partner violence, and the extent of convergence or difference between interviewers and survey participants (National Research Council, 1996). Although some research has suggested that women are likely to be more forthcoming about their experiences with violent victimization when interviewed by women who share their ethnic heritage, the impact of interviewer-respondent characteristics on survey responses has not been deeply investigated.

Studies have found that female partner victimization is more likely to be accompanied by sexual and emotional abuse (Saunders, 1988). Female victims of intimate violence also suffer more physical injuries and emotional and psychological consequences than do men (Stets and Straus, 1990).

## Income

A series of research studies over the past decades has found consistent evidence of strong relationships between poverty and the reported occurrence and severity of child maltreatment, especially neglect (Giovannoni and Billingsley, 1970; Pelton, 1981, 1994; Wolock and Horowitz, 1979, 1984). Although child maltreatment may occur in families in high income brackets, abuse and neglect seem to be concentrated among the poorest of the poor. Pelton (1994) has estimated that more than 90 percent of all reported incidents of child maltreatment occur in families below the median income (estimated at $40,611 in 1995); 40 to 50 percent of all incidents occur within families whose incomes fall above the poverty level (estimated at $15,569) but below the median income.

The absence of experimental research that can examine the impact of different forms of material and income supports on the reduction of poverty and child maltreatment rates makes it difficult to identify the pathways by which low income influences parenting behaviors and interactions with children. Stress is thought to be the dominant variable associated with the relationship between low income and caregiving behaviors, but research attention has recently focused on other factors as well, including material hardships, housing, coping and caregiving strategies, and dangerous environments (Pelton, 1994).

Severe violence toward children is more likely in poor families who have fewer economic and social resources to help with child care responsibilities, especially among those who are least able to cope with the material hardships of poverty (Gelles and Straus, 1988). Although most poor people do not use violence toward intimates, self-report surveys and official report data find that the rates of all forms of family violence, except child sexual abuse, are higher for those whose family income is below the poverty line. As noted above, poor families are more likely to be in contact with social service agencies and hence be under greater scrutiny, thereby increasing the likelihood that they will be reported for abuse or neglect. Nonetheless, the association between child maltreatment and poverty persists in self-report data as well as in official data (Straus et al., 1980; Wauchope and Straus, 1992).

In their review of studies of risk markers for domestic violence, Hotaling and Sugarman (1990) report that, although wife assault occurs across all occupational, educational, and income groups, it is more common and more severe in families with lower socioeconomic status. In addition, higher-socioeconomic-status women seem to be just as likely as lower-socioeconomic-status women to report being verbally assaulted and just as likely to have experienced minor physical violence (i.e., having something thrown at them, being pushed, shoved, slapped, or grabbed). But the frequency and severity of serious assaults appear to be linked to socioeconomic status (Hotaling and Sugarman, 1990). Pillemer and Finkelhor (1988) found no difference in elder abuse rates based on economic status.

## Race

The picture is less clear on race. Both official report data and self-report survey data often report that child abuse and violence toward women are overrepresented among minorities. Data from the National Crime Victimization Survey indicate that the rate of domestic violence is essentially the same for whites (5.4 per 1,000), blacks (5.8 per 1,000), and Hispanics (5.5 per 1,000) (Bureau of Justice Statistics, 1994). All three National Incidence Studies of Child Abuse and Neglect found no significant relationships between the incidence of maltreatment and the child's race or ethnicity (Sedlak and Broadhurst, 1996).

The two National Family Violence Surveys, however, found stronger relationships between race/ethnicity and both violence between partners and violence toward children. Although in the first National Family Violence Survey, the difference in rates between blacks and whites disappeared when income was controlled, an analysis of the larger dataset from the Second National Family Violence Survey[1] found that some differences persisted even when income was controlled (Gelles and Straus, 1988). The second survey also found significantly higher rates of domestic violence and child physical abuse among Hispanics than among non-Hispanic whites. When income, place of residence (urban/nonurban), and age were controlled, the differences disappeared for domestic violence but remained for severe physical abuse of children (Straus and Smith, 1990).

## Situational and Environmental Factors

### Personality Characteristics

Researchers have searched for personality characteristics or psychiatric disorders to explain the behavior of family violence perpetrators. Only a small

---

[1]The Second National Family Violence Survey included oversamples of both blacks and Hispanics (Gelles and Straus, 1988).

percentage of parents involved in child maltreatment are diagnosed with a psychiatric disorder (Steele and Pollock, 1974). Although no consistent pattern has emerged, identification of psychiatric disorders in perpetrators, when present, is important in determining appropriate intervention strategies, especially in cases involving depression or schizophrenia.

Although a consistent profile of parental psychopathology or a significant level of parental mental disturbance has not been supported (Melnick and Hurley, 1969; Polansky et al., 1981, 1992; Spinetta and Rigler, 1972), a set of personality characteristics associated with child maltreatment has emerged with sufficient frequency to warrant attention. These characteristics include low self-esteem, external locus of control, poor impulse control, depression, anxiety, and antisocial behavior (National Research Council, 1993a).

A number of studies have found a high incidence of psychopathology and personality disorders, most frequently antisocial personality disorder, borderline personality organization, and post-traumatic stress disorder among men who assault intimate partners (Hamberger and Hastings, 1986, 1988, 1991; Hart et al., 1993; Dutton and Starzomski, 1993; Dutton, 1994, 1995b; Dutton et al., 1994). Nonetheless, batterers appear to be a heterogeneous group, a finding that has led some researchers to develop typologies to represent different subgroups (Gondolf, 1988; Saunders, 1992). In some cases, the psychological needs of perpetrators can reflect socially constructed role expectations, especially when cultural norms can provide social permission for males to terrorize and control their partners (Warshaw, 1997). A high incidence of psychological or emotional problems among those who physically abuse an elderly relative has also been reported (Pillemer, 1986).

## Stress and Marital Conflict

A number of stressful life events, such as unemployment, financial problems, and sickness or death in the family have been identified as possibly related to violence. For example, an association between unemployment and child maltreatment has been documented by a number of researchers (e.g., Gabinet, 1983; Gelles and Hargreaves, 1981; Krugman et al., 1986; Whipple and Webster-Stratton, 1991). In another analysis, high levels of marital conflict and low socioeconomic status emerged as the primary predictors of increased likelihood and severity of wife assault (Hotaling and Sugarman, 1990). The relationship among stressful life events, the personalities of the people affected by them, and the role of stress as a factor in marital conflict and family violence remains poorly understood. For example, it is not certain whether individuals in violent relationships lack specific skills that can improve their ability to negotiate and compromise and eliminate the use of violence as a strategy to resolve conflict, or whether the sources of marital conflict in seriously or frequently violent relationships are different from those that characterize other relationships (Hotaling and Sugarman,

1990). Conflict over heavy drinking by husbands, often exacerbated by their employment or status insecurity (such as having less education than their wives) illustrates the type of interaction that may increase the use of violence as a conflict resolution strategy.

## Social Isolation and Social Support

The data on social isolation are somewhat less consistent than are the data for the previously discussed correlates. First, because so much of the research on family violence is cross-sectional, it is not clear whether social isolation precedes violence in the home or is a consequence of it. Second, social isolation has been crudely measured, and the purported correlation may be more anecdotal than statistical. Nevertheless, researchers often agree that people who are socially isolated from neighbors and relatives are more likely to be violent in the home. Social support appears to be an important protective factor. One major source of social support is the availability of friends and family for help, aid, and assistance. The more a family is integrated into the community and the more groups and associations they belong to, the less likely they are to be violent (Straus et al., 1980).

## Intergenerational Transmission of Violence

The notion that abused children grow up to be abusing parents and violent adults has been widely expressed in the family violence literature (Gelles, 1980). One review that examined self-reports of the intergenerational transmission of violence toward children concluded that the best estimate of the rate of intergenerational transmission is 30 percent (Kaufman and Zigler, 1987). Although a rate of 30 percent is substantially less than the majority of abused children, it is considerably more than the rate of 2 to 4 percent found in the general population (Straus and Gelles, 1986). A study that examined continuity and discontinuity of abuse in a longitudinal study of high-risk mothers and their children found that mothers who had been abused as children were less likely to abuse their own children if they had emotionally supportive parents, partners, or friends (Egeland et al., 1987). In addition, the abused mothers who did not abuse their children were described as "middle class" and "upwardly mobile," suggesting that they were able to draw on economic resources that may not have been available to the abused mothers who did abuse their children. A study that looked prospectively at the cycle of violence hypothesis found that physically abused and neglected children are at risk of becoming violent offenders when they grow up, compared with matched controls of the same age, sex, race, and approximate social class (Widom, 1989b).

Evidence from studies of parental and marital violence indicates that, although witnessing or experiencing violence by caregivers in one's family of origin is often correlated with later violent behavior, such experience is not the sole determining factor. When the intergenerational transmission of violence occurs, it is probably the result of a complex set of social and psychological processes and confounded with other, more discriminating risk markers, such as marital conflict and socioeconomic status (Hotaling and Sugarman, 1990).

Some studies have examined childhood sexual abuse as a risk factor for committing sex crimes as an adult. A review of 23 retrospective and 2 prospective studies concluded that experiencing childhood sexual abuse is neither a necessary nor a sufficient cause of adult sexual offending (U.S. General Accounting Office, 1996). However, one of the prospective studies did find a significant correlation between being sexually abused as a child and being arrested for prostitution as an adult (Widom and Ames, 1994).

Although experiencing and witnessing violence is believed to be an important risk factor, the actual mechanism by which violence is transmitted from generation to generation is not well understood. The role of the media, for example, may have a powerful influence in transmitting sex-role expectations, conflict resolution strategies, and images of family interactions.

**Alcohol and Drug Use**

The use of alcohol is often associated with aggression, suggesting that it may be a risk factor for family violence, but the associations among alcoholism, drug use, and family violence are poorly understood. Results of studies on alcoholism and child maltreatment have been contradictory, with some studies finding a significant relationship and others not (Hamilton and Collins, 1985; Widom, 1992). Estimates of the extent of alcoholism among abusive parents range from 18 to 38 percent, compared with estimates of 6 to 16 percent for the general population (Harford and Parker, 1994; Robins et al., 1984; Widom, 1992).

Alcohol use has been reported in 25 to 85 percent of incidents of domestic violence (Kantor and Straus, 1987). Although alcohol consumption patterns are associated with other variables related to violence (such as witnessing violence in one's home) (Kantor, 1993), the positive relationship of men's drinking to domestic violence persists even after sociodemographic variables, hostility, and marital satisfaction are statistically controlled for (Leonard and Blane, 1992; Leonard and Senchak, 1993; Hotaling and Sugarman, 1990). Men's drinking patterns, particularly binge drinking, are associated with domestic violence across all ethnic and social classes (Kantor, 1993). Alcohol abuse is also present in a large proportion of elder abuse cases (Pillemer, 1986).

**Gender Inequality and Sex-Role Expectations**

An important risk factor for violence against women appears to be gender inequality. Individual, aggregate, and cross-cultural data find that the greater the degree of gender inequality in a relationship, community, and society, the higher are the rates of violence toward women (Browne and Williams, 1993; Coleman and Straus, 1986; Levinson, 1989; Morley, 1994; Straus, 1994; Straus et al., 1980).

One review of 52 case-comparison studies did not find significant differences in measures of sex role inequality between violent and nonviolent couples (Hotaling and Sugarman, 1986). In a later analysis, the authors observe that expectations about division of labor in the household was one of four markers associated with a risk factor that they labeled "marital conflict." The other three markers were marital conflict, frequency of husband's drinking, and educational incompatibility (Hotaling and Sugarman, 1990).

## Presence of Other Violence

A final general risk factor is that the presence of violence in one family relationship increases the risk that there will be violence in others. For example, children in homes in which there is violence between their parents are more likely to experience violence than are children who grow up in homes where there is no such violence. Moreover, children who witness and experience violence are more likely to use violence toward their parents and siblings than are children who do not experience or see violence in their homes (Straus et al., 1980; Straus and Gelles, 1988; Fagan and Browne, 1994).

## Risk Factors for Victims

Early research in domestic violence and child maltreatment looked for factors that differentiated victims from nonvictims. It was suggested that personality or other personal traits of victims could provoke anger or aggression. Much of this research has been criticized on methodological grounds (e.g., Leventhal, 1981), and it has been suggested that personality traits of victims identified in some early studies were the result rather than the cause of the violence (Hotaling and Sugarman, 1990; Pittman and Taylor, 1992). Compared with research on offenders, there has been somewhat less recent research on victims of family violence that focuses on factors that increase or reduce the risk of victimization. Most research on victims examines the consequences of victimization (e.g., depression, psychological distress, suicide attempts, symptoms of post-traumatic stress syndrome) and the effectiveness of various intervention efforts.

## Children

Early research suggested that a number of factors raise the risk of a child's being abused. Low-birthweight babies (Parke and Collmer, 1975), premature babies (Elmer and Gregg, 1967; Newberger et al., 1977; Parke and Collmer,

1975; Steele and Pollock, 1974), and children with developmental or other disabilities (Friedrich and Boriskin, 1976; Gil, 1971; Steinmetz, 1978) were all described as being at greater risk of being abused by their parents or caregivers. However, a review of such studies calls into question many of these findings (Starr, 1988). One major problem is that few investigators used matched comparison groups. More recent studies did not find premature babies or children with disabilities as being at higher risk for abuse (Egeland and Vaughan, 1981; Starr et al., 1990).

The very youngest children appear to be at the greatest risk of abuse, especially the most dangerous and potentially lethal forms of violence (Fergusson et al., 1972; Gil, 1971; Johnson, 1974). Not only are young children physically more fragile and thus more susceptible to injury, but also their vulnerability makes them more likely to be reported and diagnosed as abused when injured. Older children are most likely to be underreported as victims of abuse.

## Marital Partners

Being female is the most consistent risk factor for being a victim of domestic violence (Hotaling and Sugarman, 1986). Early studies unsuccessfully attempted to find a psychological profile that put a woman at risk of being battered. Early descriptive and clinical accounts described battered women as dependent, having low esteem, and feeling inadequate and helpless (Ball, 1977; Hilberman and Munson, 1977; Shainess, 1979; Walker, 1979) and reported a high incidence of depression and anxiety among clinical samples (Hilberman, 1980). Later studies have questioned whether these victim characteristics were present before the women were battered or are the result of the victimization (Hotaling and Sugarman, 1990). Clinical studies often use small and selective samples and fail to have comparison groups.

A comprehensive review of risk factors found that the only one consistently associated with being a victim of physical abuse was having witnessed parental violence as a child (Hotaling and Sugarman, 1986). As noted earlier, this finding was modified in a later review, and the authors attribute this modification to the use of multivariate analysis that can distinguish between minor and severe violence, marital conflict, and the use of violence in the home (Hotaling and Sugarman, 1990).

## Elders

Research on elder abuse is divided on whether elder victims are more likely to be physically, socially, and emotionally dependent on their caregivers or whether it is the offender's dependence on the victim that increases the risk of elder abuse (see Pillemer and Suitor, 1992; Steinmetz, 1990). Conventional wisdom suggests that it is the oldest, sickest, most debilitated, and dependent elders who are prone to the full range of mistreatment by their caregivers. However, Pillemer and Suitor (1992) have found that the victim's dependence was not as powerful a risk factor as perceived by clinicians, the public, and some researchers. A history of violence, particularly between spouses, may be predictive of elder abuse in later life (Lachs and Pillemer, 1995).

## INTERVENTIONS

A broad set of public and private initiatives at the national, state, and local levels has generated a complex array of institutions to address the consequences and the origins of family violence, but the dimensions of this effort are difficult to observe or measure (see Table 2-2). The large majority of legal, health, and social service interventions and programs relies extensively on community resources that reflect both regional strengths and limitations. In some cases, such efforts have emerged in the absence of national legislation to determine eligibility criteria or accountability standards as a basis for federal funding, and activities have evolved in health, social service, and legal settings (such as home visitations programs and adult protective services) that were not designed with the treatment or prevention of family violence as a primary goal. In other cases, federal and congressional initiatives sought to influence the design of interventions by establishing eligibility criteria, funding direct services, and specifying key elements of program design (such as the Family Violence Prevention and Services Act, the Child Abuse Prevention and Treatment Act, and the Violence Against Women legislation). As a result, the overall "system" of family violence interventions is highly disjointed, loosely structured, and often lacks central coordinating offices or comprehensive service delivery systems.

### Fragmentation of Services

The fragmented nature of the categorical services involved in addressing different aspects of family violence has inhibited the development of a detailed picture and integrated datasets in this field. The fragmentation of services discourages research and cost analyses in assessing the impact and outcomes of family violence; it is therefore difficult to determine whether sufficient services exist in selected settings, the ways in which services address selected goals (such as identification, prevention, protection, or treatment), or the conditions under which persons in need of services do not have access to appropriate care. Victims of domestic violence, for example, may be seen by emergency department personnel, other health care providers, court officials, and battered women's shelter staff, but rarely do these service or agency staff members have an opportunity to collaborate, review, or understand the full dimensions of the victim's needs and experiences. Children who have been assaulted by relatives in their homes may have also witnessed incidents of violence between their parents, but the social

TABLE 2-2  Array of Services for Family Violence by Service Sector and Purpose

| Sector | Prevention | Case Identification/ Risk Factor Detection | Short-Term Victim Protection/Risk Assessment/Treatment | Long-Term Intervention |
|---|---|---|---|---|
| Social services | Education programs<br>Service provider training programs<br>Community coordinating councils<br>Comprehensive community services<br>Community support groups | Surveys<br>Case reports programs<br>Child protective services | Shelters<br>Batterers' treatment<br>Family preservation services<br>Parenting practices and family support | Peer support groups<br>Education and job training<br>Housing (transitional and permanent)<br>Child and elder placement |
| Health | Service provider training programs | Health reports<br>Emergency room procedures<br>Diagnostic protocols | Home visitation and family support | Mental health services for victims<br>Mental health services for offenders |
| Law enforcement | Service provider training programs | Uniform crime reports orders<br>National crime victimization surveys | Temporary restraining<br>Arrest procedures<br>Batterers' treatment programs<br>Victim advocates | Offender incarceration<br>Sentencing guidelines<br>Prosecution procedures<br>Conditions of probation and parole |

SOURCE: Committee on the Assessment of Family Violence Interventions, National Research Council and Institute of Medicine, 1998.

service agency and law enforcement personnel who respond to cases of child maltreatment may not be in a position to address other forms of violent behavior in the home.

The fragmentation of the field has led some observers to question whether there is, in fact, a unified body of research and knowledge that can inform and integrate the different dimensions of this social problem. This complicated terrain has also discouraged and impeded efforts to determine the scope of federal, state, or local treatment and prevention programs, many of which are authorized and funded through a series of statutes that lack a coherent framework or strategy. Yet the broad array of services and resources, while poorly integrated, serves an extensive population. The lack of evidence and analysis about the effectiveness of the system of interventions as a whole does not mean that individual services are not doing an adequate job in addressing the needs of individual clients and communities. But the absence of coherence in the system of family violence interventions makes it difficult to observe or understand ways in which discrete parts of this system may interact, complement, or conflict with each other.

In some cases, federal programs have provided resources to assist with organizing services, technical assistance, and data collection requirements that have helped to standardize a developing program or set of activities. Yet federal efforts lack a set of common goals or comprehensive strategy and often reflect administrative desires to meet the needs of child or adult victims in the context of existing service systems rather than initiating broad reforms focused explicitly on family violence. Furthermore, the role of the federal government has in large part been designed to strengthen and support local or state initiatives that reflect an enormous array of policy and program strategies, often through unrestricted block grants. The inherent flexibility in these types of funding mechanisms inhibits national or regional efforts to collect data on the clients, program outcomes, and measures of effectiveness.

The broad scope and desegregated nature of federal efforts in the area of family violence interventions are reflected in a 1986 report prepared by the Office of the Assistant Secretary for Planning and Evaluation in the U.S. Department of Health and Human Services (DHHS) (U.S. Department of Health and Human Services, 1986). It is the last known federal interdepartmental review of programs focused on child abuse and neglect, domestic violence, and elder abuse; it identifies nine federal departments and three independent agencies that provide services or sponsor research relevant to family violence (see Table 2-3). The 1986 report was preceded by a detailed review of DHHS services for victims of domestic violence undertaken in 1979, when legislation for a categorical program of financial assistance for the provision of services to victims of domestic violence was being considered by the Congress (U.S. Department of Health and Human Services, 1981). The 1981 report noted that no information on services for domestic violence victims had been routinely collected in prior years, because no programs within DHHS had a specific mandate to serve these victims. This

TABLE 2-3   Federal Programs That Provide Services or Sponsor Research Relevant to Family Violence

Department of Health and Human Services

Social services
  Project SHARE
  Community services block grant
  Office of Human Development services
  Coordinated discretionary funds program
  Social services block grant
  Child welfare services
  Foster care and adoption assistance
  Head Start program
  Runaway and homeless youth program
  Developmental disabilities program
  Native Americans program
  Older Americans program
  Child abuse and neglect prevention and treatment program
  National Center on Child Abuse and Neglect
  Advisory Board on Child Abuse and Neglect

Health
  Medicaid (Title XIX)
  Primary care block grant
  Maternal and child health block grant
  Alcohol, Drug Abuse and Mental Health Services block grant
  Preventive Health and Health Services block grant
  Centers for Disease Control and Prevention
  Adolescent Family Life Program
  Indian Health Service Program
  National Institute of Mental Health
  National Institute on Aging
  National Institute on Alcohol Abuse and Alcoholism
  National Institute on Drug Abuse
  National Institute on Child Health and Human Development

Income support
  Aid to Families with Dependent Children
  Supplemental Security Income Program

Department of Agriculture
  Food stamps
  Extension Service

Americorps
  The Foster Grandparent Program
  Retired Senior Volunteer Program
  Volunteers in Service to America (VISTA)

*continued on next page*

TABLE 2-3    (*Continued*)

---

Department of Defense

Department of Education

Department of Housing and Urban Development

Department of the Interior

Department of Justice
  Violence against women grants
  National Institute of Justice
  Office of Victims of Crime grants

Department of Transportation

Department of the Treasury

United States Commission on Civil Rights

General Services Administration

---

SOURCE: U.S. Department of Health and Human Services, 1986.

report describes ways in which 13 separate DHHS service programs had been used to provide assistance to victims of domestic violence, although the vast majority of the eligibility requirements for these programs did not include domestic violence.

For example, through the Social Services (Title XX) program, states receive federal funding for their child protective services programs, which provide social services designed to protect children from abuse, neglect, and exploitation. Service providers who participated in the survey that was part of the 1981 DHHS report indicated that they refer victims of spouse abuse to other service providers (such as shelters or adult protective services programs) for direct help with the problem of domestic violence (U.S. Department of Health and Human Services, 1981). As a result, multiple agencies may become involved in meeting the needs of one family, and problems of coordination and integration of services become increasingly important with the emergence of specialized services.

## Impacts and Costs

The costs associated with family violence include two key components: (1) direct costs, those of providing treatment and services, and (2) indirect costs, such as reduced productivity, diminished quality of life (including pain and suffering), and decreased ability to care for oneself or others. It is extremely difficult to estimate the range of these costs. Efforts to collect data on the dimensions of the programs and services are impeded by their desegregated nature and their reliance on different reporting measures and units of analysis. Yet it is known that the injuries and mental health problems that occur in the wake of family violence have imposed a heavy burden on a broad range of service providers, including women's shelters, schools, hospitals, mental health clinics, police stations, and district attorney's offices. Responses to reports of domestic violence or the endangerment of children, for example, involve time-consuming and costly investigations to determine program eligibility by a broad range of social service programs, including child protective services, children and family resource programs, child welfare, and foster care offices.

In cases in which injury has occurred and the victim or caregivers seek medical assistance, a wide range of health resources may be used, such as emergency department and trauma centers; various medical services, including pediatric, obstetric, and gynecological services; mental health services; oral health and nursing facilities; orthopedic, neurological, and radiological treatment programs; and community health centers. One recent study of the cost implications of treating children in a pediatric intensive care unit, for example, reported that children rendered critically ill from abuse differ markedly from other critically ill children in terms of age, severity of injury, mortality, and expenses for acute medical care (Irazuzta et al., 1997). This study further indicated that, despite the resource-intensive nature of their cases, children whose caregivers sought medical treatment for abuse-related injuries in an intensive care unit were at greater risk of death and severe residual morbidity, often because of irreversible brain injury, than the general patient population in the same unit within the time period of the study.

The legal system has been profoundly affected by the problem of family violence, especially in handling cases involving decisions about child placement, termination of parental rights, and abuse by intimate partners. Massachusetts state courts, for example, issued almost 100,000 restraining orders during the period 1992-1994; on average, once every 10 minutes in Massachusetts a victim of domestic violence seeks a restraining order against an abusive defendant (Adams, 1994). The documentation and treatment of reports of family violence, especially abuse by intimate partners, presents a significant burden on local police agencies and state and municipal courts, including the criminal, family, and juvenile justice systems (Cochran, 1994). More recently, a broad range of voluntary and quasi-public programs have emerged to deal with the aftermath and prevention of family violence, including battered women's shelter programs, child fatality review teams, children's trust fund organizations, family preservation services, and local and state coordinating councils.

The true range of costs associated with the immediate impact of family violence is simply unknown, but conservative estimates would suggest that the costs are quite large. Estimates vary widely depending on the definitions applied, the measurement of both extent and service utilization, and assumptions about the cost of service utilization (see Table 2-4). The expenses of treatment programs for child maltreatment have been estimated to cost more than $500 million annually (U.S. General Accounting Office, 1991a); these costs cover only direct services (such as medical treatment, short-term foster care, and specialized education) and do not include mental health or educational services that may be required as a long-term consequence of child abuse or neglect. The General Accounting Office estimate also does not include additional costs associated with juvenile courts, longer-term foster care, drug or alcohol treatment, adult criminal activities, foregone future earnings, and potential welfare dependence, which have been acknowledged as consequences of child maltreatment but not quantified.

TABLE 2-4    Estimated Annual Costs of Family Violence

| Study | Costs Included | Annual Cost Estimate (for U.S., unless otherwise noted) |
|---|---|---|
| Straus, 1986 | Data related to intrafamily violence | $1.7 billion |
| Daro, 1988 | Medical costs | $20 million[a] |
| | Rehabilitation and special education | $7 million |
| | Foster care | $7.1 billion |
| | Lost productivity | $658 million-$1.3 billion |
| Meyer, 1992 | Short- and long-term medical treatment and lost productivity | $5-$10 billion[b] |
| Dayaratna, 1992 | National health care costs generated as a function of $326.6 million annual health care costs for Pennsylvania Blue Shield | $6.5 billion[b] |
| Zorza, 1994 | National costs generated as a function of $506 million annual health care medical costs for New York City | $31 billion[b] |
| Miller et al., 1994 | Medical bills; out-of-pocket expenses; property losses; productivity losses at home, school, work; pain, suffering, and lost quality of life | $67 billion[b] |

[a]Includes only costs of child maltreatment.
[b]Includes only costs of partner abuse.

SOURCE: Committee on the Assessment of Family Violence Interventions, National Research Council and Institute of Medicine, 1998.

Recent estimates place the annual cost of domestic violence in the United States at between $1.7 billion (Straus, 1986) and $140 billion (Miller et al., 1994). The variation among cost estimates stems from differences in the variables selected to generate cost figures; for example, Miller's estimate includes a high set of indirect costs associated with pain and suffering, which were not included in the Straus estimates. Another major source of difference is the definition used to determine the size of the victimized population. Depending on what prevalence estimates are used, the number of cases for which costs are estimated is affected. And the larger the prevalence rate used, the higher the annual estimate of total cost. One way to narrow the wide range of cost estimates would be to generate a national estimate of the prevalence or incidence of specific types of family violence. The Centers for Disease Control and Prevention, for example, is involved in an effort to define intimate violence in a form that could be used to establish national baseline rates. An interagency task force on child abuse and neglect is conducting a similar effort to define child maltreatment so that common data elements could be established in research studies in this field.

The consequences of victimization are another variable that can generate vastly differing total costs. Cost estimates can include mental as well as physical health, long- as well as short-term treatment costs, family or social costs (such as lower productivity, absenteeism, high rates of turnover, and loss of earnings) as well as personal costs, indirect as well as direct costs, and costs of services for perpetrators as well as for victims. A model that includes emergency room costs only will generate a smaller total cost estimate than one that includes the cost of long-term mental health services to victims, which may not be accrued until months or years after an abusive incident.

Once it has been determined how many cases of family violence should be counted and what costs will be measured, the source of cost data can affect total cost estimates. Conservative estimates may rely on cost data that are relatively easy to obtain, such as the cost of medical treatment; such estimates may thus be limited to expenses directly associated with service fees. In contrast, comprehensive cost estimates may include indirect costs for which no reliable estimate is available, such as the cost of diminished productivity and the costs incurred by the need to provide volunteer advocacy services. Large differences between total cost figures associated with estimating the impact of the problem of family violence can result from the inclusion or elimination of such indirect costs.

The size of indirect cost measurements can be influenced by various estimating factors, such as the use of econometric forecasting techniques, including discount rates and future productivity costs. Applying annual productivity increase rates and discount rates will affect the total cost and result in a more sophisticated, and theoretically more accurate, estimate. The techniques used to estimate loss of productivity, usually human capital or willingness-to-pay approaches, also affect indirect cost measurements.

The more comprehensive the model, the greater the cost estimate it yields

(Table 2-4). One comprehensive model for estimating the annual cost of domestic violence includes direct costs, such as health care costs, social service costs, and criminal justice costs, as well as indirect costs, such as morbidity and mortality costs, which measure lost output when a victim is incapacitated or killed (Rice et al., 1996). Several assumptions are implicit in the model: that direct cost components can be estimated with available data on charges and expenditures for goods and services; that a discount rate of 4 percent and an average annual increase in productivity of 1 percent are appropriate in generating future costs, and that certain other costs of health and social services, such as moral support and advocacy for victims, should be excluded. The costs of these may be significant, but no reliable data exist from which to estimate them.

A cost estimate for child maltreatment for the year 1983 was developed by calculating the number of child abuse reports received, what percentage were substantiated, and what percentage actually received various types of services, including foster care (Daro, 1988). It estimated that the immediate cost of hospitalizing abused and neglected children was $20 million annually, rehabilitation and special education cost $7 million annually, and foster care costs were $460 million annually. Additional short-term costs include education, juvenile court, and private therapy costs. Longer-term costs included $14.8 million for juvenile court and detention costs, $646 million for long-term foster care, and future lost earnings of abused and neglected children of between $658 and $1.3 billion.

Extrapolating Daro's costs for 1994, Westman (1995) included estimates for hospitalization, rehabilitation and special education, foster care, social services case management, and court expenses. His cost estimate was between $8.4 and $32.3 billion each year, based on a range of $12,174 to $46,870 per maltreated child per year.

Miller et al. (1994) estimate that personal crime costs Americans $105 billion each year. Including pain and suffering, the cost rises to $450 billion. Violent crime accounts for $426 billion of the total. The authors estimate that child abuse costs $67,000 per incident, sexual abuse $99,000, and emotional abuse $27,000 for an average of $60,000 per incident of child abuse. The authors estimated that child neglect costs $9,700 per incident. Thus, the total cost of child abuse and neglect per year is estimated to be $56 billion. Miller et al. (1994) do not include in their estimate the cost for sibling violence, noncriminal violence toward parents, or noncriminal elder abuse. Thus, their cost estimate of $77 billion for child abuse and domestic violence still underestimates the total costs of family violence each year.

What is also unknown in reviewing these cost estimates is the extent to which existing expenses associated with health, social services, and legal services could be reduced if effective preventive interventions were in place. Reducing the scope of family violence and mitigating its consequences would have some impact on existing service expenses, most of which are borne by individuals or public agencies, but the size of that impact remains uncertain.

# 3

# Improving Evaluation

Improving the standards of evidence used in the evaluation of family violence interventions is one of the most critical needs in this field. Given the complexity and unique history of family violence interventions, researchers and service providers have used a variety of methods and a broad array of measures and evaluation strategies over the past two decades. This experimentation has contributed important ideas (using qualitative and quantitative methods) that have helped to establish a baseline for the assessment of individual programs. What is lacking, however, is a capacity and research base that can offer specific guidance to key decision makers and the broader service provider community about the impact or relative effectiveness of specific interventions, as well as broad service strategies, to address the multiple dimensions of family violence.

Recognizing that more rigorous studies are needed to better determine "what works," "for whom," "under what conditions," and "at what cost," the committee sought to identify research strategies and components of evaluation designs that represent key opportunities for improvement. The road to improvement requires attention to four areas: (1) assessing the limitations of current evaluations, (2) forging functional partnerships between researchers and service providers, (3) addressing the dynamics of collaboration in those partnerships, and (4) exploring new evaluation methods to assess comprehensive community initiatives.

The emerging emphasis on integrated, multifaceted, community-based approaches to treatment and prevention services, in particular, presents a new dilemma in evaluating family violence interventions: comprehensive interventions are particularly difficult, if not impossible, to implement as well as study using experimental or quasi-experimental designs. Efforts to resolve this dilemma may benefit from attention to service design, program implementation, and assessment experiences in related fields (such as substance abuse and teenage pregnancy prevention). These experiences could reveal innovative methods, common lessons, and reliable measures in the design and development of comprehensive community interventions, especially in areas characterized by individualized services, principles of self-determination, and community-wide participation.

Improving on study design and methodology is important, since technical improvements are necessary to strengthen the science base. But the dynamics of the relationships between researchers and service providers are also important; a creative and mutually beneficial partnership can enhance both research and program design.

Two additional points warrant mention in a broad discussion of the status of evaluations of family violence interventions. First, learning more about the effectiveness of programs, interventions, and service strategies requires the development of controlled studies and reliable measures, preceded by detailed process evaluations and case studies that can delve into the nature and clients of a particular intervention as well as aspects of the institutional or community settings that facilitate or impede implementation. Second, the range of interactions between treatment and clients requires closer attention to variations in the individual histories and social settings of the clients involved. These interactions can be studied in longitudinal studies or evaluations that pair clients and treatment regimens and allow researchers to follow cohorts over time within the general study group.

## ASSESSING THE LIMITATIONS OF CURRENT EVALUATIONS

The limitations of the empirical evidence for family violence interventions are not new, nor are they unique. For violence interventions of all kinds, few examples provide sufficient evidence to recommend the implementation of a particular program (National Research Council, 1993b). And numerous reviews indicate that evaluation studies of many social policies achieve low rates of technical quality (Cordray, 1993; Lipsey et al., 1985). A recent National Research Council study offered two explanations for the poor quality of evaluations of violence interventions: (1) most evaluations were not planned as part of the introduction of a program and (2) evaluation designs were too weak to reach a conclusion as to the program's effects (National Research Council, 1993b).

The field cannot be improved simply by urging researchers and service providers to strengthen the standards of evidence used in evaluation studies. Nor can it be improved simply by urging that evaluation studies be introduced in the early stages of the planning and design of interventions. Specific attention is needed to the hierarchy of study designs, the developmental stages of evaluation research and interventions, the marginal role of research in service settings, and the difficulties associated with imposing experimental conditions in service settings.

## A Hierarchy of Study Designs

The evaluation of family violence interventions requires research directed at estimating the unique effects (or net impact) of the intervention, above and beyond any change that may have occurred because of a multitude of other factors. Such research requires study designs that can distinguish the impact of the intervention within a general service population from other changes that occur only in certain groups or that result simply as a passage of time. These design commonly involve the formation of (at least) two groups: one composed of individuals who participated in the intervention (often called the treatment or experimental group) and a second group composed of individuals who are comparable in character and experience to those who participated in the intervention but who received no services or received an intervention that was significantly different from that under study (the control or comparison group). Some study designs involve multiple treatment groups who receive modified forms of the services that are the subject of the evaluation; other studies use one subject group, but sample the group at multiple times prior to and after the intervention to determine whether the measures immediately before and after the program are a continuation of earlier patterns or whether they indicate a decisive change that endures after the cessation of services; this is called a time-series design (Campbell and Stanley, 1966, and Weiss, 1972, are two comprehensive primers on the basic principles and designs of program assessment and evaluation research).

Study designs that rely on a comparison group, or that use a time-series design, are commonly viewed as more reliable than evaluation studies that simply test a single treatment group prior to and after an intervention (often called a pre-post study). More rigorous experimental designs, which involve the use of a randomized control group, are able to distinguish changes in behavior or attitude that occur as a result of the intervention from those that are influenced by maturation (the tendency for many individuals to improve over time), self-selection (the tendency of individuals who are motivated to change to seek out and continue their involvement with an intervention that is helping them), and other sources of bias that may influence the outcome of the intervention.

The importance of estimating the net impact of innovative services and determining their comparative value highlights several technical issues:

1. The manner in which the control or comparison groups are formulated influences the validity of the inference that can be drawn regarding net effects.

2. The number of participants enrolled in each group (the sample size) must be sufficient to permit statistical detection of differences between the groups, if one exists.

3. There should be agreement among interested parties that a selected outcome is important to measure, that it is a valid reflection of the objective of the intervention, and that it can reflect change over time.

4. Evidence is needed that the innovative services were actually provided as planned, and that the differences between the innovative services and usual services were large enough to generate meaningful differences in the outcome of interest.

Over the last few decades, evaluation research has developed a general consensus about the relative strength of various study designs used to assess the effectiveness (or net effects) of interventions (Figure 3-1; see also Green and Byar, 1984). The lowest level of evidence in the hierarchy is *nonexperimental designs*, which include case studies and anecdotal reports. This type of research often consists of detailed histories of participant experiences with an intervention. Although they may contain a wealth of information, nonexperimental studies cannot provide a strong base for inference because they are unable to control for such factors as maturation, self-selection, the interaction of selection and maturation (the tendency for those with more or less severe problem levels to mature at differential rates), historical influences that are unrelated to the intervention, other interventions they may have received, a variety of response biases and demand characteristics, and changes in instrumentation (the interviewer becomes more familiar with the client over the course of the study).

The next level of evidence is *quasi-experimental research designs* (levels 4 through 6 in Figure 3-1). Although these designs can improve inferential clarity, they cannot be relied on to yield unbiased estimates of the effects of interventions because the research subjects are not assigned randomly. Two research reviews of family violence interventions suggest that some trustworthy information can be extracted from quasi-experimental designs, so they are not without merit (Finkelhor and Berliner, 1995; Heneghan et al., 1996). Although quasi-experimental study designs can provide evidence that a relationship exists between participation in the intervention and the outcome, the magnitude of the net effect is difficult to determine. In other fields, quasi-experimental results are more trustworthy when the studies involve a broader evidential basis than simple pre-post designs (Cook and Campbell, 1979; Cordray, 1986).

The highest level of evidence is *experimental designs* that include controls to restrict a number of important threats to internal validity. These are the least prevalent types of designs in the family violence literature. Although, in theory, properly designed and executed experiments can produce unbiased estimates of net effects, other threats to validity emerge when they are conducted in largely uncontrolled settings. Such threats involve various forms of generalization (across persons, settings, time, and other constructs of interest), statistical problems, and logistical problems (e.g., differential attrition from measurement or noncompliance with the intervention protocol). These other threats to validity

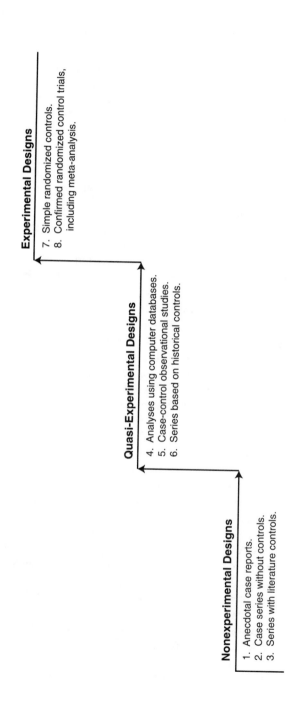

FIGURE 3-1 Hierarchy of strength of evidence in research evaluations. SOURCE: Modified from Green and Byar (1984). Copyright John Wiley & Sons Limited. Reproduced with permission.

can be addressed by replications and the synthesis of research results, including the use of meta-analysis (Lipsey and Wilson, 1993). Replication is an essential part of the scientific process; replication studies can reveal evidence from both successes and failures. The proper use of research synthesis can provide a tool for understanding variation and similarities across studies and will uncover robust intervention effects, if they are present, even if the individual studies are not generalizable because their samples are not representative, the interventions are unique, or their measures are inconsistent (Cook and Shadish, 1994; Cordray, 1993; Colditz et al., 1995).

## Developmental Stages of Research

Interventions often undergo an evolutionary process that refines theories, services, and approaches over time. In the early stages, interventions generate reform efforts and evaluations that rely primarily on descriptive studies and anecdotal data. As these interventions and evaluation efforts mature, they begin to approach the standards of evidence needed to make confident judgments about effectiveness and cost.

Current discussions about what is known about family violence interventions are often focused on determining the effectiveness or cost-effectiveness of selected programs, interventions, or strategies. Conclusions about effectiveness require fairly high standards of evidence because an evaluation must demonstrate, with high certainty, that the intervention of interest is responsible for the observed effects. This high standard of evidence is warranted to change major policies, but it may inhibit a careful assessment of what can be derived from a knowledge base that is still immature.

Of the more than 2,000 evaluation studies identified by the committee in the course of this study, the large majority consist of nonexperimental study designs. For example, one review of 29 studies of the treatment of sexually abused children indicated that more than half of the studies (17) were pre-post (also called before and after) designs that evaluated the same group of children at two or more time intervals during which some kind of professional intervention was provided (Finkelhor and Berliner, 1995). Similarly, a methodological review of intensive family preservation services programs excluded 36 of 46 identified program evaluations because they contained no comparison groups (Heneghan et al., 1996). Thus, while hundreds of evaluation studies exist in the family violence research literature, most of them provide no firm basis for examining the relative impact of a specific intervention or considering the ways in which different types of clients respond to a treatment, prevention, or deterrence intervention.

Still, nonexperimental studies can reveal important information in the developmental process of research. They can illuminate the characteristics and experience of program participants, the nature of the presenting problems, and issues associated with efforts to implement individual programs or to change systems of service within the community. Although these kinds of studies cannot provide evidence of effectiveness, they do represent important building blocks in evaluation research.

## Developmental Stages of Interventions

A similar developmental process exists on the programmatic side of interventions. Many family violence treatment and prevention programs have their origins in the efforts of advocates concerned about children, women, elderly people, and the family unit. Over several decades of organized activity, these efforts have fostered the development of interventions in social service, health, and law enforcement settings that program sponsors believe will improve the welfare of victims or control and reduce the violent behavior of perpetrators. Some programs are based on common sense and legal authority, such as mandatory reporting requirements; some are based on theories borrowed from other areas, such as counseling services for victims of trauma (Azar, 1988); and some are based on broad theories of human interaction that are difficult to operationalize, such as comprehensive community interventions. Rarely do family violence interventions result from the development of theory or data collection efforts that precede the implementation of a particular program or strategy. Significant exceptions can be found in some areas, however, such as the treatment of domestic violence (especially the use of arrest policies) and the development of home visitation services and intensive family preservation services. All these interventions were preceded by research studies that identified critical decision points in the intervention process that could be influenced by policy or service reforms (such as deterrence research in domestic violence cases) and research suggesting that families may be more responsive to services during times of crisis (such as a decision to move a child from a family setting into out-of-home placement) or change (such as the birth of a child).

Initial attempts to implement strategies are followed by refinements that include concrete descriptions of services, the development of models to differentiate types of interventions, and the emergence of theories or rationales to explain why particular approaches ought to be effective. As these models are replicated, empirical evidence and experience emerge that clarify who is best served by a particular intervention and under what circumstances. As programs mature and become better articulated and implemented, the evaluation questions and methods become more complex.

## The Marginal Role of Research in Service Settings

Most research on family violence interventions is concentrated in social service settings, in which researchers have comparatively easy access to clients and can exert greater control over the service implementation process that accompanied the development of the intervention. Research is also concentrated in the area of child maltreatment, which has a longer history of interventions than domestic violence or elder abuse. It is important to reiterate that the distribution of the evaluation studies reviewed in this report does not match the history of the programs and the interventions themselves. Some interventions, such as home visitation and family preservation services, are comparatively new and employ innovative service strategies. Because they easily lend themselves to evaluation of small study populations, they have been the subject of numerous evaluation studies. Other, more extensive interventions, such as foster care, judicial rulings on child placement, and shelter services for battered women, involve larger numbers of individuals and are more resistant to study because they are deeply embedded in major institutional or advocacy settings that are often not receptive to or do not have the resources to support research. As a result, research is often marginalized in discussions of the effectiveness of certain programs or service strategies, and the conditions that can foster empirical program evaluation studies are restricted to a fairly narrow range of program activity.

This situation appears to be changing. The growing costs of ongoing interventions have stimulated interest in the public sector in knowing more about the processes, effects, and outcomes associated with service strategies, interventions, and programs. In the site visits and workshops that were part of our study, program advocates with extensive experience with different service models expressed a receptivity to learning more about specific components of service systems that can allow them to tailor services to the individual needs of their clients and communities. Researchers have documented the variation among victims and offenders, suggesting that, in assigning cases to service categories, repetitive and chronic cases should be distinguished from those that are episodic or stimulated by unusual stress. Furthermore, inconsistent findings and uncertainties associated with the ways in which clients are referred to or selected for programs and interventions suggest that more attention should be focused on the pathways by which individual victims or offenders enter different service settings.

There is now greater interest in understanding the social, economic, legal, and political processes that shape the development of family violence interventions. At the same time, program advocates have begun to focus on the development of comprehensive community interventions that can move beyond the difficulties associated with providing professional services in institutional settings and establish resource centers that can aid parents, families, women, and children in their own communities. The development of these comprehensive and individualized interventions has stimulated further interest in knowing more about the ways in which client characteristics, service settings, and program content interact to stimulate behavioral change and lead to a reduction in child maltreatment, domestic violence, and elder abuse.

## Imposing Experimental Conditions in Service Settings

It is difficult for researchers to establish good standards of evidence when they cannot exert complete control over the selection of clients and the implementation of the intervention. But several strategies have emerged in other fields that can guide the development of evaluation research as it moves from its descriptive stage into the conduct of quasi-experimental and true experimental studies.

An important part of this process is the development of a "fleet of studies" (Cronbach and Snow, 1981) that can provide a broad and rich understanding of a specific intervention. For example, a recent report by the National Research Council and the Institute of Medicine used a variety of sources of evaluation information to examine the effects of needle exchange programs on the risk of HIV transmission for intravenous drug users (National Research Council, 1995). Several program evaluations conducted over several years made it possible for the study panel to examine the pattern of evidence about the effectiveness of the needle exchange program. Although each individual study of a given project was insufficient to support a claim that the needle exchange program was effective, the collective strengths of this fleet of studies taken together provided a basis for a firm inference about effectiveness.

The only fleet of studies identified in our review of evaluations is the Spousal Arrest Replication Program (SARP) discussed in Chapter 5. In contrast, although multiple studies have been conducted of parenting programs and family support interventions (such as lay counseling, peer group support, and parent education), their dimensions, subject samples, and instrumentation are too varied to allow strong inferences to be developed at this time.

Evaluation may lag behind the development and refinement of intervention programs, especially when there is a rush to experiment without establishing the necessary conditions for a successful endeavor. Premature experimentation can leave the impression that nothing works, especially if the problem to be addressed is complex, interventions are limited, and program effects are obscure. Yet early program experimentation studies can be helpful in describing the characteristics of clients who appear to be receptive or impervious to change, documenting the barriers to program implementation, and estimating the size, intensity, costs, and duration of the intervention that may be required. If these lessons can be captured, they are a valuable resource in moving the research and program base to a new level of development, one that can address multiple and contextual interactions.

## Flaws in Current Evaluations

The committee identified 114 evaluation studies conducted in the period 1980-1996 that have sufficient scientific strength to provide insights on the effects of specific interventions in the area of child maltreatment, domestic violence, and elder abuse (Table 3-1). This time period was selected because it provides a contemporary history of the evaluation research literature while maintaining manageable limits on the scope of the evidence considered by the committee. As noted in Chapter 1, each of the studies employed an experimental or quasi-experimental research design, used reliable research instrumentation, and included a control or comparison group. In addition, a set of 35 detailed review articles summarizes a broader set of studies that rely on less rigorous standards but offer important insights into the nature and consequences of specific interventions (Table 3-2). Most of the 114 studies identified by the committee focus on interventions conducted in the United States. As a group, these studies represent only a small portion of the enormous array of evaluation research that has been conducted.

A rigorous assessment of the quasi-experimental studies and research review papers reveals many methodological weaknesses, including differences in the nature of the treatment and control groups, sample sizes that are too small to detect medium or small effects of the intervention, research measures that are unreliable or that yield divergent results with different ethnic and cultural groups, short periods of follow-up, and lack of specificity and consistency in program content and services. The lack of equivalence between treatment and control groups in quasi-experimental studies can be illustrated in one study of therapeutic treatment of sexually abused children, in which children in the therapy group were compared with a group of no-therapy children (Sullivan et al., 1992). In a review of the study findings, the authors note that although children who received treatment had significantly fewer behavior problems at a one-year follow-up assessment, the no-therapy comparison group consisted of children whose parents had specifically refused therapy for their children when it was offered (Finkelhor and Berliner, 1995). This observation suggests that other systematic differences could exist within the two groups that affected their recovery (for example, having parents who were or were not supportive of psychological interventions).

Similarly, a review of intensive family preservation services programs indicated that, in a major Illinois evaluation of the intervention, the 2,000 families included were distributed across six sites that administered significantly different types of programs and services (Rossi, 1992). As a result, the sample size was reduced to the 333 families associated with each individual site; small effects associated with the intervention, if they occurred, could not be observed (Rossi, 1992). A later methodological review of intensive family preservation services indicated that 5 of 10 studies that used control or comparison groups had treatment groups that included fewer than 100 participants (Heneghan et al., 1996).

The quality of the existing research base of evaluations of family violence interventions is therefore insufficient to provide confident inferences to guide policy and practice, except in a few areas that we identify in this report. Never-

TABLE 3-1 Interventions by Type of Strategy and Relevant Quasi-Experimental Evaluations, 1980-1996

| Intervention | Quasi-Experimental Evaluations |
| --- | --- |
| Parenting practices and family support services **4A-1** | Barth et al., 1988<br>Barth, 1991<br>Brunk et al., 1987<br>Burch and Mohr, 1980<br>Egan, 1983<br>Gaudin et al., 1991<br>Hornick and Clarke, 1986<br>Lutzker et al., 1984<br>National Center on Child Abuse and Neglect, 1983a,b<br>Reid et al., 1981<br>Resnick, 1985<br>Schinke et al., 1986<br>Wesch and Lutzker, 1991<br>Whiteman et al., 1987 |
| School-based sexual abuse prevention **4A-2** | Conte et al., 1985<br>Fryer et al., 1987<br>Harvey et al., 1988<br>Hazzard et al., 1991<br>Kleemeier et al., 1988<br>Kolko et al., 1989<br>McGrath et al., 1987<br>Miltenberger and Thiesse-Duffy, 1988<br>Peraino, 1990<br>Randolph and Gold, 1994<br>Saslawsky and Wurtele, 1986<br>Wolfe et al., 1986<br>Wurtele et al., 1986, 1991 |
| Child protective services investigation and casework **4A-3** | |
| Intensive family preservation services **4A-4** | AuClaire and Schwartz, 1986<br>Barton, 1994<br>Bergquist et al., 1993<br>Dennis-Small and Washburn, 1986<br>Feldman, 1991<br>Halper and Jones, 1981<br>Pecora et al., 1992<br>Schuerman et al., 1994<br>Schwartz et al., 1991<br>Szykula and Fleischman, 1985<br>Walton et al., 1993<br>Walton, 1994<br>Wood et al., 1988<br>Yuan et al., 1990 |

*continued on next page*

TABLE 3-1   *(Continued)*

| Intervention | Quasi-Experimental Evaluations |
| --- | --- |
| Child placement services **4A-5** | Chamberlain et al., 1992<br>Elmer, 1986<br>Runyan and Gould, 1985<br>Wald et al., 1988 |
| Individualized service<br>programs **4A-6** | Clark et al., 1994<br>Hotaling et al., undated<br>Jones, 1985 |
| Shelters for battered women **4B-1** | Berk et al., 1986 |
| Peer support groups for battered<br>women **4B-2** | |
| Advocacy services for battered<br>women **4B-3** | Sullivan and Davidson, 1991<br>Tan et al., 1995 |
| Domestic violence prevention<br>programs **4B-4** | Jaffe et al., 1992<br>Jones, 1991<br>Krajewski et al., 1996<br>Lavoie et al., 1995 |
| Adult protective services  **4C-1** | |
| Training for caregivers **4C-2** | Scogin et al., 1989 |
| Advocacy services to prevent<br>elder abuse  **4C-3** | Filinson, 1993 |
| Mandatory reporting  requirements<br>**5A-1** | |
| Child placement by the courts **5A-2** | |
| Court-mandated treatment for<br>child abuse offenders **5A-3** | Irueste-Montes and Montes, 1988<br><br>Wolfe et al., 1980 |
| Treatment for sexual abuse<br>offenders **5A-4** | Lang et al., 1988<br>Marshall and Barbaree, 1988 |
| Criminal prosecution of child<br>abuse offenders **5A-5** | |
| Improving child witnessing **5A-6** | |
| Evidentiary reforms **5A-7** | |

TABLE 3-1 *(Continued)*

| Intervention | Quasi-Experimental Evaluations |
| --- | --- |
| Procedural reforms **5A-8** | |
| Reporting requirements **5B-1** | |
| Protective orders **5B-2** | |
| Arrest procedures **5B-3** | Berk et al., 1992a<br>Dunford et al., 1990<br>Ford and Regoli, 1993<br>Hirschel and Hutchison, 1992<br>Pate and Hamilton, 1992<br>Sherman and Berk, 1984a,b<br>Sherman et al., 1992a,b<br>Steinman 1988, 1990 |
| Court-mandated treatment for domestic violence offenders **5B-4** | Chen et al., 1989<br>Dutton, 1986<br>Edleson and Grusznski, 1989<br>Edleson and Syers, 1990<br>Hamberger and Hastings, 1988<br>Harrell, 1992<br>Palmer et al., 1992<br>Tolman and Bhosley, 1989 |
| Criminal prosecution **5B-5** | Ford and Regoli, 1993 |
| Specialized courts **5B-6** | |
| Systemic approaches **5B-7** | Davis and Taylor, 1995<br>Gamache et al., 1988 |
| Training for criminal justice personnel **5B-8** | |
| Reporting requirements **5C-1** | |
| Protective orders **5C-2** | |
| Education and legal counseling **5C-3** | |
| Guardians and conservators **5C-4** | |
| Arrest, prosecution, and other litigation **5C-5** | |
| Identification and screening **6A-1** | Brayden et al., 1993 |

*continued on next page*

TABLE 3-1    *(Continued)*

| Intervention | Quasi-Experimental Evaluations |
|---|---|
| Mental health services for child victims of physical abuse and neglect **6A-2** | Culp et al., 1991<br>Fantuzzo et al., 1987<br>Fantuzzo et al., 1988<br>Kolko, 1996a,b |
| Mental health services for child victims of sexual abuse **6A-3** | Berliner and Saunders, 1996<br>Cohen and Mannarino, 1996<br>Deblinger et al., 1996<br>Downing et al., 1988<br>Oates et al., 1994<br>Verleur et al., 1986<br>Wollert, 1988 |
| Mental health services for children who witness domestic violence **6A-4** | Jaffe et al., 1986b<br>Wagar and Rodway, 1995 |
| Mental health services for adult survivors of child abuse **6A-5** | Alexander et al., 1989, 1991 |
| Home visitation and family support programs **6A-6** | Larson, 1980<br>Marcenko and Spence, 1994<br>National Committee to Prevent Child Abuse, 1996<br>Olds, 1992<br>Olds et al., 1986, 1988, 1994, 1995<br>Scarr and McCartney, 1988 |
| Domestic violence screening, identification, and medical care responses **6B-1** | McLeer et al., 1989<br>McLeer and Anwar, 1989<br>Olson et al., 1996<br>Tilden and Shepherd, 1987 |
| Mental health services for domestic violence victims **6B-2** | Bergman and Brismar, 1991<br>Cox and Stoltenberg, 1991<br>Harris et al., 1988<br>O'Leary et al., 1994 |
| Elder abuse identification and screening **6C-1** | |
| Hospital multidisciplinary teams **6C-2** | |
| Hospital-based support groups **6C-3** | |

SOURCE: Committee on the Assessment of Family Violence Interventions, National Research Council and Institute of Medicine, 1998.

TABLE 3-2   Reviews of Multiple Studies and Evaluations

| | Type of Abuse | Citation | Focus | Studies Reviewed |
|---|---|---|---|---|
| 1. | Child abuse | Becker and Hunter, 1992 | A review of interventions with adult child molesters, intrafamilial and extrafamilial. | 27 studies |
| 2. | Child abuse | Blythe, 1983 | A review of interventions with abusive families. | 16 studies |
| 3. | Child abuse | Briere, 1996 | A review of treatment outcome studies for abused children. | 3 studies |
| 4. | Child abuse | Carroll et al., 1992 | An evaluation of school curricula child sexual abuse prevention program evaluations. | 18 programs |
| 5. | Child abuse | Cohen et al., 1984 | A review of evaluations (many completed prior to 1980) of programs to prevent child maltreatment: early and extended contact, perinatal support programs, parent education classes, and counseling programs. | 20 studies |
| 6. | Child abuse | Cohn and Daro, 1987 | Review of child neglect and abuse prevention programs. | 4 evaluations |
| 7. | Child abuse | Dubowitz, 1990 | Review of evaluations of cost and effectiveness of child abuse interventions. | 5 evaluations |
| 8. | Child abuse | Fantuzzo and Twentyman, 1986 | A review of psychotherapeutic interventions with victims of child abuse. | 30 studies |
| 9. | Child abuse | Fink and McCloskey, 1990 | Review of child abuse prevention programs. | 13 evaluations |
| 10. | Child abuse | Finkelhor and Berliner, 1995 | Review of child abuse treatment programs, characterizing them by type of study design. Included sex education, music therapy, family therapy, group therapy, and cognitive behavioral treatment. | 29 evaluations |
| 11. | Child abuse | Frankel, 1988 | Review of family-centered, home-based services for child protection. | 7 studies |
| 12. | Child abuse | Fraser et al., 1991 | Review of family and home-based services and intensive family preservation programs. | 7 studies |

*continued on next page*

TABLE 3-2    *(Continued)*

| Type of Abuse | Citation | Focus | Studies Reviewed |
|---|---|---|---|
| 13. Child abuse | Garbarino, 1986 | Review of results of child abuse prevention programs. | 5 studies |
| 14. Child abuse | Heneghan et al., 1996 | A review of 46 family preservation services program evaluations, including 5 randomized trials and 5 quasi-experimental studies. | 10 studies |
| 15. Child abuse | Kelly, 1982 | A review of integral components of behavioral treatment strategies to reorient pedophiliacs. | 32 studies |
| 16. Child abuse | Kolko, 1988 | A review of in-school programs to prevent child sexual abuse. | 15 studies |
| 17. Child abuse | McCurdy, 1995 | A review of evaluations of home visiting programs. | 10 studies |
| 18. Child abuse | McDonald et al., 1990 | Comparison review of California Homebuilder-type interventions including in-home services designed to improve parenting skills and access to community resources. | 8 in-home care projects |
| 19. Child abuse | McDonald et al., 1993 | Comparison of the findings of evaluations of foster care programs. | 27 studies |
| 20. Child abuse | National Resource Center on Family Based Services, 1986 | An evaluation of child placement prevention projects in Wisconsin from 1983-1985. | 14 projects |
| 21. Child abuse | O'Donohue and Elliott, 1992 | A review of evaluations of psychotherapeutic interventions for sexually abused children. | 11 studies |
| 22. Child abuse | Olds and Kitzman, 1990 | Review of randomized trials of prenatal and infancy home visitation programs for socially disadvantaged women and children. | 26 studies |
| 23. Child abuse | Olds and Kitzman, 1993 | Review of randomized trials of home visitation programs designed to ameliorate child outcomes including maltreatment. | 19 studies |

TABLE 3-2    (*Continued*)

| | Type of Abuse | Citation | Focus | Studies Reviewed |
|---|---|---|---|---|
| 24. | Child abuse | Pecora et al., 1992 | Review of studies of family-based and intensive family preservation programs. | 12 studies |
| 25. | Child abuse | Rossi, 1992 | Review of Homebuilders-type programs. | 9 studies |
| 26. | Child abuse | Sturkie, 1983 | Review of group treatment interventions for victims of child sexual abuse. | 18 studies |
| 27. | Child abuse | Wolfe and Wekerle, 1993 | Review of studies reporting on treatment outcomes with abusive and/or neglectful parents and children. | 21 studies |
| 28. | Child abuse | Wurtele, 1987 | Review of results of school curricula to teach children sexual abuse prevention skills. | 11 studies |
| 29. | Domestic violence | Edleson and Tolman, 1992 | Review of group batterer treatment programs for male spouse abusers. | 10 studies |
| 30. | Domestic violence | Eisikovits and Edleson, 1989 | Review of outcome studies of batterer treatment programs. | approximately 20 studies |
| 31. | Domestic violence | Gondolf, 1991 | Review of results of evaluations of court-mandated and voluntary batterer counseling programs. | 30 batterer programs studied, 6 evaluations reviewed |
| 32. | Domestic violence | Gondolf, 1995 | Review of evaluations of batterer treatment programs. | |
| 33. | Domestic violence | Rosenfeld, 1992 | Review of batterer treatment programs focusing on recidivism data. | 25 studies |
| 34. | Domestic violence | Saunders and Azar, 1989 | Review of various family violence interventions, including services to prevent child abuse and domestic abuse. | |
| 35. | Domestic violence | Tolman and Edleson, 1995 | Review of effectiveness of batterer treatment programs. | |

SOURCE: Committee on the Assessment of Family Violence Interventions, National Research Council and Institute of Medicine, 1998.

theless, this pool of evaluation studies and additional review articles represents a foundation of research knowledge that will guide the next generation of family violence evaluation efforts and allows broad lessons to be derived from the research literature. For example, research evaluations of the treatment of sexually abused children have concluded that therapeutic treatment is beneficial for many clients, although much remains unknown about the impacts and interactions associated with specific treatment protocols or the characteristics of children and families who are responsive or resistant to therapeutic interventions (Finkelhor and Berliner, 1995). The knowledge base also provides insight into the difficulties associated with implementing innovative service designs in various institutional settings and the range of variations associated with clients who receive family violence interventions in health care, social service, and law enforcement settings.

## Sample Size and Statistical Power

Studies of family violence interventions are often based on small samples of clients that lack sufficient statistical power to detect meaningful effects, especially when such effects are distributed nonrandomly across the subject population and do not persist over time. Statistical power is the likelihood that an evaluation will detect the effect of an intervention, if there is one. Two factors affect statistical power: sample size and effect size (the effect size, ES, is usually measured in terms of the mean difference between the intervention and control groups as a fraction of the standard deviation). In designing an evaluation, researchers need to consider the effect size that would be needed to achieve satisfactory statistical power (power is commonly deemed adequate when there is an 80 percent chance of detecting a hypothesized result).

Conventional statistical estimates suggest that large effects of an intervention (an effect size that exceeds 0.80) require a sample size of at least 20 individuals. This sample size is the modal size used in child abuse studies reported in a review by Finkelhor and Berliner (1995). These studies would have to posit large differences between innovative services and usual care to observe program effects. As the meaningful effect size becomes smaller, a larger sample size is needed to detect it. Medium effects (ES = 0.50) require a sample size of at least 80 individuals to observe the effect, if it exists. Small effects (ES = 0.20), which may be important in terms of understanding the types of individuals who respond positively or negatively to specific interventions, require larger sample sizes of 300 or more to observe the effects, if they exist (Cohen, 1988). Few family violence intervention studies reported to date have used samples this large.

Calculating the actual statistical power for each sample size and the "expected effect" scenario represents an important measure of the statistical adequacy of family violence studies. For example, an intervention that is expected to produce a medium effect and involves 20 clients per group has only a 46 percent chance of detecting the effect (if it exists). To reach conventional levels of power (80 percent), the sample sizes should be increased fourfold to 80 per group to detect medium and large effects. If the true effect is small, a 15-fold increase in the sample size would be necessary.

The use of multisite evaluations can increase the statistical strength of family violence intervention studies, as long as separate sites adhere to common design elements of the intervention and apply uniform eligibility and risk assessment criteria (difficulties in these areas have been identified in at least one evaluation of intensive family preservation services—see Schuerman et al., 1994). An alternative is to extend the duration of each study to allow sufficient time to accrue an appropriate sample. But expanding the time frame increases the possibility that the intervention may be revised or changes may occur in the subject population or the community.

### Lessons from Nonexperimental Studies

Limitations in the calibre of study designs, the weak statistical power of the majority of studies, and inconsistencies in the reliability and validity of measures suggest that little firm knowledge can be extracted from the existing literature about program effects of family violence interventions. However, in the committee's view, the evaluations described in Tables 3-1 and 3-2 provide information about obstacles that need to be addressed and successes that could be built on. Although pre-post, nonexperimental studies cannot provide solid inferences about net effects, they are important predecessors to the next generation of studies. These building blocks in the developmental process include experience with the stages of program implementation, awareness of the utility of screening measures and their sensitivity to change over time, estimates of the reliability and validity of selected research measures, and experience with recruitment and attrition in the intervention condition and measurement protocol.

These technical problems, which involve fundamental principles of what constitutes a good study design and methods, are similar to those that plague many studies of social policies. But they are overshadowed by other, more pragmatic issues related to subject recruitment and retention, ethical and legal concerns, and the integration of evaluation and program development. These pragmatic issues, discussed in the next section, require attention because they can interact with study design and methods to strengthen or weaken the overall strength of evaluation research.

### POINTS OF COLLABORATION BETWEEN RESEARCHERS AND SERVICE PROVIDERS

Several steps are necessary to resolve the technical challenges alluded to above. First, research and evaluation need to be incorporated earlier into the program design and implementation process (National Research Council, 1993b). Second, such integration requires creative collaboration between researchers and service providers who are in direct contact with the individuals who receive interventions and the institutions that support them. The dynamics of these collaborative relationships require explicit attention and team-building efforts to resolve different approaches and to stimulate consensus about promising models of service delivery, program implementation, and outcomes of interest. Third, the use of innovative study designs (such as empowerment evaluations, described later in this chapter) can provide opportunities to assess change associated with the impact of programs, interventions, and strategies (Fetterman et al., 1996). Drawing on both qualitative and quantitative methods, these approaches can help service providers and researchers share expertise and experience with service operation and implementation.

Numerous points in the research and program development processes provide opportunities for collaboration. Service providers are likely to be more responsive if the research improves the quality and efficiency of their services and meets their information needs. Addressing their needs requires a reformulation of the research process so that researchers can provide useful information in the interim for service providers while building a long-term capacity to focus on complex issues and conducting experimental studies.

## Knowledge About Usual Care[1]

The first point of collaboration between research and practice occurs in the development of information about the nature of existing services in the community. If the elements of service delivery that are represented by normal or usual care are not known, then the extent to which innovative interventions differ from or resemble usual care cannot be assessed. If the experimental condition does not involve a substantially greater or different amount of service, then the experiment will degrade to a test of the effects of similar service levels; it will become difficult to distinguish equivalent effects from no beneficial impact in the evaluation of the treatment under study. This type of study may lead to conclusions that the new intervention is ineffective, when in fact it does not differ significantly from usual care.

In his assessment of family preservation services, Rossi (1992) notes that, although usual care circumstances generally involve less service than is delivered in intensive family preservation programs, families who do not receive the intensive services rarely receive no service at all. Without knowing more precisely the magnitude and quality of the differences between the treatment and control conditions, estimates of effects are difficult to interpret. Findings of no difference (which are common in many social service areas) can result from insufficient

---

[1]The following sections draw on material presented in Cordray and Pion (1993).

service distinctions among conditions and groups, as well as small sample sizes (Lipsey, 1990). In some cases, degraded differences between groups play a larger role in loss of statistical power than reductions in sample size (Cordray and Pion, 1993).

## Program Implementation

A second point of collaboration between researchers and service providers occurs in developing knowledge about the nature and stages of implementation of the intervention being tested. This assessment requires attention to client flow, rates of retention in treatment, organizational capacity (how many clients can be served), and features that distinguish the treatment from usual care circumstances. Knowledge about program implementation also requires articulation of the "logic model" or "theory of change" that provides a foundation for the services that are provided and how they work together to serve the client.

The reliability and the validity of outcome measures consume a great deal of attention in the evaluation literature. Of equal importance are the reliability and the validity of the service delivery system itself and the ways in which intervention services compare with those provided in the usual-care or no-treatment conditions. Measurement of service delivery features provides a basis for transporting successful interventions to other locations, and it offers an opportunity to provide assistance to program developers in monitoring the delivery of services.

Conducting a randomized assessment of an intervention that is poorly implemented is likely to show, with great precision, that the intervention did not work as intended. But such a study will not distinguish between failures of the theory that is being tested and failures of implementation. Program designers need to identify critical elements of programs to explain why effects occurred and to assist others who wish to replicate the intervention model in a new setting. Collaboration between researchers and program staff is thus essential to incorporate attention to the experience with program design and implementation into the overall evaluation plan.

## Client Referrals, Screening, and Baseline Assessment

A third point of collaboration between researchers and service providers occurs in the development of knowledge about paths by which clients are referred, screened, and assigned to treatment or control conditions. This area focuses on knowing more about the entire context, structure, and operation of the program throughout all its stages—from the moment an individual is identified as a potential client to his or her last recorded contact with the program. Such knowledge can improve evaluations of family violence interventions by providing strategies on how to enhance sample sizes yet stay within the eligibility criteria established by the program. Research on the client selection and assessment processes can make more explicit the social, economic, legal, and political factors that affect the paths by which individuals self-select or are referred to family violence programs in health, social service, and law enforcement settings. Research on the pathways to service can reveal the extent to which service providers can adjust their programs and interventions to the specific characteristics of their clients. It can also clarify the extent of common characteristics and variation among clients.

Clients who enter these programs have varying histories of abuse, life circumstances, financial resources, and experiences with support networks and service agencies. Capturing these individual differences at the point of baseline (preintervention) assessment allows the research study to examine the extent to which interventions have different impacts with different groups of clients. At a minimum, baseline assessment (and assignment) could be used to enhance the sensitivity of the overall design by taking into account known risk factors that can be used to reduce the influence of extraneous outcome variance.

Collaborations directed at refining the assignment process can clarify the threats to validity that arise in client selection processes when randomization is not possible or cannot be maintained. Researchers who focus on devising strategies to improve client selection will need to collaborate with caseworkers, police officers, district attorneys, judges, and other individuals who routinely work with victims at key points in the usual circumstances. Such collaborations can lead to novel approaches to assigning individuals to service conditions, which currently are not well documented in the research literature.

Discussions between researchers and practitioners can also identify important considerations that arise from the need to look at the population who are served versus those who were eligible for service but were not included in the study design. Science-based efforts to maintain rigorous and consistent eligibility criteria can sometimes result in an incomplete picture of the characteristics of the general client base, which are often familiar to the community of service providers. When clients who have multiple problems (such as substance abuse, chronic health or mental health disorders, family emergencies, or criminal histories) are routinely screened out of a study, for example, a program may appear to be effective for the service population when in reality it is being assessed for only a limited portion, and possibly the most receptive portion, of the client population. Conversely, when eligibility standards are less strict, an intervention may appear to be ineffective for the general population who receive services (who may not actually need the intervention that is provided). The creation of specific cohorts within a study design can facilitate analysis of the relative impact of the intervention in high- and low-risk groups, but such efforts require general consensus about characteristics and histories that can provide consistent markers to justify assignment to different groups.

Discussions of random assignment in evaluations of service interventions often raise concerns about the fairness or safety of denying services to some individuals for the purpose of devising a control condition. Control group issues are especially difficult in assessing ongoing interventions that try to serve all comers. Although withholding services to victims of violence for the purpose of devising a control condition is not justifiable, the rejection of random or controlled assignment of clients is not warranted. Since most intervention studies involve comparisons with usual-care circumstances, those who are assigned to this control group will receive the types and levels of services that they would have received in the absence of the intervention condition. As such, control clients receive customary services, but they do not receive services with untested benefits or uncertain risks, which may be superior or inferior to the standard of usual care.

In other situations, randomization can be employed in cases in which there is uncertainty about the nature of services to be provided. This "tie-breaker" approach has been used in law enforcement studies in which the officer in charge could randomly assign borderline cases to a treatment or control group as part of the design of the research study (Lipsey et al., 1981).

Descriptive evaluation studies identify key issues, such as the likely scope of the treatment population and the likely sources of referrals for these clients (Lipsey et al., 1981). Such studies can also help identify factors in the sociopolitical context of family violence interventions that influence service design and implementation. These "pipeline" studies can be an important part of the program and evaluation planning process (Boruch, 1994) and represent opportunities for researcher and service provider collaborations that are not well documented in the research literature.

In testing the impact of new service systems, the use of wait-list controls is another option that can be considered in the study design. For example, the Women's Center and Shelter of Greater Pittsburgh reported that they could not meet the request for services in their community. In this instance, a wait-list control may have been justified in the evaluation of the impact of shelter services. However, this approach does not resolve the problem and tensions associated with using limited fiscal resources to study, rather than extend, existing services. A variation of the use of wait-list controls is an approach that relies on a triage process to identify those most in danger, provide full services for them, and use random assignment for those in less danger. This approach may be most tolerable when a waiting list for services and a wait-list control group (or step) design can be used.

Another approach to experimental assessment involves the use of alternative forms of service, which can be distinguished in terms of their intensity, duration, or comprehensiveness. Individuals in need of services would receive (in a controlled fashion) alternative service models or administrative procedures. This approach is less appealing when alternative service models cannot be easily distinguished, since decreases in variation will influence the researchers' ability to detect small but meaningful impacts and relative differences among alternative treatment systems. The absence of differences in studies of alternative forms of service can be interpreted as showing that interventions do not have their intended effects (i.e., they are unsuccessful) or that both approaches are equally effective in enhancing well-being. The absence of a framework for assessing change over time will impede efforts to distinguish between no beneficial effects and equivalent effects.

## The Value of Service Descriptions

Collaborative research and practice partnerships can highlight significant differences between new services and usual-care services, which are generally a matter of degree. Treatment interventions may differ in terms of frequency (number of times delivered per week), intensity (a face-to-face meeting with counselors versus a brief telephone contact), or the nature of the activities (goal setting versus establishment of a standard set of expectations). Documenting these differences is critical for planning and interpreting the outcome and replication, since they establish the strength of the intervention.

The value of service descriptions is enhanced by identifying key elements that distinguish interventions from comparison groups as well as ones they have in common. Such descriptions should include information about the setting(s) in which service activities occur; the training of the service provider; the frequency, intensity, and/or duration of service; the form, substance, and flexibility of the program (e.g., individual or group counseling); and the type of follow-up or subsequent service associated with the intervention.

Most family violence interventions are poorly documented (Heneghan et al., 1996; Rossi, 1992). For example, in 10 evaluation studies of intensive family preservation services reported by Heneghan et al. (1996), all 10 described (in narrative form) the types of services that were provided, but only 5 provided data on the duration of services; 3 provided data on the number of contacts per week; and 3 provided limited, narrative information on services provided in the usual-care conditions. In a different study, Meddin and Hansen (1985) found that the majority of abuse cases that were substantiated received no services at all (see Chapter 4). This point highlights the importance of knowing more about significant differences between service levels in the treatment and comparison groups, so that innovative projects do not duplicate what is currently available.

The flexibility in services is also an issue in assessing differences in service levels. Some services are protocol driven, whereas others can be adjusted to the needs of specific clients. The most respected intervention evaluations use consistent program models that can be replicated in other sites or cities. However, most interventions in social service, health, and law enforcement settings aim to be responsive to individual client needs and profiles rather than driven by protocols because of the variation in the individual experiences of their clients. Safety planning for battered women, for example, varies tremendously depending on whether a woman plans to stay in an abusive relationship, is planning to leave, or has already left. Staff, clients, and researchers can collaborate to prepare multiple protocols for a multifaceted intervention that reflects the context and setting of the service site.

Finally, many intervention efforts presume that a social ill can be remedied through the application of a single dose of an intervention (e.g., 3 weeks of rehabilitation). Others rely on follow-up activities to sustain the gains made in primary intervention efforts. Careful description of differences in follow-up activities should be given as much attention as is given to describing the primary intervention.

## Explaining Theories of Change

In the early stages of development, the fundamental notions or theoretical concepts that guide a program intervention are not always well articulated. However, the service providers and program developers often share a conceptual framework that reflects their common understanding of the origins of the problem and the reasons why a specific configuration of services should remedy it. Extracting and characterizing the theory of change that guides an intervention can be a useful tool in evaluating community-based programs (Weiss, 1995), but this approach has not been widely adopted in family violence evaluations.

Program articulation involves a dynamic process, involving consultation with program directors, line staff, and participants throughout the planning, execution, and reporting phases of the evaluation (Chen and Rossi, 1983; Cordray, 1993; U.S. General Accounting Office, 1990). Causal models provide a basis for determining intermediate outcomes or processes that could be assessed as part of the overall evaluation plan. If properly measured, these linkages can provide insights into why interventions work and what they are intended to achieve.

## Outcomes and Follow-up

Front-line personnel often express concerns that traditional evaluation research, which relies on a single perspective or method of assessment, may measure the wrong outcome. For example, evaluations of shelters for battered women may focus on the recurrence of violence, which is usually dependent on community sanctions and protection and is out of the victim's and the shelter's control. The reliance on single measures can strip the entire enterprise, as well as victims' lives, of their context and circumstances. Another issue of concern is that outcomes may get worse before they get better. For instance, health care costs may increase in the short term with better identification and assessment of family violence survivors.

An important strategy is to measure many and different outcomes, immediate and long-term outcomes, multiple time periods, both self-report and observational measures, and different levels of outcomes. The absence of consensus about the unique or common purposes of measurement should not obscure the central point that the identification of relevant domains for measuring the success of interventions requires an open collaborative discussion among researchers, service providers, clients, sponsors, and policy makers.

Another key to improving data collection, storing, and tracking capabilities is the development of coordinated information systems that can trace cases across different service settings. Three national data systems for child welfare data collection provide a general foundation for national and regional studies in the United States: in the Department of Health and Human Services, the Administration on Children and Families' Adoption and Foster Care Analysis and Reporting System (AFCARS); the federally supported and optional Statewide Automated Child Welfare Information Systems (SACWIS); and the National Center on Child Abuse and Neglect's National Child Abuse and Neglect Data System (NCANDS), a voluntary system that includes both summary data on key indicators of state child abuse and neglect indicators and detailed case data that examine trends and issues in the field. Researchers are now exploring how to link these data systems with health care and educational datasets, using record-matching techniques to bring data from multiple sources together (Goerge et al., 1994a). This type of tracking and record integration effort allows researchers to examine the impact of settings on service outcomes. Using this approach, Wulczyn (1992), for example, was able to show that children in foster care with mothers who had prenatal care during their pregnancy had shorter time periods in placement than children whose mothers did not have prenatal care. Similarly, drawing on foster care datasets and the records of state education agencies, Goerge et al. (1992) reported that 28 percent of children in foster care also received various forms of special education. Fostering links between datasets such as NCANDS and AFCARS and other administrative record sets will require research resources, coordination efforts, and the use of common definitions. Such efforts have the potential of greatly improving the quality of program evaluations.

## Community Context

The efficacy of a family violence intervention may depend on other structural processes and service systems in the community. For instance, the success of batterer treatment (and the evaluation of attrition rates) is often dependent on the ability of criminal justice procedures to keep the perpetrator in attendance. Widespread unemployment and shortages in affordable housing may undermine both violence prevention and women's ability to maintain independent living situations after shelter stays. Evaluation outcomes therefore need to be analyzed in light of data collected about the community realities in which they are embedded.

A combination of qualitative and quantitative data and the use of triangulation can often best resolve the need to capture contextual factors and control for competing explanations for any observed changes. Triangulation involves gathering both qualitative and quantitative data about the same processes for validation, and complementing quantitative data with qualitative data about other issues not amenable to traditional measurement is recommended. Agency records can be analyzed both quantitatively and qualitatively.

At a minimum, regardless of the measures that are chosen, the ones selected ought to be assessed for their reliability (consistency) and validity (accuracy). There is a surprising lack of attention to these issues in the family violence field, although a broad range of measures is currently used in program evaluations (Table 3-3).

## THE DYNAMICS OF COLLABORATION

Strengthening the structural aspects of the partnership between researchers and service providers will change the kinds of relationships between them. Creative collaborations require attention to several issues: (1) setting up equal partnerships, (2) the impact of ethnicity and culture on the research process, (3) safety and ethical issues, and (4) concerns such as publishing and publicizing the results of the evaluation study and providing services when research resources are no longer available.

### Equal Partnerships

Tensions between service providers and researchers may reflect significant differences in ideology and theory regarding the causes of family violence; they may also reflect mutual misunderstandings about the purpose and conduct of evaluation research. For front-line service providers, evaluation research may take time and resources away from the provision of services. The limited financial resources available to many agencies have created situations in which finances directed toward evaluation seem to absorb funds that might support additional services for clients or program staff. Evaluations also have the potential to jeopardize clients' safety, individualization, and immediacy of access to care.

Recent collaborations and partnerships have gone far to address these concerns. Community agencies are beginning to realize that well-documented and soundly evaluated successes will help ensure their fiscal viability and even attract additional financial resources to support promising programs. Researchers are starting to recognize the accumulated expertise of agency personnel and how important they can be in planning as well as conducting their studies. Both parties are recognizing that, even if research fails to confirm the success of a program, the evaluation results can be used to improve the program.

True collaborative partnerships require a valuing and respect for the work on all sides. Too often the attitude of researchers in the past has been patronizing

TABLE 3-3   Outcome Measures Used in Evaluations of Family Violence
Interventions

| Type of Violence | Instrument | Subject of Outcome Measure | | |
| | | Victim | Perpetrator | Other |
| --- | --- | --- | --- | --- |
| Child Abuse | Adolescent-Family Inventory Events | | X | |
| | Adult/Adolescent Parenting Inventory | | X | |
| | Chemical Measurement Package | | X | |
| | Child Abuse Potential Inventory | | X | |
| | Child and Family Well-Being Scales | X | X | |
| | Child Behavior Checklist | X | | |
| | Conflict Tactics Scales | X | X | |
| | Coopersmith Self-Opinion Inventory | | X | |
| | Coping Health Inventory | | X | X |
| | Family Adaptability and Cohesion Scales | X | X | X |
| | Family Assessment Form | X | X | X |
| | Family Environment Scale | | X | X |
| | Family Inventory of Life Events and Changes | X | X | X |
| | Family Systems Outcome Measures | | | X |
| | Home Observation | | | X |
| | Kent Infant Development Scale | X | | |
| | Maternal Characteristics Scale (Wright) | | X | |
| | Minnesota Child Development Inventories | X | | |
| | Parent Outcome Interview | | X | |
| | Parenting Stress Index | | X | |
| Domestic Violence | Adult Self-Expression Scale | X | X | |
| | Conflict Tactics Scales | X | X | |
| | Depression Scale CES-D | X | X | |
| | Quality of Life Measure | X | | |
| | Rosenberg Self-Esteem Scale | X | X | |
| | Rotter Internal-External Locus of Control Scale | X | X | |
| | Social Support Scale | X | | |
| Elder Abuse | Anger Inventory | | X | |
| | Brief Symptom Inventory | X | X | |
| | Rosenberg Self-Esteem Scale | X | X | |

SOURCE: Committee on the Assessment of Family Violence Interventions, National
Research Council and Institute of Medicine, 1998.

toward activists, and front-line agency personnel have been suspicious of researchers' motives and commitment to the work. Honest discussion is needed of issues of parity, all the possible gains of the enterprise for all parties, what everyone would like out of the partnership, and any other unresolved issues. Both sides need to spend time observing each other's domains, in order to better realize their constraints and risks.

The time constraints associated with setting up partnerships, especially those associated with short deadlines for responding to requests for proposals, need attention. Rather than waiting for a deadline, service providers and researchers need to support a plan for assessing the effects of interventions early in their development.

Viable collaborations also involve the consumers of the service at every step of the evaluation process. Clients can suggest useful outcome variables, the contextual factors that will modify those outcomes, elements of theory, and strategies that will maximize response rates and minimize attrition. They can help identify risks and benefits associated with the intervention and its evaluation.

Finally, collaboration that leads to a common conceptual framework for the evaluation study and intervention design is an essential and productive process that can identify appropriate intermediate and outcome measures and also reconcile underlying assumptions, beliefs, and values (Connell et al., 1995).

## The Impact of Ethnicity and Culture

Ethnicity and culture consistently have significant impact on assessments of the reliability and validity of selected measures. Most measures are tested on populations that may not include large representation of minority cultural groups. These measures are then used in service settings in which minorities are often overrepresented, possibly as a result of economic disadvantage.

The issues of ethnicity and cultural competence influence all aspects of the research process and require careful consideration at various stages. These stages include the formation of hypotheses taking into account any prior research indicating cultural or ethnic differences, careful sampling with a large enough sample size to have enough power to determine differential impact for different ethnic groups, and strategies for data analysis that take into account ethnic differences and other measures of culture.

Improving cultural competence involves going beyond cultural sensitivity, which involves knowledge and concern, to a stance of advocacy for disenfranchised cultural groups. The absence of researchers who are knowledgeable about cultural practices in specific ethnic groups creates a need for greater exposure to diverse cultural practices in such areas as parenting and caregiving, child supervision, spousal relationships, and sexual behaviors. This approach requires greater interaction with representatives from diverse ethnic communities in the research process as well as agency services to foster a cultural match with the participants (Williams and Becker, 1994).

In analyzing of the effect of social context on parenting, caregiving behaviors, and intimate relationships, greater attention to culture and ethnicity is advisable. Evaluating the role of neighborhood and community factors (including measures such as social cohesion, ethnic diversity, and perceptions by residents of their neighborhood as a "good" or "bad" place to raise children) can provide insight into the impact of social context on behaviors that are traditionally viewed only in terms of individual psychology or family relationships.

## Safety and Ethics

Safety concerns related to evaluation of family violence interventions are complex and multifaceted. Research confidentiality can conflict with legal reporting requirements, and concern for the safety of victims must be paramount. Certificates of confidentiality are useful in this kind of research, but they simply shield the researcher from subpoena and do not resolve the problems associated with reporting requirements and safety concerns. Basic agreements regarding safety procedures, disclosure responsibilities, and ethical guidelines need to be established among the clients, research team, service providers, and individuals from the reporting agency (e.g., child or adult protective services) to develop strategies and effective relationships.

## Exit Issues

Ideally the research team and the service agency will develop a long-term relationship, one that can be sustained, through graduate student involvement or small projects, between large formal research studies. Such informal collaborations can help researchers in establishing the publications and background record needed for large-scale funding. Dissemination of findings in local publications is also helpful to the agency.

Formal and informal collaboration requires that all partners decide on authorship and the format of publication ahead of time. Multiple submissions for funding can attract resources to carry out some aspects of the project, even if the full program is not externally funded. The collaboration also requires thoughtful discussions before launching an evaluation about what will be released in terms of negative findings and how they will be used to improve services.

One exit issue often not addressed is the termination of health or social services in the community after the research is completed. Innovative services are often difficult to develop in public service agencies if no independent source of funds is available to support the early stages of their development, when they must compete with more established service strategies. Models of reimbursement and subsidy plans are necessary to foster positive partnerships that can sustain services that seem to be useful to a community after the research evaluation has been completed.

## EVALUATING COMPREHENSIVE COMMUNITY INITIATIVES

Family violence interventions often involve multiple services and the coordinated actions of multiple agencies in a community. The increasing prevalence of cross-problems, such as substance abuse and family violence or child abuse and domestic violence, has encouraged the use of comprehensive services to address multiple risk factors associated with a variety of social problems. This has prompted some analysts to argue that the community, rather then individual clients, is the proper unit of analysis in assessing the effectiveness of family violence interventions. This approach adds a complex new dimension to the evaluation process.

As programs become a more integrated part of the community, the challenges for evaluation become increasingly complex:

1. Because participants receive numerous services, it is nearly impossible to determine which service, if any, contributed to improvement in their well-being.

2. If the sequencing of program activities depends on the particular needs of participants, it is difficult to tease apart the effects of selectivity bias and program effects.

3. As intervention activities increasingly involve organizations throughout the community, there is a growing chance that everyone in need will receive some form of service (reducing the chance of constituting an appropriate comparison group).

4. As program activities saturate the community, it is necessary to view the community as the unit of analysis in the evaluation.

5. The tremendous variation in individual communities and diversity in organizational approaches impede analyses of the implementation stages of interventions.

6. An emphasis on community process factors (ones that facilitate or impede the adoption of comprehensive service systems), as opposed to program components, suggests that evaluation measures require a general taxonomy that can be adapted to particular local conditions (Kaftarian and Hansen, 1994).

Conventional notions of what constitutes a rigorous evaluation design are not easily adapted to meet these challenges. Hollister and Hill (1995), after a careful review of the technical requirements of conventional evaluation techniques, conclude that randomization is not feasible as a means of assessing the impact of comprehensive community initiatives; they also conclude that the alternatives to randomization are technically insufficient. Weiss (1995) reiterates these points, noting that community-based programs are particularly difficult to evaluate using conventional control groups because it is unlikely that a sufficient number of communities could be recruited and assigned to the experimental and control conditions. Those with an interest in arresting the spread of violence are likely to have already installed ameliorative efforts. If all communities willing to volunteer for such an experiment have initiated such efforts, the amount of programmatic difference between communities is likely to be too small to allow for the detection of effects. Using nonrandomly assigned comparison communities engenders similar problems and adds another—selectivity bias—that is particularly difficult to account for using conventional statistical procedures (Hollister and Hill, 1995).

Weiss (1995) proposes an alternative evaluation model, based on clarifying the theories of change that explore how and why an intervention is supposed to work. The evaluation should start with the explicit and implicit assumptions underlying the theory guiding the intervention efforts; this theory is generally based on a series of small steps that involve assumptions about linkages to other activities or surrounding conditions. By creating a network of assumptions, it is possible to gather data to test whether the progression of actions leads to the intended end point. Examining the steps and progression through each phase also provides a better understanding of how interventions work and where problems arise.

Connell and Kubisch (1996) note that this perspective provides some basic principles to guide collaborative evaluations. First, the theory of change should draw on the available scientific information, and it should be judged plausible by all the stakeholders. Second, the theory of change should be doable—that is, the activities defined in the theory can be implemented. Third, the theory should be testable, which means that the specification of outcomes follows logically from the theory. A greater reliance on the use of measures or indicators, in turn, follows from the theory-based specification of outcomes.

This approach is consistent with the evaluation of single interventions. Theories of change are established by relevant stakeholders, important outcomes are selected on the basis of activities embodied in these theories, and logical expectations are established for declaring that the intervention has achieved its collective goals. What is different in the evaluation of community-based interventions is the standard of evidence that is established. In the traditional evaluation, the standard focuses on meeting technical and logical criteria surrounding the validity of the causal claim. In the theory of change model, the logical consequences of programmatic activities and actions, as judged by the stakeholders, are the standard of evidence.

A related approach is the use of empowerment evaluation to encourage self-assessment and program accountability in a variety of community-based interventions (Fetterman et al., 1996). Empowerment evaluations allow programs to take stock of their existing strengths and weaknesses, focus on key goals and program improvements, develop self-initiated strategies to achieve these goals, and determine the type of evidence that will document credible progress. Such evaluations represent opportunities to encourage collaboration between research and practice while providing interim data that can lead to program improvements.

The measurement issues for community-based studies are complex and invoke the use of specialized research designs. If comparable archival records are available, approaches such as an interrupted-time-series design could be used to strengthen the calibre of these assessments. But community-to-community variation in record keeping diminishes hope that such designs could be employed, except as case studies.

The evaluation challenges that emerge from large-scale community-based efforts are formidable. The approach detailed by Connell and Kubisch (1996) seems promising in that theories of interventions can help to establish lines of reasoning and lines of evidence that can be developed and probed; with careful thought, the effects of community-based interventions may be demonstrated.

The emphasis on innovative methodological approaches, in which evaluation designs are built into the program from its very inception, requires the development of a research capacity that is flexible, creative, and able to integrate both quantitative and qualitative research findings. What is not yet known are the circumstances that are conducive to these synthesis efforts; the extent to which they can be successful in identifying relevant and interim community process factors as well as child, family, and community outcomes in the prevention and treatment of family violence; and the relative effectiveness of such approaches when compared to traditional service delivery system efforts.

## CONCLUSION

Evaluation studies in the area of family violence are usually small in scale, likely to be underpowered, and subject to a long list of rival interpretations because of study designs that include threats to validity, such as the lack of appropriate control groups, small study samples, unreliable research measures that have not been tested across diverse social classes and ethnic and cultural groups, short follow-up periods, and inconsistencies in program content and service delivery. Limited evidence exists in this field about what works, for whom, and under what conditions. Furthermore, program development and service innovation have exceeded the capacity of the service system to conduct meaningful evaluation and research studies on existing programs, interventions, and strategies or integrate such research into service delivery efforts.

It is not clear whether this state of affairs is due to limited funding, short time horizons for studies that prevent the accumulation of a sufficient sample size, or the absence of the pre-evaluation research necessary to describe usual-care services and the nature of the intervention. This characterization is comparable to that of other fields of violence research.

At numerous points in the research and program development processes, there are opportunities for greater collaboration between service providers and researchers. Developing knowledge about what works, for whom and under what conditions requires attention to four areas: (1) describing what is known about services that are currently available within the community, (2) documenting the theory of change that guides the service intervention, (3) describing the stages of implementation of the service program, and (4) describing the client referral, screening, and baseline assessment process. The size and sensitivity of individual studies could be enhanced by greater attention to the referral and screening processes and the workloads of staff in service agencies. More useful evaluation information could be gathered by paying closer attention to the information needs of staff. Creative study designs that incorporate principles of self-determination and mutual understanding of the goals of research in the design of evaluation of research studies could be developed through collaboration among researchers, front-line workers, and program developers. Team-building efforts are needed to address the dynamics of collaboration and to foster greater opportunity for functional partnerships that build a common respect for research requirements and service information needs.

Understanding the interventions from the perspective of those who develop or use them could go a long way toward illuminating the strengths and weaknesses of existing services. The development of measurement schemes that faithfully reflect the theories and processes underlying interventions is a promising area of greater collaboration. The use of community measures and the role of social context, including the impact of social class and culture, deserve further analysis in evaluating family violence interventions.

# 4

# Social Service Interventions

State and municipal governments and nongovernmental entities provide a broad range of social services designed to prevent or treat family violence. These services include counseling and advocacy for victims of abuse; family and caregiver support programs; alternative living arrangements, including out-of-home placement for children, protective guardianship for abused elders, and shelters for battered women; educational programs for those at risk of abusing or being abused; intensive service programs to maintain families at risk of losing their child; and individual service programs in both family and placement settings.

Social service interventions may consist of casework as well as therapeutic services designed to provide parenting education, child and family counseling, and family support. Social service interventions also may include concrete services such as income support or material aid, institutional placement, mental health services, in-home health services, supervision, education, transportation, housing, medical services, legal services, in-home assistance, socialization, nutrition, and child and respite care. The scope and intensity of casework, therapeutic services, and concrete assistance to children and adults in family violence interventions are often not well documented, and they may vary within and between intervention programs. As a result, similar interventions (such as parenting practice and family support services) may offer very different kinds of services depending on the resources available in the community and the extent to which the clients can gain access to available services.

Some social service interventions (such as child protective services) are directly administered by state agencies; some services (such as parenting education and family support programs) are funded by government agencies but are provided by public or private services; other services (such as advocacy services for battered women) rely on grass roots support or local voluntary agencies. All of these interventions are designed to address the social support and safety needs of individuals and families, but they often have different focal points in meeting the needs of their clients. Their goals include the protection of children and vulnerable adults; the enhancement of parents' ability to support and care for their children; the preservation of families; and the development of resources and networks to enhance family functioning, the safety of women, and the care of children and the elderly.

Although treatment and prevention interventions for child maltreatment, domestic violence, and elder abuse have drawn on a series of theoretical frameworks over the past three decades, the connections between interventions and research are often uncertain and ambiguous. Their development has involved trial-and-error experiments in which ideas gain prominence for a short time, only to fade when disappointing results are documented (Wolfe, 1994). The interventions have focused on different levels—the individual, the family, the neighborhood, and the social culture—each providing a different set of outcomes of interest, complicating the tasks of designing interventions and evaluating their effects.

In addition to shifts in theoretical frameworks and relevant outcomes, evaluations of social service interventions have been complicated by two other significant factors: (1) variations in programs that are viewed as a single intervention and (2) differences in the population of children or adults who receive the social services. Conflicting results in evaluation research studies thus may reflect these program differences (such as the intensity or scope of services or the training of service personnel) or variations in the personal histories or types of problems experienced by the clients served.

This chapter reviews social service interventions and the available evaluations of them, using the selection criteria discussed in Chapter 1, first for child maltreatment, then for domestic violence, and finally for elder abuse.

Although this discussion of social service approaches to addressing family violence identifies specific interventions, these are far from distinct strategies. There is substantial overlap in the specific services provided by each intervention—which raises the critical cross-cutting question of which elements in this set of interventions are most effective in preventing and treating family violence. Nevertheless, the specific interventions discussed in this chapter have been identified by the field, and the evaluation literature has evolved from these services as they are identified. For this reason, the committee has retained these somewhat arbitrary distinctions. Although the interventions are described in discrete categories, the individual interventions are part of a continuum of services available to victims and their families. The interventions discussed in one section may therefore be relevant in other sections of the chapter and to interventions discussed in the chapters on legal and health care interventions.

## CHILD MALTREATMENT INTERVENTIONS

Research points to the interaction of multiple factors in the maltreatment of children; the interaction of these factors has been described in a variety of theoretical models that have evolved over the past decade (National Research Council, 1993a,b). Current models include (a) the ecological models of Belsky and Garbarino, based on the original conceptions of Urie Bronfenbrenner (Belsky, 1980; Garbarino, 1977); (b) the transitional model, which regards child maltreatment and maladaptive parenting as extreme ends of a continuum of interactions among social and cultural forces, parenting roles, and individual behavior (Wolfe, 1991, 1994); and (c) the transactional model of Cicchetti (Cicchetti and Carlson, 1989), based on Sameroff and Chandler's (1975) formulations, which focus on interactions among risk and protective factors in the social environment of the family. All three approaches share underlying assumptions that individual characteristics of the child or parent are insufficient to explain the nature and emergence of child maltreatment; each group of models uses a different set of assumptions to examine the interactive processes, perceptions, stresses, and social supports in the family environment.

Theorists have considered specific factors that appear to play a significant role in the different models: social isolation (DePanfilis, 1996; Kennedy, 1991; Ammerman, 1989), stress (Fanshel et al., 1992; Kennedy, 1991), mental health disorders (McCord, 1983), lack of knowledge about child development and rearing (Wolfe, 1987), contributing child behavior (including the lack of knowledge of self-protective behaviors) (Fanshel et al., 1992), and social and individual characteristics such as poverty and substance abuse. Three decades of research and practice have shifted the focus of treatment and prevention interventions away from models based solely on individual pathology toward broader social ecological models, with a new emphasis on the social context of parent-child relationships (Wolfe, 1994).

Although the focus of concern is the child victim, interventions in this area often target the parent (usually the mother), under the assumption that behavior change in the parent will protect the child. Such activities include parent support groups, parent education, home visiting, mental health, and other concrete social support and therapeutic services. Programs targeting children include skill-building around resistance to maltreatment, conflict management skills, and therapeutic interventions. Table 4-1 lists some major outcomes expected from social service interventions, many of which lack reliable measures. Most treatment and prevention interventions do not include data related to child maltreatment as an outcome measure, and those that do usually rely on reports of child abuse and neglect rather than observations of parent-child interactions.

Many of the outcomes highlighted in the table are interrelated; any single intervention may have several intended outcomes for parents, for children, or for both. The relationships among outcomes, such as changes in mental health,

TABLE 4-1    Expected Outcomes of Social Service Interventions for Child
Maltreatment

| Child Outcomes | Parent Outcomes |
|---|---|
| Enhanced child development and well-being | Improved parenting skills, knowledge of child development, and more realistic expectations for child behavior |
| Fewer child hospitalizations and fewer emergency room visits | More stimulating home environment |
| Lower injury and death rates and reduced child accident rate | Reduced use of corporal punishment |
| Amelioration of symptoms of maltreatment | Increased use of community services and enhanced social support |
| Ability to recognize dangerous and potentially dangerous situations | Fewer and more widely spaced pregnancies (for young parents) |
| Knowledge of and appropriate use of self-protective behaviors | Reduced stress |
| Reduction in reports of child abuse and neglect Reduction in out-of-home placements | |

SOURCE: Committee on the Assessment of Family Violence Interventions, National Research
Council and Institute of Medicine, 1998.

parenting skills, use of community and other support services, child development, child maltreatment reports, and injury and death rates, are still poorly
understood.  Changes in cognitive or social skills may or may not be accompanied by behavioral changes (such as use of community resources); both are
thought to be highly influenced by social context and cultural forces.  For example, individuals are unlikely to seek out formal or informal services that have
consistently been unavailable or unreliable in their family networks or neighborhoods.

Six social service interventions for child maltreatment are reviewed in the
sections that follow:  (1) parenting practices and family support services, (2)
school-based sexual abuse prevention, (3) child protective services investigation
and casework, (4) intensive family preservation services, (5) child placement
services, and (6) individualized service programs.  The sections are keyed to the
appendix tables that appear at the end of the chapter.

## 4A-1:  Parenting Practices and Family Support Services

Child neglect is the most common form of child maltreatment reported to child protective service agencies (National Center on Child Abuse and Neglect, 1996b). Researchers have suggested that families who are socially isolated and lack social support may be more prone to neglect than matched comparison samples (Belsky, 1980, 1993; Belsky and Vondra, 1989; Bronfenbrenner 1979; Cicchetti, 1989; Rizley and Cicchetti, 1981; Thompson, 1994, 1995; Wolfe, 1987, 1991). A number of strategies for intervention have been described and evaluated in the research literature, including (1) individual social support interventions, such as lay counseling, in-home education and parent aide programs, and parent education support group interventions; (2) multiservice interventions that match services to the specific needs of families; (3) risk assessment interventions that assess the strength of the family social support systems; (4) social skills training that seeks to improve a family's ability to gain access to appropriate resources and services (see Table 4-2); and (5) intensive family preservation services, which provide family support counseling and referrals during periods of crisis. These interventions are discussed below in terms of what is known about the outcomes associated with different strategies. Another strategy for preventive intervention, the home visitation program, is usually administered by public health departments and is discussed in Chapter 6 in our review of health care interventions.

Variations in the selection of relevant outcomes as well as differences in the service and evaluation designs make it difficult to compare the results of social service interventions in the area of child maltreatment. There is a lack of consensus about the definition of neglect (Dubowitz et al., 1993; Hegar and Youngman, 1989; Zuravin, 1991), the goal of the intervention, key constructs that should be assessed in evaluating outcomes (Cameron, 1990; Gottlieb, 1980), the tools that can accurately measure the presence or absence of neglectful behavior, and the meaning of social support. Most of the evaluations in this area use relatively limited sample sizes, and few have control group comparisons (DePanfilis, 1996).

The variety of outcomes measured includes maltreatment and placement rates, client motivation to change neglecting conditions, childrearing practices, parents' personal care, and child outcomes in domains such as cognitive, language, verbal, and social skills (DePanfilis, 1996). Although reducing child maltreatment is the ultimate goal for most interventions, proxy outcomes, such as measures of improved child health and emotional and social adjustment, are often used to measure an intervention's effectiveness. Official reports of child abuse and neglect are often viewed as unreliable indicators, because incidents may not be reported to authorities, or may be falsely reported, or because surveillance bias may affect reports in treatment families who are in close contact with social services programs.

In addition, variations in the components, duration, and intensity of treatment services and the length of follow-up periods confound efforts to identify particularly promising interventions. Controlled designs of multiservice inter-

TABLE 4-2    Range of Family Support Interventions

| Strategy | Description |
| --- | --- |
| Social network models | Used to evaluate the quantity and quality of a family's linkages with formal and informal supportive resources outside the family system. Each model is structured somewhat differently, but all seek to identify intervention targets for strengthening the social network of families. |
| | Examples include: |
| | The Eco Map (Hartman, 1978) |
| | The Social Network Map (Tracy, 1991; Tracy and Whittaker, 1990) |
| | Index of Social Network Strength (Gaudin, 1979) |
| | Pattison Psychosocial Inventory (Hurd et al., 1981) |
| | Social Network Form (Wellman, 1981; Wolf, 1983) |
| Individual social support | Operates from a family empowerment philosophy and includes multiple types of social support mixed with professional interventions. Services may include casework services, support groups, parent training, support by lay therapists or parent aides, memberships in recreational centers, transportation, and homemaker services. Individually planned service mixes seek to match services to the specific needs of families. |
| Parent education and support groups | Offer information and role modeling as well as social support to impoverished families. Parent groups provide information on basic child care skills, problem solving, home management, and social interaction skills. |
| Social skills training | Seeks to increase the effectiveness of other interventions geared to serve specific social support functions. Researchers have suggested that neglectful parents are often handicapped by a lack of social skills that might enable them to utilize community support services. |

SOURCE: Modified from DePanfilis (1996).

ventions have not been used to clearly document which program components are effective for which specific presenting problems.

**Quasi-Experimental Evidence**

Table 4A-1 lists 15 evaluations on increasing social support that meet the committee's criteria for inclusion. The table includes studies that examine parenting education and social support interventions for families that experience different types of stress, as well clinical interventions that focus more explicitly on providing mental health services for parents involved in known cases of child maltreatment.

*Reduced reported maltreatment.*    Three quasi-experimental evaluations with reports of child maltreatment as an outcome measure indicate no statistically significant difference in the rate of reports of abuse and neglect for experimental versus comparison groups following treatment (Barth et al., 1988; Barth, 1991; Wesch and Lutzker, 1991). A fourth study initially indicated fewer reports of abuse/neglect in the treatment program than a comparison group (Lutzker et al., 1984), but this result was not maintained in the follow-up study (Wesch and Lutzker, 1991).

Some evaluators have used the standardized Child Abuse Potential Inventory (CAPI) as a proxy outcome to assess the likelihood that parents will abuse their children again. Two evaluations of the Child Parent Enrichment Project, for example, found that treatment-group parents had significantly lower CAPI scores post-treatment, relative to pretreatment and relative to control parents (Barth et al., 1988; Barth, 1991).

*Parental competence and skills.*    Another outcome thought to enhance child well-being is improved parental competence.  Seven of nine studies testing gains in parenting competence  indicate positive effects of interventions to reduce child neglect (Burch and Mohr, 1980; Egan, 1983; Gaudin et al., 1991; Hornick and Clarke, 1986; Larson, 1980; National Center on Child Abuse and Neglect, 1983a; Schinke et al., 1986).  One study did not find enhanced parenting skills in treatment groups relative to comparison groups (Resnick, 1985). A second study of parenting skills at home and in laboratory observation of parent-child interactions, which was the only study to explicitly include fathers, also found no reliable change pre- to postintervention.  The authors noted that aversive behavior scores for fathers in the treatment group did not differ significantly from scores of the nondistressed fathers in the no-treatment control group (Reid et al., 1981). Methodological factors, such as the use of observed effects versus self-report data and reliance on project-developed instruments rather than standardized assessment tools, discourage the comparison of these results with other studies.

An evaluation was conducted of an intervention designed to change parental perceptions and expectations, to teach relaxation procedures to mediate stress and anger, and to train parents in problem-solving skills (Whiteman et al., 1987).  The results indicate that all three individual intervention strategies improved parents' scores on affection, discipline, and empathy indexes relative to no-treatment control parents.  A composite intervention, which combined all three strategies, produced the largest change in index scores.

Findings from less rigorous studies, which did not meet the committee's selection criteria, examined the effect of teaching social skills to parents at risk of neglect. Three studies report that parent support groups that offer social skills and problem-solving training are more successful with neglectful parents than programs offering more general content on child development (Daro, 1988; Gaudin et al., 1991, 1993). In a study of the Homebuilders program, the behavioral intervention to teach social skills was identified as an essential component (Kinney et al., 1991).

*Parental mental health.*   New theoretical models that emphasize the interactions among social context, mental health, and family functioning have emerged in interventions for child maltreatment, focusing on the need to improve parental self-esteem, stress management, and the regulation of impulsive behaviors in order to enhance parental (usually the mother's) abilities to manage children through everyday care and discipline (Wolfe, 1994). Since parental apathy and impulsivity are commonly associated with caregiver behaviors in cases of child neglect (Polansky, 1981), a number of studies hypothesize that improving parents' mental health will result in reduced child neglect. The relevant outcome in this approach is the intervention's ability to produce beneficial changes in the parents' mental health relative to comparison groups, including reduction of depression and negative effects of life stress and enhanced self-esteem. Six studies report at least short-term improvements in scores on standardized measures for treatment parents in these areas (Barth et al., 1988; Barth, 1991; Brunk et al., 1987; Egan, 1983; Resnick, 1985; Schinke et al., 1986). However, the only study that included long-term follow-up reported that treatment gains were not maintained after a one-year interval, and the hypothesized connection between short-term competence enhancement and long-term prevention of maltreating behaviors lacked empirical support (Resnick, 1985).

*Social support.*   Social support has been described as the social relationships that provide (or can potentially provide) material and interpersonal resources that are of value to the recipient (Thompson, 1994). The absence or presence of social support and involvement in social networks has been identified as an important risk factor for abusive families, especially in cases of neglect. Social support can provide a variety of services that help reduce stress in family life, including individual and family counseling, advice on parenting practices, child and respite care, financial and housing assistance, sharing of tasks and responsibilities, skill acquisition, and access to information and services.

A number of evaluations use social network assessment tools to determine if interventions can reduce social isolation for neglectful families, thereby decreasing propensity for neglectful behavior (Barth et al., 1988; Barth, 1991; Gaudin et al., 1991, 1993; Resnick, 1985; Schinke et al., 1986). Two found no beneficial results in social support (Barth et al., 1988; Barth, 1991); two others found improved social support for families receiving treatment (Gaudin et al., 1991;

Schinke et al., 1986). A sixth study found initial improvement in social support that deteriorated over time (Resnick, 1985).

These results have not yet been able to suggest that network assessments will lead to more effective interventions or improved treatment outcomes (DePanfilis, 1996). However, one less rigorous recent study suggests that collecting data on perceived social support, the reported frequency of use, and satisfaction with different types of support may provide better indicators of social support than structural features alone (Tracy and Abell, 1994).

Some research has focused on the role of "natural helpers"—individuals who supplement the efforts of formal social service agents and who have connections to the values and norms of the community in the social environment of distressed families (Collins and Pancoast, 1976; Thompson, 1994, 1995). The efficacy of natural helpers in counteracting the multiple stresses of disadvantaged communities is not well understood; some research has suggested that creating a web of social support for families at risk of abuse or neglect may require connections with self-help groups (such as Parents Anonymous) or family support centers that are especially knowledgeable about the problems of child maltreatment and can provide counseling and advice outside the context of everyday social relationships (Thompson, 1994).

*Home environments.* One evaluation looked at improvements in home environments as a proxy for decreased likelihood of child neglect with mixed results (Larson, 1980). Larson found improvements in treatment group families.

## Implications

Social service interventions designed to improve parenting practices and provide family support have not yet demonstrated that they have the capacity to reduce or prevent abusive or neglectful behaviors significantly over time for the majority of families who have been reported for child maltreatment. Although parental behavior can be modified in terms of stress, empathy, anger control, and child discipline, confidence in these and other proxy outcomes (such as improved parental skills and altered perceptions of child behavior) requires greater understanding of the key attributes of parental competence that relate to child maltreatment. Several interventions have demonstrated an ability to improve parental competence in the short term, but whether these gains can be maintained over long periods under stressful conditions and across different periods of the child's development is not certain. The intensity of the parenting and social support services required may be greater than initially estimated in order to address the fundamental sources of conflict, stress, and violence that occur repeatedly over time in the family environment, especially in disadvantaged communities. Focusing as they do on single incidents and short periods of support, the interventions in this area may be inadequate to deal with problems that are pervasive, multiple, and chronic.

The use of social networks to build and sustain parental competence is a separate area that requires further analysis. Although a parent's use of social networks to support family functioning can be influenced through interventions, there is not enough evidence to indicate whether changes in social networks can create changes in parenting practices that endure over time and result in reduced child maltreatment. The evidence, although intriguing, does not yet provide clear indications as to which types of families are most likely to benefit from parental education and family support services as opposed to mental health services designed to address depression, lack of empathy, and impulsive behavior in both parents and children. Neither does the research base yet clarify whether enriching the supply of community resources will lead to expanded use of support services by families at risk of child maltreatment. Consistent dialogues between researchers and practitioners could facilitate greater awareness of the need to match families with individualized interventions.

### 4A-2: School-Based Sexual Abuse Prevention

Sexual abuse prevention programs are organized around the theory that children can be taught to avoid abuse or to protect themselves from further abuse by reporting threatening or abusive situations and employing other learned self-protective behaviors (Daro and McCurdy, 1994). Most child sexual abuse prevention education is classroom-based, brief in duration, and includes training on concepts of body ownership, types of touching, and skills to avoid or escape sexually abusive situations. Children are encouraged "to tell." Curricula may also include assertiveness training for older youths (Barth and Derezotes, 1990). Some programs include a parental component, although such efforts are rarely evaluated (Reppucci and Haugaard, 1988). Formats include skits, puppet shows, songs, films, videos, and story and coloring books.

Table 4A-2 lists 14 evaluations in this area that meet the committee's criteria for inclusion. In general, these evaluations lack long-term follow-up data and rely on proxy outcomes, such as an increase in children's knowledge and skills (Carroll et al., 1992). The evaluations indicate that, although most programs can provide positive changes in cognitive skills and program-specific prevention behavior, especially when they draw on age-appropriate materials and special teacher training, the size and duration of this effect for children at different developmental stages remain generally unknown. Two programs that included 1- to 6-month follow-up found that children retained "flight" responses to situational lures (Harvey et al., 1988; Kolko et al., 1989). However, the evaluations have not included long-term follow-up studies that could demonstrate that these changes constitute a sexual abuse prevention effect for the general population of children, reduce the risk of sexual abuse to the vulnerable children who receive the training, or mitigate the consequences of sexual abuse when it occurs by encouraging reports to an adult. The studies demonstrate that children can retain prevention information, but retention may be influenced by age at exposure, length of training, and inclusion of review sessions. Moreover, there is some question about children's ability to translate knowledge into actual behavior and whether increased knowledge or learned self-protective behaviors do protect children from sexual abuse by family members.

### 4A-3: Child Protective Services Investigation and Casework

The primary duty of state- or county-administered child protective services (CPS) agencies is to investigate and either substantiate or dismiss reports of child maltreatment; these casework management services (as opposed to treatment and prevention services) account for the large majority of the CPS budget in most communities. In the course of an investigation, social workers are charged with a dual responsibility: protecting the safety of the child and maintaining the family if that course is consistent with child protection. Short-term interventions in this area include provision of casework services, concrete and therapeutic interventions, referral to community-based services, and short-term placements during the investigation phase. Services provided after investigation include concrete services, education, referral to community-based agencies, crisis intervention, treatment, and temporary or permanent placement in substitute care if necessary (National Center on Child Abuse and Neglect, 1996a).

There is wide variation in the duration, timing, and kinds of CPS interventions offered to maltreated children and their families, from no services to support, counseling, and placement services (Meddin and Hansen, 1985). Some reviews of the effectiveness of social casework intervention with troubled families in general (not just child protective services) have indicated limited evidence of the effectiveness of casework intervention (Lindsey, 1994), noting that the caseworker often has little ability to change the structural and institutional barriers (such as unemployment, dangerous neighborhoods, poor housing) that confront many of their clients, limiting the scope of the intervention to smaller-scale problems.

There are no evaluations of child protective services that meet the committee's criteria for inclusion. Thus, several decades of experience with different types of CPS interventions remain relatively unexamined in the research literature, and the impacts of case identification and investigation procedures and practices are unknown. In the absence of a research base, policy makers rely on anecdotes and media accounts to formulate guidelines for casework interventions. The available studies analyze how type of abuse and degree of risk influence rates of case investigation, substantiation, and child placement as a result of investigation (Barth et al., 1994; English and Aubin, 1991; Murphy et al., 1991). At present, child sexual abuse is the most likely type of abuse to be investigated;

neglect is the least likely to be investigated and substantiated, although the large majority of reported cases involve allegations of neglect.

## 4A-4:  Intensive Family Preservation Services

Once child maltreatment has been substantiated, assuming resources are available, caseworkers design a service plan.  Many localities have adopted an array of services referred to as intensive family preservation services, which are designed to avert child placement in substitute care and, if possible, keep the family intact through the provision of therapeutic and concrete services, such as home appliance repairs and temporary rent subsidies.

Interventions in this area are short term and crisis oriented.  Prior to referral for services, a child must be assessed as at imminent risk of removal from the family.  Although specific components of these services vary, there are some common features (Fraser et al., 1991; Wells and Biegel, 1992).  Generally, they are brief (4-6 weeks), intense, home-based, therapeutic, and concrete; the caseloads tend to be small.  In keeping with the 1980 Adoption Assistance and Child Welfare Act (Public Law 96-272), the programs are shaped by the philosophy that, as long as their safety can be reasonably ensured, the best place for children to live is in their own homes.  Family preservation strategies are also guided by the theory that families are more responsive to change during periods of crisis and are more likely to engage in services at such times (Heneghan et al., 1996; Kinney et al., 1977; Edna McConnell Clark Foundation, 1985).

The outcome measures used in evaluations of intensive family preservation services are (1) prevention of child removal and (2) reduction in the length of stay in placement outside the home.  Some studies count any type or length of placement in measuring outcome (Feldman, 1991), whereas other studies do not consider placement with a relative or other temporary placement (Pecora et al., 1992).  The use of administrative data on placements excludes other indices of success, such as a reduction in the number of runaway episodes (Bath and Haapala, 1993).  And, although placement is a primary outcome measure, it is not always indicative of service failure (Nelson 1988; Tracy, 1991; Wells and Biegel, 1992).

### Quasi-Experimental Evidence

Table 4A-4 lists 14 evaluations in this area that meet the committee's criteria for inclusion (the use of a comparison or control group in the conduct of the study).  Some investigators found small or temporary effects on families (Feldman, 1991; Schwartz et al., 1991; Dennis-Small and Washburn, 1986; Pecora et al., 1992).  Others reported that the majority of families who receive services improved significantly and maintained improvements for 6 months to a year

(Bergquist et al., 1993; Halper and Jones, 1981; Walton et al., 1993; Walton, 1994; Wood et al., 1988). Still others found no difference in the number of episodes of out-of-home placements for families who received services over comparison families, but they do report shorter placement episodes (AuClaire and Schwartz, 1986; Schwartz et al., 1991).

In a methodological assessment of an identified field of 46 evaluations, 36 were excluded from further consideration because they used no comparison groups (Heneghan et al., 1996). Four of the remaining group of 10 studies were also found to be methodologically unacceptable because of poorly defined assessment of risk, inadequate descriptions of the interventions provided, and nonblinded determination of the outcomes. The methodological review of 10 evaluation studies by Heneghan et al. (1996) concluded that rates of out-of-home placements were 21 to 59 percent among families who received intensive family preservation services and 20 to 59 percent among comparison families. The relative risk of placement was significantly reduced by services in only two studies; one of these sites had the highest rate of placement for both treatment and comparison groups.

## Implications

Although intensive family preservation services may delay placement for many families in the short term (Schwartz et al., 1991; Pecora et al., 1992), there is little evidence to date that the services resolve the underlying family dysfunction that precipitated the crisis or improve the child's well-being or the family's functioning. The use of placement rates as a primary outcome is problematic, since it is a "program-based" measure that may not fully capture the range of positive effects of the intervention (Heneghan et al., 1996). Attention to other child and family outcomes, such as child development, maternal-child interactions, episodes of maltreatment, and injury rates, might demonstrate more conclusively that these services provide better child and family outcomes than foster care, but these effects have not been tested in the evaluation literature.

At best, a 30-day intervention can be expected only to stabilize the immediate crisis that places the child at imminent risk. Dramatic results cannot be expected in this area given the number and magnitude of the problems faced by many families and the variability in the services that are provided to them (Schuerman et al., 1994). The results suggest that longer-term interventions may be required to sustain changes initiated by the intensive family preservation services and that the differential effects for different types of families need more attention.

Evaluations in this area are confounded by differences in the types of abuse and characteristics of families and children referred for services. Targeting services to families who are most likely to benefit from them is an important goal. However, it is uncertain whether improved targeting will significantly reduce child placement rates, because those families who are most likely to benefit may not be the same as those who are most at risk for child removal.

Several major issues require consideration in assessing the effectiveness of these interventions. First is the issue of targeting: Do the programs actually serve children at imminent risk of placement? Many studies do not define what is meant by imminent risk and programs vary regarding the concept of "placement" (Feldman, 1991; Tracy, 1991; Wheeler et al., 1992; Schuerman et al., 1994; Fraser et al., 1991; Yuan et al., 1990; Schwartz et al., 1991). As a result, it has been difficult to establish valid comparisons of results across studies. Furthermore, the decision about what constitutes imminent risk is usually based on the subjective judgment of the caseworker (Rossi, 1992; Tracy, 1991; McCroskey and Meezan, 1993).

Several studies question the utility of imminent risk as an eligibility criterion for the programs (Ensign, 1991; Rossi, 1992; Schuerman et al., 1994; Yuan et al., 1990). They also do not account for the spontaneous remission of symptoms, as families reestablish their equilibrium after the abatement of the crisis that triggered the intervention (Jones, 1991; Rossi, 1992). Until standardized definitions and objective assessment tools are adopted to measure services, placement, and risk, tests of the efficacy of an intervention strategy using this criterion will remain difficult.

## 4A-5: Child Placement Services

In some cases, removal of the child from the home becomes unavoidable. Placement settings include foster care, therapeutic foster care, residential group care, and psychiatric hospitalization. Recently kinship care, or placement with a relative, has been included in this array of services. For teenagers who have remained in alternative care to adulthood, interventions have been designed to foster safety and self-sufficiency in the transition from foster care to independent living.

The number of children taken from their homes as a result of investigations is not clear (Table 4-3). One study of 169 investigations indicated that 59.7 percent of the substantiated cases were offered no services, that placement (13 percent) and counseling (11 percent) were the most frequently offered services for cases that did receive attention, and that for those children placed, services prior to placement were considered by social workers only one-third of the time (Meddin and Hansen, 1985). A more recent study found that 56 percent of all indicated cases were closed the same day they were officially substantiated (Salovitz and Keys, 1988). Estimates of the number of out-of-home placements as a result of maltreatment range from 1 to 15 percent for substantiated cases (American Humane Association, 1979; Runyan et al., 1981; National Center on Child Abuse and Neglect, 1996c; English, 1994).

An increased focus on the nature and effectiveness of placement services for

TABLE 4-3  Responses to Reports of Child Maltreatment by Child Protective Services

| Citation | Substantiated Cases Offered Services (%) | Substantiated Cases Resulting in Out-of-Home Placement/ Dependency Proceedings (%) |
|---|---|---|
| Meddin and Hansen, 1985 | 60 | 13 |
| Salovitz and Keys, 1988 | 44 | |
| National Committee to Prevent Child Abuse, 1991 | 78 | |
| Tjaden and Thoennes, 1992 | 75 | 21 |
| McCurdy and Daro, 1994 | 19 state reports vary from 29-100; average 60 | |
| English, 1994 | | 15 |

SOURCE: Committee on the Assessment of Family Violence Interventions, National Research Council and Institute of Medicine, 1998.

maltreated children has emerged in the past 10 years. Although out-of-home placements represent a small percentage of all services for children reported and substantiated for maltreatment, recent data from the U.S. General Accounting Office (1993) indicate a 55 percent increase in placement from 1985 to 1991. Adolescents ages 12 to 18 were the largest group in placement in 1986; by 1995, children under age 5 are the largest group in placement (Goerge et al., 1994b). Rapid growth in the numbers of children who are placed outside the home is evident in urban centers associated with the onset of the drug epidemic, although the rate of placement relative to numbers of cases handled by the child welfare system has remained relatively stable. The entry and length of stay fluctuates over time and between population subgroups, the number of infants entering foster care has increased dramatically, and infants have longer lengths of stay than children who enter at older ages (Goerge et al., 1994b).

**Quasi-Experimental Evidence**

Table 4A-5 lists the four evaluations in this area that meet the committee's criteria for inclusion. Effectiveness of foster care has generally been measured in two ways: (1) whether or not the placement is permanent and (2) the level of the child's or adult's ability to function upon leaving foster care. Two studies reviewing long-term outcomes indicate that children who are removed from their homes fare no worse on proxy variables for development and social adjustment than their maltreated peers who are left at home (Runyan and Gould, 1985; Wald et al., 1988). A study of infants in residential treatment showed short-term improvements in height and weight and interaction skills, a decline in psychomotor development pre- to postintervention, and a decline in interaction skills 5 months later (Elmer, 1986). A fourth study reported that foster parent retention and satisfaction with their foster children's behavior can be enhanced by providing training, support, and increased stipends (Chamberlain et al., 1992), but it is uncertain whether such changes lead to improvements in the children's functioning as well.

Research on foster care outcomes generally consists of follow-up studies of youth in foster care with little comparison group analysis, weak retrospective designs, and small sample sizes, with significant attrition rates of subjects across studies (Royse and Wiehe, 1989). A review of 27 less rigorous evaluations of foster care found a variety of poor outcomes (including failure to complete high school, public assistance, homelessness, and frequent use of alcohol and drugs) for adults who grew up in foster care (McDonald et al., 1993). However, there was significant variation in the methodology and results of the studies included in the review. Many of these studies compared foster care children to those who lived with their biological families without considering the issue of maltreatment. Longitudinal studies of children in foster care (Fanshel and Shinn, 1978; Fanshel, 1992; Runyan and Gould, 1985; Widom, 1991) found generally favorable outcomes for children; the authors found no evidence that foster care alone was responsible for a significant portion of social adjustment problems, including crime and delinquency, encountered by child victims of maltreatment. Other studies have found less positive long-term outcomes for adults who were children in foster care: their educational attainment is below average (Palmer, 1976; Zimmerman, 1982; Festinger, 1983; Jones and Moses, 1984); their unemployment is higher than in the general population (Festinger, 1983; Barth, 1990; Jones and Moses, 1984; Zimmerman, 1982); and housing for many is marginal or unstable (Russell, 1984; Harari, 1980; Jones and Moses, 1984; Susser et al., 1987; Sosin et al., 1991).

Since those studies were completed, the Independent Living program has been initiated in many states, specifically targeting youth ages 16 to 18 leaving foster care. The purpose of this program is to help prepare foster children for the transition to independence, including specific training in employment, education, and other basic living skills. Studies conducted on youth leaving foster care in the 1990s may reveal different results.

**Implications**

A key question for foster care research studies is whether out-of-home placement for children who have experienced abuse or neglect creates a separate source of additional harm or benefit for their development. The evaluation research base is not sufficient to provide clear answers, but longitudinal studies suggest many children who reside in foster care fare neither better nor worse than those who remain in homes in which maltreatment has occurred. However, the changing character of children in foster care over the last decade, with the trend toward increased placement of children under age 5, requires new studies to examine whether the age, length, or stability of placement is correlated with beneficial or adverse outcomes, especially when children in placement are compared with young children who have been maltreated but remain with their families. Prior research has shown that the younger the child is at placement, the less likely the child will return home.

Comparing family foster care to residential services (a group home or center-based form of placement) suggests that children in foster care are better able to function in less restrictive post-discharge environments and are more often discharged to family or relative care. Foster care appears to offer significant cost advantages compared with residential treatment (Hawkins et al., 1985, 1989; Rubenstein et al., 1978). But there is some question as to whether children in foster care and residential treatment are comparable in terms of their mental health and experience with trauma (Barth et al., 1994). Interpretation of the data on whether placement in foster care is permanent is made difficult by the need to average across all children in placement (Shyne and Shroeder, 1978; Wiltse, 1985).

Although residential services are widely used as an intervention for older and more disturbed youth who cannot live with their families, they have not been assessed to determine their effectiveness. There is little empirical evidence available to identify which characteristics of an after-care intervention are effective, although such services are widely acknowledged as important (Whittaker and Pfieffer, 1994; Jenson et al., 1986).

## 4A-6: Individualized Service Programs

Out-of-home placements may not necessarily signal the end of service provision to the child victim; in some cases, intensive programs are designed to prevent the need for other, more costly, or perhaps stigmatizing interventions. Individualized service programs have been developed to identify flexible and intensive intervention plans that meet children's needs and provide services in the least restrictive environment, either with their biological families or not. These programs emphasize consideration of the total environment in which the maladjusted behavior occurs rather than focusing solely on the child's behavior.

The majority of the research in this area is descriptive or focuses on implementation issues (Burchard et al., 1993; Burchard and Clarke, 1989; Duchnowski et al., 1993; Van Den Berg, 1993; Dollard et al., 1994). Most evaluations are anecdotal, drawing on nonstandardized measures and data-gathering procedures and small, nonrandom samples; they lack control or comparison groups and clear specification of program components and procedures (Bates et al., 1995).

Table 4A-6 lists the three evaluations in this area that meet the committee's criteria for inclusion. Two studies that measured the comparative success of individualized service interventions against subsequent reports of child maltreatment and removal of the child did not show positive results (Hotaling et al., undated; Jones, 1985). Both found that children receiving individualized services were just as likely to live out of the home and their families were just as likely to be the subject of maltreatment reports as comparison families receiving routine community services.

One of the most rigorous studies of individualized service interventions compared 109 children in foster care who received individualized services to children who did not (Clark et al., 1994). Both groups had significantly improved scores on measures of emotional and behavioral adjustment, but children who received individualized services had significantly improved scores on certain dimensions (such as withdrawal of attention). The treatment group had significantly fewer days of incarceration and fewer felony convictions than the comparison group.

The very nature of individualized service interventions makes them difficult to evaluate, and the evaluations difficult to compare. Because each family in the treatment group is theoretically receiving the mix of services designed to address its particular needs, repeated iterations would be required to identify the "best" or "most effective" mix of services for a particular kind of family. Trying to generalize from one study population to another with different characteristics and problems would require increasingly complex methodology. The most effective approach may be to design methodologically sound evaluations of each individual service plan, and then design evaluations to test varying service packages.

## DOMESTIC VIOLENCE INTERVENTIONS

Today, there are approximately 1,800 programs in the United States for victims of violence by spouses and intimate partners; approximately 1,200 of these programs are shelters (Plichta, 1995). Shelter programs emerged in the 1970s in response to grass roots concerns about the need to provide places of safety and emotional support for battered women and their children. The shelter movement has evolved to include a broad array of related social services, including 24-hour hotlines, counseling, job training, medical and legal assistance, referrals to drug and alcohol treatment, and housing assistance. This combination of crisis intervention and social support has emerged in a variety of settings, including religious organizations, women's organizations, hospitals, and community development programs. Individual social workers, psychologists, and clinics also provide services to victims of domestic violence.

This section describes social service interventions designed for battered women and evaluations of such interventions. Mental health programs for battered women and children who witness domestic violence are discussed in the chapter on health interventions. Programs for male perpetrators of domestic violence are discussed in the chapter on legal interventions, since the client referrals to these programs are largely administered through the courts.

As in the field of child abuse, variation in the outcomes identified complicates the task of designing and implementing evaluations of services for battered women. Although the ultimate goal is to foster violence-free lives, it is often unrealistic to expect a brief intervention focused on the victim to create a situation in which a batterer is no longer violent. Interim outcomes are therefore often used to judge the effectiveness of interventions—such as greater empowerment and increased options for victims, improved life skills (including improved communication and self-assertive skills), and more effective use of available community services. Even these proxies, however, are difficult to quantify in a standardized way (Table 4-4). Given the difficulty of precisely defining desired outcomes of interventions for domestic violence and the even greater difficulty of quantifying them, only a small number of quasi-experimental evaluations of such interventions exist. Some evaluations that did not meet the committee's criteria for inclusion nonetheless are discussed below because they are valuable in their attempt to clarify issues in outcome measurement and program implementation.

TABLE 4-4  Expected Outcomes of Social Service Interventions for Domestic Violence

| Outcome | Data Source |
| --- | --- |
| Absence of violence | Interviews with survivors, former perpetrators<br>End of relationship with perpetrator<br>Police reports<br>Medical/hospital records |
| Empowerment | Interviews with survivors<br>Discrete actions (e.g., adopting safety plan)<br>Improved measure of self-sufficiency, self-reliance<br>Improved mental health |
| Effective use of community services | Caseworker records |
| Self-sufficiency | Interviews with victims<br>Discrete actions accomplished (e.g., obtaining a job, pursuing education, finding housing) |

SOURCE: Committee on the Assessment of Family Violence Interventions, National Research Council and Institute of Medicine, 1998.

Four interventions are described in the sections that follow: (1) shelters for battered women, (2) peer support groups for battered women, (3) advocacy services for battered women, and (4) domestic violence prevention programs. The sections are keyed to the appendix tables that appear at the end of the chapter.

### 4B-1: Shelters for Battered Women

No national data exist on the number or the characteristics of clients who are served by various shelter programs. Individual state data on waiting lists and turn-away rates indicate that the resources are inadequate to meet the needs of victims of domestic violence (National Research Council, 1996).

Women who go to shelters tend to be from lower socioeconomic groups. Women with more economic resources may not appear in shelter samples because they are able to pay for temporary shelter or rely on housing provided by friends or relatives; they may seek other services through private means. The racial makeup of shelter users seems to reflect the regional location of the shelters. It may be that women who use shelter services are experiencing the most serious violence at home and therefore do not represent other women who are victimized (Berk et al., 1986).

Most studies of shelters and the outcomes of shelter stays are descriptive. The committee found no evaluations that compared outcomes for women using shelters with outcomes for battered women not using shelters. Several studies do compare women's pre- and post-shelter experiences or compare groups of shelter residents based on services provided either during or after the shelter stay. Recruiting samples of battered women to study can be difficult. Some researchers advertise for subjects, creating a sample that is subject to self-selection bias. Most studies have drawn samples from women who seek help at a shelter or elsewhere (for example, the courts). The use of such samples makes it impossible to have a control group of women who have not sought services, so that a quasi-experimental evaluation is not possible.

One potentially important outcome measure for programs is the victim's progression through stages of change. Housing, education or job training and acquisition, economic self-sufficiency, child care, safety, and other issues need to be resolved before a woman can completely separate from an abusive partner on whom she has been emotionally or financially dependent. Work is currently under way on a tool for the measurement of one conceptualization of the stages of change women experience on their way to leaving a violent relationship (Brown, 1997). This may prove to be an important instrument for assessing programs for victims of violence. Should such an instrument be developed, it will be critical to evaluate whether it is a valid and meaningful measure for all women or only certain groups.

Table 4B-1 lists the only evaluation in this area that meets the committee's criteria for inclusion. It found that, for some women, shelters appeared to limit new incidents of violence in the 6 weeks following shelter stays (Berk et al., 1986). Another larger but not controlled study found that shelters play a pivotal role in helping women seek appropriate support services (Gondolf and Fisher, 1988).

Beyond traditional shelters, transitional housing programs, which provide not only shelter but also continued advocacy and counseling services to residents, allow women to gradually make the transition from violent home, to emergency shelter, to marshaling the skills and resources necessary to eventually live independently. These transitional programs have not yet been rigorously evaluated; anecdotal information from service providers and victims indicates that the opportunity for an extended period of safe, low-cost housing, support services including child care and health services, and opportunities for generating an independent source of income are critical to the goal of violence-free, independent living.

### 4B-2:  Peer Support Groups for Battered Women

The most common auxiliary service offered to battered women in the social service context is peer or support group counseling. These programs may be offered through a shelter, social service agency, religious group, or other community organization. The groups are facilitated by professional therapists, paraprofessionals, or victim advocates and generally focus on identification of feelings about being victimized, education about domestic violence, and skill-building and self-protective behaviors (Walker, 1979; Dutton, 1992). Few such services have been evaluated (Taylor, 1995), and none meets the committee's criteria for inclusion.

### 4B-3:  Advocacy Services for Battered Women

Advocacy services are typically provided to battered women by shelter staff or trained lay persons in the community, who include self-identified survivors of domestic violence themselves. The role of the advocate is to inform the client of her legal, medical, and financial options, to validate her feelings of being victimized, to facilitate her access to community resources, to assist her in goal setting and making choices, and to provide emotional support. Advocacy services may be provided in-person either in a shelter, in a community agency, or by telephone hotline. Advocacy services are frequently offered by communities in conjunction with emergency shelter and more formal individual counseling or support groups.

Table 4B-3 lists two evaluations in this area that meet the committee's criteria for inclusion. The outcome measures used include standardized mental health instruments and nonstandardized measures of social support and access to community resources. Neither study found a connection between the use of advocacy services and the cessation of violence. Tan et al. (1995) conclude that short-term advocacy may not be sufficient given the severe life difficulties that battered women face.

An emerging intervention for battered women extends traditional advocacy services into weeks and months beyond the crisis period during which services are commonly available. One less rigorous study found that women significantly improved their scores for appraisal support (finding someone to talk to about one's problems); there was also some evidence of an increase in self-esteem by the end of the program (Tutty, 1995). Although this evaluation does not meet the criteria for a quasi-experimental evaluation, it is the first to use qualitative and quantitative methods to review follow-up services.

The evaluations reviewed do not indicate that short-term advocacy services for battered women reduce the risk of future violence to the victims. However, advocacy programs do appear to improve other outcome measures, such as increased social support for the victim and enhanced self-esteem and feelings of empowerment. Future research should focus on how these outcomes are associated with long-term safety for battered women. More research and experimentation with longer-term advocacy models are needed.

### 4B-4: Domestic Violence Prevention Programs

Domestic violence prevention efforts generally consist of school-based programs on dating and on domestic violence in intimate relationships. Such programs focus on gender roles, expectations, and personal safety as well as legal statutes regarding relationship violence. Community-wide efforts have begun recently in some areas to build this movement through specific strategies to educate men and women about domestic violence and to create a community norm that reduces social tolerance of and provides sanctions for violent behavior (including restrictions on gun ownership).

Table 4B-4 lists four evaluations in this area that meet the committee's criteria for inclusion. These evaluations test students' knowledge about and attitudes on relationship violence before and after the prevention program, as well as personal experience with dating violence (Jones, 1991; Jaffe et al., 1992; Krajewski et al., 1996; Lavoie et al., 1995).

These studies found generally positive changes associated with prevention programs. Two found increased levels of knowledge in participants relative to no-training controls (Jones, 1991; Krajewski et al., 1996). A third found that all students improved their knowledge of and attitudes about dating violence (Lavoie et al., 1995). Although Krajewski et al. and Lavoie et al. found more definitive attitude effects than Jones, all three studies identified differential effects on boys and girls, with girls showing more positive attitudinal and knowledge effects.

No longitudinal studies exist to document whether these programs, which may change knowledge or attitudes about violence between intimates, have any long-term impact on domestic violence. As with school-based programs to prevent child sexual abuse, future research will need to test the relationship between knowledge gain, attitudinal change, and behaviors that can reduce or prevent violence.

## ELDER ABUSE INTERVENTIONS

Elder abuse has recently emerged as an area of interest to researchers and service providers. A wide range of preventive approaches is suggested by theory and risk factors, including programs that promote good mental health (reducing depression), independence, and social contact; buffer stressful life events; and resolve conflict without violence. Support groups and training that emphasize elder rights and advocacy, outreach efforts to inform minority communities, financial management programs, and instructional sessions in behavior management for caregivers of Alzheimer's patients have been proposed as ways to reduce the potential for abuse or neglect. Most programs have been conducted on a small scale without specification of outcome measures and without the procedures or resources necessary for good evaluation.

Interventions in elder abuse mirror the experience with child maltreatment and domestic violence. Social service programs designed to prevent maltreatment of elders include adult protective services agencies, casework and provision of concrete and therapeutic services, individualized service programs, training for caregivers, advocacy services, family counseling, and out-of-home placement services.

Three interventions are described in the sections that follow: (1) adult protective services, (2) training for caregivers, and (3) advocacy services to prevent elder abuse. There are few evaluations in this area that meet the committee's criteria for inclusion. Therefore, some of the information presented in the sections below is derived from descriptive information of existing programs. The sections are keyed to the appendix tables that appear at the end of the chapter.

### 4C-1: Adult Protective Services

All 50 states have some form of adult protective service program to investigate referrals of cases of abuse or neglect of the elderly, although such programs are comparatively recent interventions in some regions (Byers et al., 1993; Quinn, 1985; Tatara, 1995). If a vulnerable adult appears to lack the capacity to consent to service, agencies are frequently empowered to initiate guardianship proceedings. These agencies are designed to provide short-term, crisis-oriented interventions, usually lasting no more than 90 days (Fredriksen, 1989).

In addition to investigation and case management, many state agencies can provide concrete services, such as income support or material aid, institutional placement, mental health services, in-home health services, supervision, education, transportation, housing, medical services, legal services, in-home assistance, socialization, nutrition, respite care, and casework. These services may be offered both to the victim and to the abuser if the caseworker feels that such support may lessen the risk for future abuse (Quinn et al., 1993; Illinois Department on Aging, 1990).

Most state protective services agencies have the legal authority to intervene in emergency situations to remove the victim or abuser from the home, to institutionalize the victim, or to appoint a guardian to manage the victim's affairs. The decision to take any of these actions rests on the agency's determination that the victim is mentally or physically incapable of protecting herself without this intervention.

There are no evaluations of adult protective services interventions that meet the committee's criteria for inclusion. One less rigorous study found that the intervention most likely to result in reduced risk for the victim was the placing of a cognitively impaired victim into long-term care (Quinn et al., 1993). Unimpaired victims of physical abuse, emotional abuse, or exploitation tend to remain in the community and to remain at high risk for future abuse.

A survey of types of social service interventions available in 335 area agencies on aging is illustrative (Blakely and Dolon, 1991). Almost half of the sample (181 agencies) offered information and referrals on elder abuse, reported cases of suspected elder abuse to adult protective services agencies, and worked to increase public awareness of the problem. A similar number (182 agencies) report serving as advocate for victims of elder abuse, and 178 provide educational programs to elder clients and to relevant professional groups and lawmakers to enhance awareness of the problem. Slightly fewer agencies reported such activities as direct services to clients, receiving referrals of elder abuse cases from adult protective services, case management services, participation in state or community task forces focused on elder abuse, demonstration projects, and sponsoring or conducting research. Agencies reported their most successful activities as public education, legal assistance and ombudsman services, respite and other caregiver services, and influencing legislation.

### 4C-2: Training for Caregivers

It has been suggested that lack of understanding of the needs and care of the elderly by caregivers may contribute to mistreatment (Kinderknecht, 1986). As with new parent training offered to families at risk for child abuse and neglect, education for caregivers for the elderly can reduce the risk of violence stemming from unmet expectations or misunderstanding of physical and behavioral changes that may be attributed to meanness or "acting-up" (Kinderknecht, 1986). Like new parents, caregivers may require extensive information about hygiene, nutrition, medication, and routine needs of elderly family members in order to care for them properly (Ansello et al., 1986).

Table 4C-2 lists the only evaluation in this area that meets the committee's criteria for inclusion. This evaluation of a training program for caregivers of elderly family members showed relatively little change over time for any group on the participants' self-esteem or level of anger. Training was associated with a slight reduction in the reported costs of providing care at a rate that approached statistical significance. Both the control and the delayed training group showed increased symptoms of distress over time, and the training group reported a definite decrease in symptoms (Scogin et al., 1989).

### 4C-3: Advocacy Services to Prevent Elder Abuse

Advocacy services to identified abused elders include companionship, legal, financial, health care advice, and referral to community services. The goal may be referrals to available community services, or efforts may be made to elicit joint responses from the health, social services, and legal fields.

Table 4C-3 lists the only evaluation in this area that meets the committee's criteria for inclusion. The Elderly Abuse Support Project of Rhode Island's Department of Elderly Affairs provides assistance, support, and advocacy to elderly victims of abuse in the utilization of the criminal justice system. Trained volunteers spent an average of two hours a week with the victims, providing information and encouragement in pressing charges, obtaining restraining orders, providing transportation and/or accompaniment to police stations or to the court, and assisting with completion of reports and forms (Filinson, 1993). Several major limitations in the study prevent a conclusive statement about the intervention, including the small sample size, a possible mismatch between the control and treatment groups (particularly with reference to substance abuse by the perpetrators), and systematic bias in the completion of the forms. The results did suggest that the volunteer program, in comparison with the conventional system, could lead to more ambitious goal-setting, greater achievement of goals, and more extensive monitoring of cases. However, with regard to facilitating utilization of the criminal justice system, the primary goal of the project, there was no difference between the intervention or control cases.

Victim Services, Inc., in cooperation with the New York City Police Department, is currently conducting an evaluation of a joint community policing and social service response to elder abuse. In the evaluation, completed in September 1997, 400 complainants who reported elder abuse incidents in public housing to the New York City Police Department were randomly assigned to one of four treatment conditions (Davis and Taylor, 1995): home visits from a joint police and social service team after the complaint; a letter sent to complainants describing elder abuse services available in the community; a public education campaign targeting specific public housing units; and a no-treatment control condition.

## CONCLUSIONS

The most extensive area of study in evaluations of social service interventions for family violence is the field of child maltreatment research. A knowledge base has developed that focuses primarily on parenting practices and family support services, school-based sexual abuse prevention programs, intensive family preservation interventions, and individualized service programs for children in the child welfare system. In contrast, widely used social services such as child protective services, kinship care, and other out-of-home placement services provided through the child welfare system have not been the focus of evaluation studies that could provide significant insights into the benefits or harms associated with these interventions.

Areas that have received extensive study focus on program-specific outcomes, such as reports of child maltreatment or out-of-home placement rates. In general, important outcomes in other domains, such as those related to child health and development and level of family functioning, are unexamined, although they are increasingly the focus of studies of interventions related to parenting practices and family support. The research base in this area, which has had the longest period of development in the area of family violence, has not yet achieved consensus on the key measures of child or family well-being or parenting practices that would allow separate studies to compare their results over time.

The research reviewed in this chapter suggests the following:

- Social service interventions designed to improve parenting practices and provide family support have not yet demonstrated that they have the capacity to reduce or prevent abusive or neglectful behaviors significantly over time for the majority of families who have been reported for child maltreatment.
- The intensity of the parenting, mental health, and social support services required may be greater than initially estimated in order to address the fundamental sources of instability, conflict, stress, and violence that occur repeatedly over time in the family environment, especially in disadvantaged communities. Focusing as they do on single incidents and short periods of support, the interventions in this area may be inadequate to deal with problems that are pervasive, multiple, and chronic.
- Although a parent's use of social networks to support family functioning can be influenced through interventions, there is not enough evidence to indicate whether changes in social networks can create changes in parenting practices that endure over time and result in reduced child maltreatment rates. The evidence, although intriguing, does not yet provide clear indications as to which types of families are most likely to benefit from parental education and family support services as opposed to mental health services designed to address depression, lack of empathy, and impulsive behavior in both parents and children.
- Evaluations of child sexual abuse prevention interventions show some

evidence that school-based programs can provide positive changes in knowledge and attitudes related to prevention behavior. However, the size and duration of this effect for children at different developmental stages remain generally unknown, and there is no evidence tracing these outcomes either to reductions in sexual abuse involving family members or to mitigated effects of such abuse.

• Intensive family preservation services for families that have experienced child maltreatment may delay child placement for many families in the short term, but there is little evidence to date that the services resolve the underlying family dysfunction that precipitated the crisis or improve the child's well-being or the family's functioning. Although it is possible that intensive family preservation services may provide better child and family outcomes for some children and families than foster care, these effects have not been tested in the evaluation literature. Service providers do not have an effective screening method to determine which children or families who have been reported for maltreatment would benefit from intensive services designed to prevent child placement.

• Longitudinal studies suggest that many children who reside in foster care fare neither better nor worse than those who remain in homes in which maltreatment has occurred. However, the changing character of children in foster care over the last decade, with the trend toward increased placement of children under age 5, requires new studies to examine whether the age, length, or stability of placement is correlated with beneficial or adverse outcomes, especially when children in placement are compared with young children who have been maltreated but remain with their families.

• Child maltreatment prevention programs focused on improvements in parenting practices, family support resource centers, and informal social support systems show promise of influencing cognitive and problem-solving skills and child discipline behavior. However, it is not certain if such gains can be established for families who experience multiple sources of stress (such as domestic violence, substance abuse, unemployment, and violent neighborhoods) or whether such gains can be sustained over time once the intervention has ended. The emerging research base suggests that interventions designed to strengthen parenting practices and family functioning require serious attention to the crises and unpredictable nature of problems that occur in the homes of families in disadvantaged neighborhoods to counteract pressures that encourage the use of violence in resolving family disputes and parent-child relationships.

In the area of domestic violence, evaluation studies have focused on the role of shelters and advocacy services for battered women, and domestic violence prevention programs. Little is known about the role of informal or formal support services for victims of domestic violence who choose not to rely on shelters, crisis intervention programs, or advocacy services in seeking to reduce or prevent the use of violence in their intimate relationships. The only study of battered women's shelters that met the committee's criteria for inclusion indicates that shelters can have an immediate effect on limiting incidents of violence—probably a result of reducing exposure and access between the victim and batterer. Longer-term outcomes pertaining to violence, relationship issues, and independent living await documentation. The research base is not yet strong enough to indicate whether other types of support programs, including transitional housing, peer group support, and advocacy services are effective in improving the health, safety, and well-being of the clients who use them.

For elder abuse, there is no research base to inform decisions about how best to address social service interventions. The two studies of elder abuse interventions reviewed by the committee, focused on training for caregivers and on advocacy services to prevent elder abuse, suggest that caregiver training had mixed results and that advocacy services did not succeed in facilitating utilization of the criminal justice system.

Despite the proliferation of services available, evaluations of social service interventions have lacked the rigor and specificity needed to identify which services, or combinations of services, are most effective with which types of victims and offenders. Resources that can contribute to the future development of rigorous service evaluations include

- improved characterization of the services provided in an intervention, including description of the intensity, frequency, length, and scope of the program as well as the training of service personnel;
- the development of consensus about the relevant outcomes and the use of consistent measures of client, family, and community characteristics that can facilitate comparative analyses across studies;
- the identification of subgroups that may benefit from, or be resistant to, certain types of interventions and the identification of cohorts within study samples;
- the inclusion of comparison groups in evaluation studies that can indicate when support programs can make a difference in child, adult, or family outcomes among groups that experience common, different, and multiple stressors in their social environments; and
- the clarification of the theoretical frameworks that guide service interventions.

**APPENDIX TABLES BEGIN ON NEXT PAGE**

TABLE 4A-1  Quasi-Experimental Evaluations of Parenting Practices and Family Support Services

| Intervention | Citation | Initial/Final Sample Size<br>Duration of Intervention<br>Follow-up |
|---|---|---|
| Child Parent Enrichment Project (CPEP), Contra Costa, California.  Clients received pre- and postpartum services from parenting consultants for 2 hours per week for 6 months. | Barth et al., 1988 | N(X) = 24/10<br>N(O) = 26/7<br><br>Randomly assigned comparison group received standard community services<br><br>6 months |
| Two and 5-year follow-up evaluations of CPEP, Contra Costa, California. | Barth, 1991 | N(X) = 97<br>N(O) = 94<br><br>6 month and 2- and 5-year follow-up |
| Parent training (PT), multisystemic therapy (MT) provided to 43 families, in which one parent had been investigated for child abuse or neglect but not child sexual abuse.  Therapy sessions lasted 1.5 hours per week for 8 weeks. | Brunk et al., 1987 | N(PT) = 22/17<br>N(MT) = 21/16<br><br>8 weeks |
| Positive Parenting, a weekly group educational developmental treatment program for abusing parents. | Burch and Mohr, 1980 | N(X) = 45/21<br>N(O) = 41/10<br><br>4 months |
| Instruction in a combination of stress management or cognitive restructuring skills and child management instruction focused on the acquisition of cognitive and behavioral skills.  Offered by the Panel for Family Living in Tacoma, Washington. | Egan, 1983 | N(stress management) = 11;<br>N(child management) = 11;<br>N(combination) = 9<br>N(O) = 10<br><br>6 weeks |

| Data Collection | Results |
|---|---|
| Child Abuse Potential Inventory, Depression Scale, State-Trait Anxiety Inventory, Pearlin Mastery Scale, Social Support Scale, use of prenatal care, birth outcome, infant temperament | CPEP participants showed advantages in prenatal care, birth outcomes, better reports of child temperament, and better indicators of child welfare. CPEP mothers tended to report better well-being. No significant differences demonstrated in levels of support. Reports of child abuse were similar for both groups. |
| Same as above | No advantages for self-report measures measured at 1-year posttest. Reports of child abuse similar for both groups. Some indication of greater success with families with less severe problems. |
| Symptom-90 Checklist, Child Behavior Checklist, Family Environment Scales, Family Inventory of Life Events and Changes, treatment outcome questionnaire developed for the project, parent-child interaction system rated by evaluator | Parent training was more effective than multisystemic therapy at reducing identified social problems. Families who received either treatment showed decreased parental psychiatric symptomology, reduced overall stress, and a reduction in severity of identified problems. |
| Written test based on the program | Abusing parents who became part of an educational developmental treatment program showed significant and positive changes in potential stress factors, isolation factors, knowledge of child development, attitudes, and values compared with the control group. |
| State-Trait Anxiety Inventory, Recent Events Survey, Family Environment Scale, role play interview, parent-child observation | Improvements in positive affect between parent and child were noted for stress management parents. Stress management parents also reported less negative affect associated with negative life events. Parents who received the child management component were more likely to talk to their child during a role-playing disciplinary situation, were less likely to verbally attack their child, and were more likely to reinforce their child's good behavior. |

TABLE 4A-1 *(Continued)*

| Intervention | Citation | Initial/Final Sample Size / Duration of Intervention / Follow-up |
|---|---|---|
| The Social Network Intervention Project (SNIP) was designed to provide support network intervention services to neglectful families, including personal networking, mutual aid. | Gaudin et al., 1991 | N(X) = 28/34 N(O) = 21/17  Comparison group received traditional agency services  2-23 months, median 10 |
| Supportive home helpers, spending an average of 17.5 hours per month with each client in person (12.3 hours) or on the phone for families with high-risk or abusing mothers. | Hornick and Clarke, 1986 | N = 55  A matched comparison group received routine services  12 months |
| Project 12-Ways, a multiple setting behavioral management program including parent-child interaction training, health maintenance and nutrition assistance, home safety training, counseling, job finding counseling, and referral for treatment of substance abuse. | Lutzker et al., 1984 | N(X) = 51 N(O) = 46  1 year |
| Perinatal Positive Parenting provided parent training and information on child care and development, community support groups for new parents, home visits by trained volunteers, and a "warm line" to call for support and information in Royal Oak, Michigan for first-time mothers. | National Center on Child Abuse and Neglect, 1983a | 139 treatment mothers and 27 control mothers completed the BNPI; 97 treatment and 58 control mothers completed the A/API |
| Pride in Parenthood, a program for first-time parents including biweekly support group meetings for young parents in urban Norfolk, Virginia. | National Center on Child Abuse and Neglect, 1983b | N(X) = 27/15 N(O) = 26/15  2 years |

| Data Collection | Results |
|---|---|
| Childhood Level of Living Scale, Child Neglect Severity Scale, Indicators of Caretaking Environment Scale, Social Network Assessment Guide, Adult Adolescent Parenting Inventory | SNIP families reported improvement on all measures compared with the control families. Reincidence of one type of maltreatment occurred during the period of the intervention for 27 (79.4%) of SNIP families and two types of maltreatment for the other 7 (20.6%) SNIP families. This compares unfavorably with the untreated families. |
| Cattell's 16 Personality Factor Test, Coopersmith's Self-Opinion Form, Nurturance and Parent Observation Scales, Parent Attitude/Belief Scales, Parent Behavior Rating Scales, Client Satisfaction Questionnaire | Results showed a trend toward improvement on outcomes measures for both treatment groups. The group receiving lay therapy improved only slightly more than the group receiving standard treatment; however, there was significantly less attrition in the lay therapy group. Lay therapy involved more direct client contact than standard treatment and was significantly more costly. |
| Reports of child abuse and neglect | The 1-year follow-up on recidivism showed a 21% rate of child abuse and neglect for the treatment group and a 31% rate for the comparison group. |
| Bavolek Adult/Adolescent Parenting Inventory (A/API), Broussard Neonatal Perception Inventory (BNPI) | No significant differences between treatment and control groups on the BNPI and A/API. |
| BNPI, A/API | Treatment parents improved their scores on outcome measures from pre- to posttest, control families did not. |

TABLE 4A-1  *(Continued)*

| Intervention | Citation | Initial/Final Sample Size<br>Duration of Intervention<br>Follow-up |
|---|---|---|
| Social learning theory counseling, child management training offered to parents of distressed families by the Oregon Social Learning Center. | Reid et al., 1981 | N(X) = 27 distressed/ abusive families<br><br>N(O) = 27 nondistressed families<br><br>4 weeks<br><br>12-month follow-up |
| Comparison of two programs for single mothers living on government assistance in Ontario, Canada. Both programs offered 14 weeks of weekly, 2.5 hours of service. Opportunity for Advancement (OFA) is an esteem-building and socially supportive group treatment. New Directions for Mothers (NDM) provides life skills training and parenting skills training. | Resnick, 1985 | N(OFA) = 18/10<br>N(NDM) = 18/10<br>N(O) = 18/13<br><br>14 weeks |
| Twelve 1-hour weekly sessions on stress reduction/management offered to 70 adolescent mothers in a public school continuation program. | Schinke et al., 1986 | N(X) = 33<br>N(O) = 37<br><br>12 weeks<br><br>3-month follow-up |
| Project 12-Ways, a multiple setting behavioral management program including parent-child interaction training, health maintenance and nutrition assistance, counseling for home safety training, job finding, and referral for treatment of substance abuse. | Wesch and Lutzker, 1991 | N = 232<br><br>A subset of study participants received only routine agency services |

| Data Collection | Results |
|---|---|
| In-home observations of family interaction | Treatment data suggest that intensive training in parenting skills can be highly effective in reducing the level of parent-child conflict in abusive homes. |
| Parental Attitudes Research Instrument, The Way I See It, social network analysis, videotaped observations of parent-child interaction, report of utilization of treatment facilities, CES Depression Scale, Child Behavior Checklist | No evidence for a connection between short-term competency enhancement and long-term prevention of disorder. |
| Rosenberg Self-Esteem Scale, Beck Depression Inventory, Generating Options Test, Self-Reinforcement Attitudes Questionnaire, Social Support Inventory, Personal Support Scale, Parenting Sense of Competence Scale, Good Care Scale, Pearlin Mastery Scale, behavioral role play | Study findings noted posttest and 3-month follow-up improvements among preventive intervention subjects relative to test-only control subjects on measures of personal and social support, cognitive problem solving, self-reinforcement, parenting competence and care, and interpersonal performance. |
| Subsequent child abuse and neglect charges, rate and severity of recidivism, out-of-home placement | Both treatment and standard service groups experienced decreases in child abuse and neglect. |

TABLE 4A-1  (*Continued*)

| Intervention | Citation | Initial/Final Sample Size<br>Duration of Intervention<br>Follow-up |
| --- | --- | --- |
| Cognitive restructuring intervention to change the perceptions, expectations, and appraisals of the parent regarding the child as well as the stresses encountered by the parent; relaxation procedures to alleviate stress and anger; problem-solving skills to reduce hostile response of parents; a "package" of interventions that includes the first three modalities. | Whiteman et al., 1987 | N(cognitive restructuring) = 8<br><br>N(relaxation) = 12<br><br>N(problem solving) = 11<br><br>N(package) = 11<br><br>N(O) = 13<br><br>6 sessions |

SOURCE: Committee on the Assessment of Family Violence Interventions, National Research Council and Institute of Medicine, 1998.

| Data Collection | Results |
| --- | --- |
| Affection Scale, Discipline Scale, Empathy Scale | Results indicated a reduction in anger measures among subjects exposed to the experimental interventions. The composite treatment resulted in the strongest degree of anger alleviation. |

TABLE 4A-2 Quasi-Experimental Evaluations of School-Based Sexual Abuse Prevention

| Intervention | Citation | Initial/Final Sample Size<br>Duration of Intervention<br>Follow-up |
|---|---|---|
| Sexual abuse prevention training offered to children aged 4-5 and 6-10 at a day care center in a suburb of Chicago, covering good and bad touching and reinforcing assertive behavior. | Conte et al., 1985 | N = 50/40<br><br>3 hours |
| Sexual abuse training program offered to 1st and 2nd grade children in a Denver, Colorado, elementary school. | Fryer et al., 1987 | N(X) = 24/23<br>N(O) = 24/21<br><br>20 minutes per day for 8 days |
| Good Touch, Bad Touch, a sexual assault prevention curriculum offered to kindergarten children from four schools in rural Georgia. | Harvey et al., 1988 | N = 90/71<br><br>A subset of study participants were part of a no-training control group.<br><br>3.5-hour sessions for 3 days<br><br>7-week follow-up |
| Feeling Yes, Feeling No, a sexual abuse prevention curriculum offered to students in 21 elementary schools in a southeastern suburb. Comparison of teacher and child training, child-only training, and teacher-only training. | Hazzard et al., 1991 | N(teacher and child training) = 6 classrooms;<br>N(child training) = 13 classrooms;<br>N(teacher training) = 13 classrooms;<br>N(O) = 8 classrooms<br><br>N = 399 students<br><br>3 sessions<br><br>6-week and 1-year follow-up |

| Data Collection | Results |
| --- | --- |
| Interview to test knowledge of sex abuse | Children in the prevention training group significantly increased their knowledge of prevention concepts whereas children in the control group did not. Older children learned more than younger children. Both younger and older children had greater difficulty learning prevention concepts of an abstract nature than concepts of a specific nature. |
| Simulation of abduction scenario to test children's reaction | The effectiveness of a primary prevention program based on age-appropriate, experiential, and interactive instruction was empirically documented. |
| Test focused on differentiation between good and sexually abusive touches in pictures and vignette | Relative to the control group, at both 3-week posttest and 7-week follow-up, children participating in the prevention program demonstrated more knowledge about preventing abuse and performed better on simulated scenes involving sexual abuse. The results indicated that children as young as kindergarten age can be taught skills to prevent sexual abuse. |
| State-Trait Anxiety Inventory for Children, video taped vignette test, parent questionnaire, What I Know About Touching Questionnaire | Treatment children exhibited significantly greater knowledge and better ability to discriminate safe from unsafe situations on the video measure than control children at posttesting. These gains were maintained at the 6-week follow-up. Children's knowledge gains and prevention skills on the video measure were maintained at the 1-year follow-up. A 1-session "booster shot" program further enhanced children's safety discrimination skills on the video measure. |

TABLE 4A-2  (*Continued*)

| Intervention | Citation | Initial/Final Sample Size<br>Duration of Intervention<br>Follow-up |
|---|---|---|
| Teacher training workshop on child sexual abuse. | Kleemeier et al., 1988 | N(X) = 26<br>N(O) = 19<br><br>6 hours<br><br>6-week follow-up |
| Red Flag, Green Flag, a sexual abuse prevention curriculum for 3rd grade students that offers teachers, children, and parents personal safety lessons and personal safety strategies in Washington County, Pennsylvania. | Kolko et al., 1989 | N(X) = 296/191<br>N(O) = 41/30<br><br>2 sessions over 2 weeks<br><br>2-week and 6-month follow-up |
| Training workshop for elementary school teachers on preventing child sexual abuse in Ottawa, Canada. | McGrath et al., 1987 | N(X) = 38<br>N(O) = 95<br><br>2 days<br><br>2-month follow-up |
| Red Flag, Green Flag, a sexual abuse prevention program. Study compared the results of the program taught to children at home by parents who received instruction with a control no-instruction parent group in a midwestern metropolitan area. | Miltenberger and Thiesse-Duffy, 1988 | N(X) = 24<br><br>35 minutes<br><br>2-month follow-up |

| Data Collection | Results |
| --- | --- |
| Teacher Knowledge Scale, Teacher Opinion Scale, Teacher Vignettes Measure, Teacher Prevention Behavior Measure, teacher rates of reporting sexual abuse of their students | Relative to controls, trained teachers demonstrated significant increases from pre- to posttesting in knowledge about child sexual abuse and pro-prevention opinions. On a post-test-only vignettes measure, trained teachers were better able than control teachers to identify indicators of abuse and suggest appropriate interventions. Over a 6-week follow-up period, trained teachers read more about child abuse than control teachers but did not differ on other behavioral dimensions such as reporting suspected abuse cases. |
| Child self-report, parent self-report, teacher self-report | Results indicated greater gains in general knowledge and prevention skills at posttraining and 6- month follow-up for trained compared with control children. Some improvements were made by trained teachers and parents of trained children. |
| Written instruments based on teacher's knowledge of child abuse | The workshop had a strong effect on the teachers' knowledge about child abuse, school practices, and the existence of policy. |
| Discrimination between good and bad touches in pictures and vignettes | Results of this study demonstrated that the program, when used by parents to teach children aged 4-7, did not produce changes in personal safety knowledge or skills. A behavioral skills training program did produce the desired acquisition of knowledge and skills. Maintenance of the gains was seen only in the group aged 6-7 at the 2-month follow-up. |

TABLE 4A-2  (*Continued*)

| Intervention | Citation | Initial/Final Sample Size<br>Duration of Intervention<br>Follow-up |
|---|---|---|
| WHO preschool program to teach children to recognize potentially victimizing situations. Includes a program for children and training for teachers. | Peraino, 1990 | N(X) = 23/10<br>N(O) = 23/9<br><br>3 weekly 15-minute sessions<br><br>1-hour training for teachers<br><br>6.5-week follow-up |
| Extra training for teachers before using a child abuse awareness curriculum with their classes. | Randolph and Gold, 1994 | N(X) = 21<br>N(O) = 21<br><br>3 2-hour sessions<br><br>3-month follow-up |
| "Touch," a film designed to teach children self-protection skills, followed by a class discussion with children from kindergarten, 1st, 5th, and 6th grades. | Saslawsky and Wurtele, 1986 | N(X) = 33<br>N(O) = 34<br><br>50 minutes<br><br>3-month follow-up |
| Two 5-minute skits written and rehearsed by medical students about child sexual abuse prevention offered to children in grades 4 and 5 in three public schools in a southeastern city. | Wolfe et al., 1986 | N(X) = 145<br>N(O) = 145<br><br>5 minutes plus discussion |

| Data Collection | Results |
| --- | --- |
| Interview questionnaire with puppet scenarios | Results showed that preschoolers who received the program scored significantly higher at posttest than did the control group. Follow-up testing demonstrated retention of learned concepts. |
| Teacher Knowledge Scale, Teacher Opinion Scale, Teacher Vignette Measure, Teacher Behavior Prevention Measure | A 3-month follow-up survey indicated that trained teachers were more likely to have engaged in certain behaviors related to the training (e.g., talking with children and reporting suspected cases of abuse). |
| Paper and pencil questionnaire, child interviews | Children who viewed the film had significantly greater knowledge about sexual abuse and enhanced personal safety skills compared with controls; older children achieved higher scores on both assessments compared with younger children. These gains were maintained at the 3-month follow-up assessment. |
| Evaluation questionnaire | Relative to controls, children who received the program showed an overall increase in knowledge of correct actions to take in the event of potential or actual abuse. |

TABLE 4A-2 *(Continued)*

| Intervention | Citation | Initial/Final Sample Size<br>Duration of Intervention<br>Follow-up |
|---|---|---|
| "Touch," a film designed to teach children self-protection skills, followed by a class discussion; a behavioral skills training program (BST) to teach safety skills, and a third treatment that combined the first two provided to children in elementary grades attending a public school in a small rural town in eastern Washington. | Wurtele et al., 1986 | N("Touch") = 19/17<br>N(BST) = 15/14<br>N(combination) = 19/18<br><br>50 minutes<br><br>3-month follow-up |
| Token Time, a personal safety curriculum for preschoolers taught by parents to their children in a YMCA preschool in a Colorado community. | Wurtele et al., 1991 | N = 52<br><br>A subset of subjects was randomly assigned to a delayed-training control group.<br><br>1 hour, 48 minutes |

SOURCE: Committee on the Assessment of Family Violence Interventions, National Research Council and Institute of Medicine, 1998.

| Data Collection | Results |
| --- | --- |
| Personal safety questionnaire, "What If" situations test | In comparison with the control presentation, the BST program, alone or in combination with the film, was more effective than the film alone in enhancing knowledge about sexual abuse. Posttreatment group comparisons suggested the superiority of the BST program for enhancing personal safety skills. Older children performed significantly better than did younger children. The knowledge and skill gains made directly after treatment were maintained for the 3 months between posttest and follow-up assessments. |
| "What If" situations test, personal safety questionnaire, parent perception questionnaire | The results suggest that parents can teach their preschoolers personal safety skills, and that the program can be implemented in the home. |

TABLE 4A-4  Quasi-Experimental Evaluations of Intensive Family Preservation Services

| Intervention | Citation | Initial/Final Sample Size Duration of Intervention Follow-up |
|---|---|---|
| Four weeks in-home service, two families per caseworker, intensive caseworker involvement, structural family therapy approach focus on alternatives to out-of-home placement. Families served for an average of 5 weeks with 14 hours of face-to-face contact offered to families with adolescents aged 12-17 approved for placement by Hennepin County, Minnesota, child protective services managers. | Au Claire and Schwartz, 1986  Schwartz et al., 1991 | N(X) = 55/22 N(O) = 58  4 weeks  12- to 16-month follow-up |
| Families First, a family systems therapy provided for 4-6 weeks with therapists on call 24 hours per day. Therapists provided advocacy and support in meeting basic needs and coordinating other services, and they provided parenting skills, mood management, communication skills training, and individual and family counseling to families of children in three California counties referred to child protective services for abuse or neglect. | Barton, 1994 | N(X) = 75 N(O) = 75  Comparison group received traditional county services.  4-6 weeks  1-year follow-up |
| Families First Program provided 4-6 weeks of intensive services such as parenting skills training, financial management, transportation, and job skills training to families with children at risk of imminent placement in Michigan. | Bergquist et al., 1993 | N(X) = 225 N(O) = 225  4-6 weeks  1-year follow-up |
| Home-based family services intervention provided by the DePelchin Children's Center, designed to solve family problems and reduce recurrence of abuse and neglect, offered to families with a child at risk for removal but not in immediate danger. Intervention compared with a group of families receiving standard community services from the Texas Department of Human Services (DHS). | Dennis-Small and Washburn, 1986 | N(X) = 87 N(O) = 85  Treatment group received services from the state DHS or a private contracted agency. Control group received standard protective services.  3-14 months |

| Data Collection | Results |
| --- | --- |
| Out-of-home placement history, postservice placement tracking, client treatment record, social worker perceptions | An overall comparison of placement episodes for home-based service and comparison group clients showed no differences in the number of placement episodes (of any length of stay). However, the two groups differed significantly on all other placement activity measures. Home-based service clients spent 1,500 fewer days in placement and had shorter average lengths of stay than did comparison group clients. |
| Family Adaptability and Cohesion Scales (FACES II), Family Inventory of Life Events and Changes (FILE), cost of services, rate of out-of-home placement | Both experimental and comparison groups showed reduction in stress over time. The experimental group showed greater improvement in communication skills than the comparison group. Costs of in-home therapy were significantly lower than the costs of out-of-home foster care. |
| Placement rates in foster care | When compared with similar families who did not receive services, children were consistently placed out-of-home at a much lower rate at 3-, 6-, and 12-months postintervention. |
| Frequency of removals, rate of recidivism, costs of services to families | Children were removed from their homes in 6 (14.6%) of the 41 families served by the intensive intervention and in 9 (9.6%) of the 46 families served by the DePelchin Children's Center. Twenty-one (24.7%) children receiving standard services were removed from the home. Standard services were less expensive than the two experimental interventions. |

TABLE 4A-4  (*Continued*)

| Intervention | Citation | Initial/Final Sample Size Duration of Intervention Follow-up |
|---|---|---|
| Homebuilders programs offered to families referred to Family Preservation Service (FPS) in five New Jersey counties. | Feldman, 1991 | N(X) = 117 N(O) = 97<br><br>Comparison group received traditional services<br><br>4-6 weeks<br><br>1-year follow-up |
| Counseling, homemakers' services, day care, medical, legal, and other family support services provided to families with children at risk of placement. | Halper and Jones, 1981 | N(X) = 60 N(O) = 60<br><br>2-25 months<br><br>1-2 year follow-up<br><br>Comparison group received one-third in-person services as treatment group |
| Homebuilders program, providing 36 hours of in-person and telephone contact in 4-8 weeks for families in Utah and Washington with one or more child at risk of imminent placement. | Pecora et al., 1992 | N(X) = 581 N(O) = 26<br><br>4-8 weeks, 36 hours<br><br>1-year follow-up |
| Families First Program, providing short-term in-home services to families referred for child abuse or neglect. Services include both therapeutic and concrete services. | Schuerman et al., 1994 | N(X) = 995 N(O) = 569<br><br>Comparison group received routine community services.<br><br>Varied for all clients |

| Data Collection | Results |
|---|---|
| Family Environment Scale, Life Event Scale, Interpersonal Support Evaluation List, Goal Attainment Scaling, Child Well-Being Scales, Parent Outcome Interview, Work Environment Scale, placement data, measures of agency effort | By the end of the 1-year follow-up, 42.7% (50) of the 177 FPS families had at least one of their children who was a target of the FPS intervention enter placement. In the control group, 56.7% (55) of the 97 families receiving traditional services had a child enter placement. There was no statistically significant difference between the groups in the number of placements experienced or cumulative time in placement. |
| Placement rates, reports of abuse and neglect, interviews with 27 subjects, Polansky's Childhood Level of Living Scale | Nine of the experimental families (15%) were reported to the Central Registry for abuse or neglect after they were referred to the project. Eight control families (15%) were reported. |
| Placement rates, Child Welfare League of America Family Risk Scales, FACES II | The treatment success rates of the Homebuilders program matched or exceeded those of other Intensive Family Preservation Services or family-centered programs using comparable intake criteria. Twelve-month follow-up data indicate treatment success rates decline over time. |
| Achievement rating by case workers, placement rates, subsequent reports of maltreatment, family and child functioning | Results offer little evidence that Family First resulted in lower placement rates. Experimental group experienced placement of children at a rate slightly higher than the control families. Results also find no evidence that Family First decreased risk of subsequent harm to children or improved case-closing rates when compared with standard services. |

TABLE 4A-4 (*Continued*)

| Intervention | Citation | Initial/Final Sample Size / Duration of Intervention / Follow-up |
|---|---|---|
| Social learning program including training in parenting skills, parent sensitization to child needs, and coping skills training offered to client families of the Cascade County, Oregon, Social Services Child Protective Service Unit. Included families with children aged 3-12 who were considered at risk for placement because of abuse. | Szykula and Fleischman, 1985 | N(X) = 24<br>N(O) = 24<br><br>Not discussed |
| In-home family-based services provided for at least 90 days, with three visits per week per family by caseworker, oriented toward the provision of concrete services and focused on skills training. | Walton et al., 1993 | N(X) = 57<br>N(O) = 53<br><br>Comparison group received routine reunification services.<br><br>90 days<br><br>1-year follow-up |
| Intensive family support services over a 30-day period provided to families referred to child protective services in Lucas County, Ohio, judged to be at least a moderate risk for placement. | Walton, 1994 | N(X) = 74/69<br>N(O) = 74/65<br><br>30 days<br><br>6-month follow-up |

| Data Collection | Results |
|---|---|
| Rate of out-of-home placement | The results indicate that this intervention reduced out-of-home placements for approximately 50% of typical child protective services caseloads. |
| Total number of days the child spent in the home during the treatment and follow-up periods. | After a 90-day service period, 93% of 57 families assigned to receive intensive intervention were reunited, compared with 28% of the 53 control families. Impacts endured for upward of 12 months following the cessation of direct intervention services. |
| Six-month follow-up survey developed for project, interview with participants, Index of Parental Attitudes, Children's Restrictiveness of Living Environments Instrument, review of case histories, Caseworker Survey, Daily Service Activity Record | When compared 6 months after case determination, families in the experimental group had fewer cases opened. The cases that were opened more often opened to the child's own home and were opened for shorter periods of time. Caregivers from the experimental group seemed more likely to use the array of services available, viewed the agency as more responsive and supportive, appeared more willing to express their needs, and utilized services more often than comparison families. |

TABLE 4A-4  *(Continued)*

| Intervention | Citation | Initial/Final Sample Size; Duration of Intervention; Follow-up |
|---|---|---|
| Families First Program in Davis, California, provided home-based, intensive services to families in which at least one abused or neglected child was at risk for placement. | Wood et al., 1988 | N(X) = 26 families/ 34 children<br>N(O) = 24 families/ 32 children<br><br>Comparison group received routine community services<br><br>4-6 weeks<br><br>1-year follow-up |
| Homebuilders model family therapy, life skills training, concrete services. | Yuan et al., 1990 | N(X) = 143<br>N(O) = 150<br><br>Service for varying periods<br><br>6-month follow up |

SOURCE:  Committee on the Assessment of Family Violence Interventions, National Research Council and Institute of Medicine, 1998.

| Data Collection | Results |
|---|---|
| Cost of placements, rate of placement, family functioning as measured by FACES II | One-year follow-up data indicate in-home treatment was successful at reducing out-of-home placement and lowering placement costs compared with comparison group. |
| Placement costs, family functioning, service use | No significant differences in placement rates between the project group and the comparison group. 75% of the project families and 82% of their children were not placed; 80% of the comparison group and 83% of their children were not placed. Approximately 23% of the families in each group had an investigation of abuse/neglect subsequent to their referral to the study. |

TABLE 4A-5  Quasi-Experimental Evaluations of Child Placement Services

| Intervention | Citation | Initial/Final Sample Size Duration of Intervention Follow-up |
|---|---|---|
| Enhanced stipends, training, and support provided to foster parents of 72 children in three Oregon counties. | Chamberlain et al., 1992 | N(enhanced support, stipend, and training [ES&T]) = 31 N(enhanced stipend [IPO]) = 14 N(O) = 27 |
| Residential treatment for abused and high-risk infants. | Elmer, 1986 | N(X) = 31 N(high-risk comparison group) = 31 N(O) = 31 <br><br> 3-month follow-up at 5-month posttreatment |
| Foster care. | Runyan and Gould, 1985 | N(X) = 114 N(O) = 106 <br><br> Comparison group of victims of child maltreatment who were left in the family home |
| Foster care of children in San Mateo, California, removed from home because of abuse and or neglect. | Wald et al., 1988 | N(X) = 76 N(O) = 76 |

SOURCE: Committee on the Assessment of Family Violence Interventions, National Research Council and Institute of Medicine, 1998.

| Data Collection | Results |
| --- | --- |
| Parent daily report, dropout/retention rates of foster parents, staff impressions measure of foster parents' skills and discipline | During the 2-year project, 12 of the 72 participating families (16.6%) (9.6% of ES&T group, 14.3% of the IPO group) discontinued providing foster care compared with the state average dropout rate of 40%. Parents in ES&T group reported significantly fewer problem behaviors in their foster children over time. |
| Bayley Scales Infant Development, Barnard Feeding and Teaching Scales, anthropometric development measures, reunification with families | At Time Two (end of Center residence), experimental children had gained more height for age, scored lower on the psychomotor scale, and stayed relatively equal to the comparison children on the motor scale. By Time Three, physical measurements were the same for the groups, the experimental group maintained its standing with the Bayley scales, scored lower on the interactions scale, but surpassed the comparison children. |
| Rate of subsequent juvenile delinquency | Foster children committed 0.050 crimes per person per year after age 11 years, cohort comparison children committed 0.059. Foster children were more likely than their comparison cohort to have committed a criminal assault. |
| Pre- and postintervention physical exams of children; interviews with caretakers, children, social workers; Wechsler Primary Scale of Intelligence; Wechsler Intelligence Scale for Children; school records of academic performance; teacher ratings of children; Child Behavioral Scale developed for project; Social Competence Instrument developed for project; reports of abuse and neglect; foster placement rates | Foster children received somewhat better physical care and missed less school than children left at home. The foster children demonstrated higher scores in overall socioemotional well-being. |

TABLE 4A-6  Quasi-Experimental Evaluations of Individualized Service Programs

| Intervention | Citation | Initial/Final Sample Size Duration of Intervention Follow-up |
|---|---|---|
| Fostering Individualized Assistance Program (FIAP) provides assessments, planning, case management, and support services to children in foster care because of abuse and neglect. FIAP compared with standard practice. | Clark et al., 1994 | N(X) = 47<br>N(O) = 62<br><br>Randomly assigned comparison group received standard foster care system services<br><br>18 months |
| Weekly visits by trained home visitors and nurse or social worker, child care, day camp, respite care, goods and services, referrals to other community services provided to families with young children who were reported as abused or neglected by school personnel. Cases were resolved as unfounded by protective services. | Hotaling et al., undated | N(X) = 39<br>N(O) = 39<br><br>Comparison group received baseline services<br><br>Weekly, for 2 years |
| Intensive services including individual, group, or family counseling; financial services; medical services; help with housing; psychological evaluation and treatment; education in home management and nutrition; tutoring and remedial education; vocational counseling; homemaker services; and day care offered to families served by a New York City program with at least one at-risk child under 14 who was not an active case under child protective services. | Jones, 1985 | N(X) = 175/80<br>N(O) = 68 |

SOURCE: Committee on the Assessment of Family Violence Interventions, National Research Council and Institute of Medicine, 1998.

| Data Collection | Results |
| --- | --- |
| Child Behavior Checklist, Youth Self-Report, days in out-of-home placement, juvenile crime court records | Both FIAP and standard practice subjects improved in emotional and behavioral adjustment measures. There was a significant improvement in the behavioral adjustment of the FIAP children in permanency placements in contrast to the standard practice group. The FIAP group had less runaways than the standard practice group. The FIAP youth spent less time in incarceration than the standard practice group. |
| Subsequent child abuse and neglect reports, number of families' unmet needs, improved social support, improved parent-child interaction, reduction in parental stress | Fifty-six percent of treatment families compared with 64% of control families were reported for child maltreatment over the 2-year study period. The experimental group did report fewer family problems and lower stress but did not report greater social support. Overall, the treatment group did not show improvements in parent-child relations compared with control groups. |
| Child Welfare Information Services foster care history data, State Central Registrar of substantiated complaints of child maltreatment, Special Services for Children information on clients served, agency case records, in-person interviews | Forty-six percent of the control children and 34% of the experimental children entered foster care during the study. Control children entered foster care sooner than experimental children. |

TABLE 4B-1  Quasi-Experimental Evaluations of Shelters for Battered Women

| Intervention | Citation | Initial/Final Sample Size<br>Duration of Intervention<br>Follow-up |
| --- | --- | --- |
| Battered women's shelter. | Berk et al., 1986 | N = 155 |
| | | Some survey participants chose to use shelter services, some did not |

SOURCE: Committee on the Assessment of Family Violence Interventions, National Research Council and Institute of Medicine, 1998.

| Data Collection | Results |
| --- | --- |
| Reports of violence, shelter stays | Shelters can reduce the risk of new violence for a woman who is taking control of her life in other ways.  Otherwise, shelters may have no impact or may even trigger retaliation from abusive spouses. |

TABLE 4B-3  Quasi-Experimental Evaluations of Advocacy Services for Battered Women

| Intervention | Citation | Initial/Final Sample Size Duration of Intervention Follow-up |
|---|---|---|
| Service of trained advocates for 10 weeks after shelter exit, 4-6 hours per week provided to residents of a domestic violence shelter in a midwestern city. | Sullivan and Davidson, 1991 | N = 41<br><br>A subset of participants was randomly assigned to a no-treatment control condition |
| Service of trained advocates for 10 weeks after shelter exit, 4-6 hours per week provided to residents of a domestic violence shelter in a midwestern city. | Tan et al., 1995 | N(X) = 71<br>N(0) = 75 |

SOURCE:  Committee on the Assessment of Family Violence Interventions, National Research Council and Institute of Medicine, 1998.

| Data Collection | Results |
| --- | --- |
| Subject interviews, Conflict Tactics Scales, Effectiveness of Obtaining Resources Scale designed for program | Four women reported experiencing further abuse within 10 weeks after leaving shelter. This was not related to either experimental condition. Women in the experimental condition reported being more successful in accessing resources. |
| Social Support Scale, Conflict Tactics Scales, Index of Psychological Abuse, Quality of Life Measure, Depression Scale CES-D, Effectiveness of Obtaining Resources Scale | The experimental intervention expanded the social network of women; women in the treatment group felt more effective in obtaining resources than the women who did not have advocates. |

TABLE 4B-4  Quasi-Experimental Evaluations of Domestic Violence
Prevention Programs

| Intervention | Citation | Initial/Final Sample Size Duration of Intervention Follow-up |
|---|---|---|
| A high school program to prevent wife assault and dating violence. | Jaffe et al., 1992 | N = 737<br><br>Delayed posttest for some participants at 6 weeks |
| Minnesota School Curriculum Project is a domestic violence awareness curriculum taught at the junior high school level, including teacher training. | Jones, 1991 | N = 560<br><br>A subset of the study participants was assigned to a matched no-treatment control group |
| "Skills for Violence Free Relationships," a prevention curriculum about women abuse presented to 7th grade health education students. | Krajewski et al., 1996 | N = 239<br><br>A subset of the study participants was assigned to a no-treatment control group |
| Comparison of short and long forms of a dating violence prevention curriculum for 10th graders. Short form was two classroom sessions (120-150 minutes). The long form added a film on dating violence and a letter-writing exercise to a fictional victim and a fictional aggressor. | Lavoie et al., 1995 | N(L) = 238<br>N(S) = 279<br><br>1-month follow-up |

SOURCE:  Committee on the Assessment of Family Violence Interventions, National
Research Council and Institute of Medicine, 1998.

| Data Collection | Results |
| --- | --- |
| London Family Court Clinic Questionnaire on Violence in Intimate Relationships | Twenty-two of 48 test items showed statistically significant changes immediately after the intervention. Females had more positive significant changes than males; males showed some undesired direction changes. Positive changes decreased by half at 6-week posttest. |
| True/false knowledge questions about domestic violence | Relative to control students, treatment students improved scores on the posttest over three points. There was little change for their group on the attitude test posttreatment. Girls had higher attitude improvement scores than boys. |
| Inventory to test knowledge and attitudes about woman abuse | Significant differences were found between experimental and control groups from pretest to posttest on both knowledge and attitude inventories. This impact did not remain stable at posttest. Females showed greater change in attitude over time. |
| Paper and pencil test | Positive pre- and posttests and experimental versus control group gain in knowledge and attitude scores indicate that a short program modified attitudes and knowledge about dating violence. |

TABLE 4C-2 Quasi-Experimental Evaluations of Training for Caregivers

| Intervention | Citation | Initial/Final Sample Size<br>Duration of Intervention<br>Follow-up |
|---|---|---|
| A combination of didactic presentations, group discussions, role playing, education about the aging process, problem solving, stress management, utilization of community resources, anger management, and guided practice for caretakers of elderly relatives who were at risk for abusing the elderly relative in their care. | Scogin et al., 1989 | N(X) = 56<br>N(delayed treatment comparison) = 16<br>N(O) = 23 |

SOURCE: Committee on the Assessment of Family Violence Interventions, National Research Council and Institute of Medicine, 1998.

TABLE 4C-3 Quasi-Experimental Evaluations of Advocacy Services to Prevent Elder Abuse

| Intervention | Citation | Initial/Final Sample Size<br>Duration of Intervention<br>Follow-up |
|---|---|---|
| Volunteer advocates provided assistance and support to victims of elder abuse in the utilization of the criminal justice system to clients of the Elder Abuse Unit of the Department of Elderly Affairs in Rhode Island. | Filinson, 1993 | N(X) = 42<br>N(O) = 42 |

SOURCE: Committee on the Assessment of Family Violence Interventions, National Research Council and Institute of Medicine, 1998.

| Data Collection | Results |
| --- | --- |
| Brief Symptom Inventory (BSI), Anger Inventory (AI), Rosenberg Self-Esteem Scale (RSPS), cost of care index | Results indicated little change over time for either group on the AI or RSPS inventories. Training was associated with a slight reduction in the cost of providing care. The training group reported a significant decrease in symptoms over time on the BSI, whereas the comparison groups reported an increase in distress over time. |

| Data Collection | Results |
| --- | --- |
| Improving self-esteem, seeking legal action, relocating victim or perpetrator, increasing social supports, access services | The findings indicate that the volunteer advocate program, in comparison with the conventional system, can lead to more ambitious goal setting, greater achievement of goals, and more extensive monitoring of cases. |

# 5

# Legal Interventions

The current array of legal interventions to address family violence includes service interventions, procedural and jurisprudential reforms, and efforts to build capacity and expertise in legal and social institutions to invoke legal sanctions—whether threatened or actual. Legal interventions, which include both the criminal and the civil justice systems, have several goals: identifying cases to bring abusers and their victims under the control and protection of legal and social institutions; addressing procedural and evidentiary problems in criminal prosecution; expanding the array of civil interventions to protect victims of abuse; reducing further violence by offenders; and increasing the range of social and legal controls affecting individuals, families, and communities.

Unlike patient-centered or client-centered health and social service interventions, the criminal justice system must also represent society's interests. Its desired outcomes are independent, and at times they may differ from, and even appear to conflict with, those of the people who have been abused. Legal interventions must take into account the issues of due process and concern for the rights of victims as well as those accused of wrongdoing, seeking a balance among interventions to enhance victim protection, facilitate the prosecution of offenders, and preserve the state's interest in fair procedures.

Legal interventions for the treatment and prevention of family violence often focus on procedural changes in law enforcement—such as arrest policies and practices, civil orders of protection, and court standards for the admissibility of evidence—rather than the provision of direct services to clients. The evaluation of such procedural reforms is made difficult by the variations in state and county jurisdictions that influence local law enforcement policies and practices. In evaluating these interventions, many researchers define success as a reduction in recidivism—a program-specific goal that the criminal justice system seldom accomplishes for any other type of offense. This emphasis on a single, hard-to-achieve measure may diminish attention to changes in other important domains, such as individual and public health; child, adult, and family functioning; public safety; equity and fairness; social support and the use of community services; and costs (Worden, 1995).

Family violence treatment and prevention interventions in law enforcement settings have received far less attention in the evaluation research literature than social service interventions (see Table 1-2); less than one-quarter of the studies (21 of 114 studies) selected by the committee for review in this report involve legal interventions. The large majority of these 21 studies focused on domestic violence (18 studies); within this subset, 7 studies examined the impact of spousal arrest policies. This is one of few areas in the family violence research literature in which replication studies have appeared (discussed in section 5B-3). These replication studies have created a database that shows real promise for secondary analyses not only for domestic violence but also for child maltreatment. For example, one recent study that focused on children who witness domestic assaults conducted a secondary analysis of the spousal assault research database to examine the characteristics and prevalence of children in the homes where police officers intervened in response to domestic violence cases (Fantuzzo et al., 1997).

In general, however, evaluations of the effectiveness of legal interventions suffer from problems similar to those in the areas of social service and health care: small study samples, ethical and legal problems in implementing experimental designs and in reporting discovered abuse, the constraints of confidentiality statutes, inadvertent effects caused by the research project, and the complexity of independent variables in multiple and overlapping interventions.

Neither research on the immediate effects of legal reforms nor assessments of the recurrence or cessation of abuse have been routinized for these interventions. Accordingly, policies and procedures reflect ideology and stakeholder interests more than empirical knowledge. With some exceptions (such as the research on arrest policies and domestic violence), the available evaluations are more descriptive than analytic. Experimental or longitudinal studies on the effectiveness of current interventions are rare. The current empirical literature is limited by the kinds of methodological shortcomings discussed in Chapter 3.

Despite the absence of research on their effectiveness, legal interventions are thought by many to play an important role with regard to family violence. For example, as noted later in this chapter, treatment interventions are sometimes provided to offenders solely as a result of arrest and court intervention, and their impact may be influenced by the quality and intensity of court oversight. This chapter reviews legal interventions and the available evaluations of them, first for child maltreatment, then for domestic violence, and finally for elder abuse.

## CHILD MALTREATMENT INTERVENTIONS

In the 1960s, following the passage of legislation that established eligibility for federal funds for child protective services programs, nearly every state adopted mandatory reporting laws, child abuse registries, expanded and newly empowered child protection agencies, and training for personnel in social, legal, and medical agencies. The emergence of child sexual abuse as a social crisis in the 1980s resulted in skyrocketing prosecutions and new evidentiary and procedural rules for such cases (Melton et al., 1995; Weisberg and Wald, 1984). Detailed procedures were put into place to detect, investigate, adjudicate, and resolve cases of child maltreatment—through supervision of families, removal of children from the home, and termination of parental rights.

There was initially strong resistance by child welfare advocates and service providers to the criminal justice system's growing role in these cases, largely based on the assumption that it either could not or would not consider the best interests of the child in making decisions. This resistance abated somewhat as the criminal justice system began to adapt to the special needs of children, establishing special courts to focus on family matters, and child welfare and mental health agencies acknowledged the deterrent role of legal restraints and sanctions on offenders.

Eight legal interventions for child maltreatment are reviewed in the following sections: (1) mandatory reporting requirements, (2) child placement by the courts, (3) court-mandated treatment of child abuse offenders, (4) treatment for sexual abuse offenders, (5) criminal prosecution, (6) improving child witnessing, (7) evidentiary reforms, and (8) procedural reforms. The sections are keyed to the appendix tables that appear at the end of the chapter.

### 5A-1: Mandatory Reporting Requirements

Prior to the medical recognition of the battered child syndrome in 1962 (Kempe et al., 1962), family violence reporting laws did not exist in federal or state statutes. Following a national advocacy effort focused on the protection of children who were physically abused, all 50 states had adopted laws by 1967 requiring health and other professionals to report suspected child abuse and neglect. Since the creation of child protective services systems and the enactment of mandatory reporting laws, increasing numbers of cases have been reported to child protection agencies without a comparable increase in the resources to support adequate investigation and response to these reports. Whether these objectives have actually been achieved is uncertain, although the number of cases reported to child protection agencies has increased significantly.

The overall change since 1976 has been a growth of 331 percent, from an estimated 10 children reported per 1,000 in 1987 to 43 children reported per 1,000 in 1994 (National Center on Child Abuse and Neglect, 1996a,b). The rapid escalation in reported cases has had a significant impact on the investigation and substantiation rates and disposition practices of social service agencies. The 1988 National Incidence Study indicated that only 40 to 50 percent of all reported cases of child maltreatment were substantiated (Sedlak, 1991). By 1994, the rate of substantiated or "indicated" reports had dropped to about 37 percent (National Center on Child Abuse and Neglect, 1996b). This imbalance has encouraged discretionary decisions in which service providers, especially in health settings, seek to provide their clients access to their own treatment programs in lieu of public services (Zellman, 1990, 1992; Brosig and Kalichman, 1992). These findings have prompted a search for revisions in the reporting requirements, to establish certain conditions under which well-trained reporters could exercise more flexibility in filing reports, provide a treatment or intervention plan in lieu of a child protective services investigation, yet maintain informal oversight of cases by child welfare officials (Finkelhor and Zellman, 1991).

The mandatory reporting laws were adopted in the belief that they would reveal cases of child maltreatment that were previously undetected and would provide a means for children and families to receive appropriate services prior to the occurrence of serious injuries, thus enhancing child safety and well-being. In reviewing the research literature on this intervention, the committee found no evaluations of mandatory reporting of child maltreatment that meet its criteria for inclusion (use of a comparison or control group in conduct of the study). Research on this topic is generally descriptive—no quasi-experimental studies have been conducted that could provide guidance to policy officials and service providers.

Designing a study on mandatory reporting with a control group is difficult for several reasons: the universal and mandatory nature of current reporting systems inhibits the formation of an appropriate comparison or control group, uncertainties exist about the appropriate outcomes to measure, and separating the outcomes of mandatory reporting from the outcomes of subsequent services is an immensely complex task. For example, should mandatory reporting be evaluated on the number of cases that are substantiated, on the number of cases that receive some other intervention because of the reporting, on improved state datasets, or on child health and well-being indicators, including child mortality and injury rates?

Mandatory reporting requirements were adopted without evidence of their effectiveness; no reliable study has yet demonstrated their positive or negative effects on the health and well-being of children at risk of maltreatment, their parents and caregivers, and service providers. Several studies have identified significant variations in reporting practices among service providers (especially health professionals) and the presence of a large number of service providers who use discretionary judgment in deciding whether to report suspected cases, especially under circumstances in which a child or family is receiving treatment or intervention services. Nonexperimental research studies have indicated that the filing of a report disrupts therapy in relatively few cases, and that a therapeutic relationship can survive and at times benefit if the therapist confronts and reports abusive behavior (Watson and Levine, 1989; Weisz, 1995).

The objectives and potential benefits of mandatory reporting include (1) increasing detection before violence escalates (when families might be more receptive to social support services), (2) relieving victims and family members of the reporting burden (and thus enhancing their safety), (3) enhancing health care provider response to family violence by fostering greater coordination among service systems, (4) punishing perpetrators, and (5) improving documentation, data collection, and knowledge about the epidemiology of family violence, which can enhance the evaluation of interventions and encourage communities to increase resources for prevention and treatment programs (Hyman et al., 1995; Hampton and Newberger, 1985).

Experience with reporting practices has raised a number of concerns about the adverse impact and unintended consequences of reporting requirements on children, their parents and caregivers, and service providers in both health care and social service settings:

(1) discouraging clients who do not want involvement with the law enforcement system from seeking social services and health care;

(2) risking retaliation by the abuser against victims who reveal abuse;

(3) creating expectations of services and protection that cannot be met;

(4) flooding the social services system with reports that involve minor cases of child maltreatment;

(5) interfering with provider-client relationships and rapport, especially in areas that involve trust, safety, goal setting, deterrence, and treatment;

(6) encouraging inadequate responses by providers, especially from those who do not understand their reporting responsibilities or who may abdicate responsibility for ongoing care once a report has been made;

(7) fostering poor case detection and data collection practices, including noncompliance, biased compliance, and false positive reporting, as well as confusion about what must be reported; and

(8) encouraging greater surveillance bias, including class or ethnic bias in reporting, because of the disproportionate reporting of low-income and minority communities who rely on public services (whose care providers are more likely to file reports) rather than private care (whose care providers are likely to use greater discretion in determining whether a report should be filed) (Besharov, 1994; Hyman et al., 1995; Hampton and Newberger, 1985).

Some critics have indicated that legal reporting requirements have weakened the protection of children by diverting administrative resources away from services for children and families in serious trouble in favor of investigation of minor cases (Besharov, 1994). The tendency to perceive family violence as criminal behavior has also raised concerns about the bias or stigma associated with reporting practices. There is concern that reporting requirements have stimulated false positive cases with damaging effects on some parents, children, and families, although the size of this impact is not known. Finally, many research investigators and sponsors believe that the reporting requirements represent an impediment to the conduct of population-based studies of child maltreatment (National Research Council, 1993a).

The effectiveness of mandatory reporting therefore needs to be examined within the broad dimensions of family violence and the impact of reporting practices on child and family access to services as well as on data collection. More important, the impact of mandatory reporting laws should be judged by the ways in which they interact with other services to help protect children and adults from abuse and neglect and to mitigate their consequences. When criminal acts can be substantiated, mandatory reporting practices can result in the prosecution of cases that would not otherwise be detected. Mandatory reporting requirements can also diminish the use of discretionary judgment and exact an unknown price on the ability of service professionals to control the timing, nature, and scope of disclosures of child maltreatment to legal authorities. These impacts may or may not be harmful to children at risk and their families, depending on the circumstances and severity of the maltreatment that is disclosed.

At this time, significant doubts exist about the ability of social service agencies to respond adequately to initial reports of suspected cases. These doubts suggest that greater caution is required before expanding the use of mandatory reporting requirements in protecting adult victims of maltreatment, especially in the areas of domestic violence and elder abuse.

## 5A-2: Child Placement by the Courts

Juvenile courts (sometimes called family courts) can issue an order of protection, order services and treatment for the family, temporarily remove the child from the home, or, as a last resort, terminate parental rights and provide permanent placement for a child whose care is overseen by the child welfare system. This section deals with the role of the courts in making such decisions; the evaluations of placement outcomes (such as foster care and group homes) are covered in Chapter 4.

The actions of juvenile courts are generally limited to cases of parental abuse and neglect (Bulkley et al., 1996). If the abuse or neglect is substantiated, the judge has a number of options, including requiring the parents to participate in treatment or cooperate with caseworkers as a condition of keeping the child at home; issuing a protective supervision order that allows parents to retain custody under certain conditions or under the supervision of the child protective services agency; removing the child from the home temporarily; giving custody of the child to the agency or other persons; and terminating parental rights to end the legal relationship between parent and child.  Alternative dispositions to the termination of parental rights have been developed as well; for example, some courts award guardianship to third parties in lieu of termination, who provide care and parental support but who do not legally supplant the relationship of the natural parents.  The courts can also establish timetables and deadlines to require public agencies to determine a service plan for the child.

Although statutory bases for termination of parental rights differ by state, in all cases the burden of proof is the standard of clear and convincing evidence, a higher standard than in other civil proceedings.  The burden of proof is on the petitioner—usually the government agency charged with child protection, but it can be others, such as family members, guardians ad litem, prospective adoptive parents, and others specified by state statute.  There is a presumption in favor of maintaining the parent-child relationship and preservation of family ties (*Santosky v. Kramer,* 455 US 745, 71 L Ed 2d 599, 102 S Ct 1388, 1982).  Testimony must include evidence that termination of parental rights would be in the best interest of the child.  The parents are entitled to due process, notice, and an opportunity to be heard and represented by counsel.  The justifications for termination of parental rights in child sexual abuse cases have included refusal to participate in or make progress in treatment, and failure to acknowledge responsibility or to take steps toward rehabilitation (Bross, 1995).

The gravity of parental rights hearings has given rise to other procedural and service interventions designed to protect the child's interests in resolving the conflict between the risks of continued involvement with abusive parents and permanent separation from them.  For example, the position of court-appointed special advocates (CASAs) has developed to represent the child's interests in custody negotiations; they are typically attorneys or trained lay volunteers who either function independently or work in conjunction with attorneys and case-workers.  Comparing a CASA lay volunteer model with a model using staff attorneys in a juvenile unit of the court, one descriptive study found that the use of CASAs resulted in more services obtained for children and reduced the time that the child spent in the home of the family of origin (Poertner and Press, 1990).  They concluded that lay volunteer CASAs could represent children in juvenile court as well as trained court attorneys.

The effectiveness of the juvenile court system in child maltreatment cases has not been formally evaluated.  The courts have the ability to protect children by exercising the power to remove them from the home or to mandate treatment and services.  Juvenile courts also have the ability to provide oversight and in-home monitoring and can act both to help the child and family and to punish the offender (Bulkley et al., 1996).  The disadvantages of the juvenile court system include the removal of the child rather than the offender from the home; the lack of due process protections for those accused of abuse comparable to criminal court procedures; the risk of unnecessary intervention with families; long, indefinite, or multiple out-of-home placements; and unnecessary removal of some children without adequate preventive or treatment services (Bulkley, 1988).

Evaluations of the effectiveness of the juvenile court system should consider what relevant outcomes constitute the most important indicators of its success or limitations. Examples include: the extent to which children's placement status remains uncertain or unstable during periods of court oversight; patterns of service utilization associated with cases in the juvenile court system compared with those that are administered by the social services agencies alone; and long-term measures of child health and well-being and family support associated with cases that are handled by juvenile courts. Such studies could compare the long-term outcomes of siblings or neighborhood children who were reported for maltreatment but were not referred for court attention to those of children whose cases received significant involvement by the juvenile court. Such studies could help clarify which characteristics of maltreatment cases are likely to stimulate court referrals and examine the disparities that exist in caseloads handled by judicial, social services, and health agencies.

### 5A-3: Court-Mandated Treatment for Child Abuse Offenders

The courts can mandate parents to treatment as a condition for keeping or regaining custody of their children. In Chapter 4, we discussed types of treatment and treatment outcome studies of parenting practices and family support services (4A-1). Here we deal with the impact on treatment of its being mandated through the courts rather than being voluntary.

Practitioners are divided on the wisdom of mandating treatment. Those who favor it believe that the threat of legal sanctions will encourage participation in treatment by parents who would otherwise refuse services. Those who question the wisdom of mandatory treatment emphasize the importance of client motivation for involvement in treatment and fear that court mandates may increase resistance to treatment. There has been very little empirical research to help settle this debate.

Table 5A-3 lists two evaluations in this area that meet the committee's criteria for inclusion. One study compared parents ordered to a treatment program with those who voluntarily entered treatment (Wolfe et al., 1980). They found that court-ordered parents were more likely to complete the treatment program. However, the other study found no such differences in treatment completion between voluntary and court-mandated parents (Irueste-Montes and Montes, 1988). Both groups attended and completed treatment at similar rates and showed similar improvements in their interactions with their children. The researchers conclude that mandating treatment does not increase resistance to participation. Although they did not ask all court-mandated participants whether they would have voluntarily entered treatment, informal comments by some of these parents suggested that they would have dropped out of the 3-year program or refused treatment altogether had the legal sanctions not been in place. Court oversight of treatment referrals thus seem to facilitate completion rates for offenders who would be unlikely to voluntarily participate in treatment programs. Whether completion results in improved parent-child interactions or positive child outcomes remains generally unknown in the research literature.

### 5A-4:  Treatment for Sexual Abuse Offenders

Treatment programs for sex offenders seem to be increasing in number, and adults who sexually abuse children are often offered treatment as part of or in lieu of other sanctions by the court.  Such programs seek to normalize sexual preferences and enhance social functioning, working from the assumptions that deviant sexual acts result from an attraction to inappropriate partners or behaviors and that social deficits restrict access to appropriate partners and cause stress in the offender, both of which increase the likelihood of offensive behavior (Marshall and Barbaree, 1988).

Although some efforts have been made to classify offenders in terms of their relationship to the target child, research studies cannot yet distinguish clearly between sexual offenses that involve familial relationships and those that do not. For example, one study classified two treatment groups as "incest offenders"— men who exclusively molested either their own daughters or granddaughters or who molested female children for whom they were serving as surrogate fathers, such as stepdaughters, adopted daughters, and daughters of a common-law wife— and "molesters of nonfamilial children"—men who molested children who were not their own and for whom they were not serving as the surrogate father (Marshall and Barbaree, 1988).  Such distinctions are ambiguous in the research literature, however; sex offender programs often do not classify treatment groups according to the nature of the relationships between the victim and the offender.

A 1994 survey found 710 sex offender programs in the United States, a 139 percent increase in programs since 1986 (Freeman-Longo and Knopp, 1992). The vast majority (573) of the programs were outpatient or community-based; 90 were prison-based; and the remaining 47 were other residential-based programs.

Three general approaches are used in treating sex offenders:  cognitive-behavioral, psychotherapeutic, and organic (also called biological or physical). Today, the cognitive-behavioral approach predominates (Freeman-Longo and Knopp, 1992) and consists of a number of cognitive and skills training methods, behavior control techniques, and, more recently, relapse prevention strategies borrowed from the field of addiction treatment (Marshall et al., 1991).  The psychotherapeutic approach includes individual, group, and family counseling. The organic approach includes surgical castration, hormonal and other pharmacological treatments, and psychosurgery.

There is no consensus in the research as to whether treating sex offenders reduces recidivism (U.S. General Accounting Office, 1996).  It is generally believed that the recidivism rate for incest offenders is low compared with that of other child molesters (Furby et al., 1989). It has also been suggested that incest is related to family dynamics and opportunism rather than to inappropriate sexual preferences, suggesting that behavior modification treatment programs may be less effective with incest offenders (Quinsey et al., 1993). One study suggests that post-treatment recidivism rates vary widely with different offender characteristics, including type of offense; the growing body of literature on the treatment of sex offenders may therefore not be applicable to incest offenders (Furby et al., 1989).

Table 5A-4 lists two evaluations in this area that meet the committee's criteria for inclusion. One study matched a treated and untreated group of child molesters, all of whom admitted their crimes and requested treatment (Marshall and Barbaree, 1988). Treatment consisted of cognitive-behavioral outpatient services. The treatment group had far lower recidivism rates than the control group on both official and unofficial measures.

The other study compared the effectiveness of a multimodal inpatient treatment for incest offenders and heterosexual pedophiles. The treatment programs included group psychotherapy, social skills training, anger management, psychodrama, film discussion of victims, and stress inoculation (Lang et al., 1988). Both groups showed improvement, and incest offenders showed greater improvement than pedophiles on trait anxiety, fear of negative evaluation, social skills deficits, indirect hostility, and irritability. By the end of a 3-year follow-up, 7 percent of the incest offenders and 18 percent of the pedophiles had reoffended. The small sample size and lack of an untreated control group make it impossible to attribute changes to the treatment. In fact, the recidivism rates reported in this study are similar to those of the untreated control group rates in the Marshall and Barbaree (1988) study.

Several reviews of less rigorous studies have shown some promising results from multicomponent, cognitive-behavioral treatment approaches, particularly with child molesters (Becker and Hunter, 1992; Marshall et al., 1991; Martens, 1992). Reviews of studies of psychotherapeutic approaches concluded that counseling was insufficient by itself to change the behavior of sex offenders (U.S. General Accounting Office, 1996). Organic treatments have shown some evidence of effectiveness, but no consensus exists about which drug is most effective or about the duration of positive effects (U.S. General Accounting Office, 1996). Marshall et al. (1991) suggest that organic treatments should not be viewed as a means for reducing reoffending in and of themselves, but they may be appropriate as a means of reducing an offender's sex drive until cognitive-behavioral treatments can begin to build self-control.

Although cognitive-behavioral approaches and other forms of treatment appear to show some positive outcomes of treatment for sex offenders, more rigorous characterizations of the types of offenders involved in treatment are needed before the effectiveness of treatment programs in reducing repeat sexual offenses can be determined for incest offenders and others who are involved in ongoing familial relationships with their victims. For incest reoffending, attention is required to the circumstances in which offenders are referred to or request treatment, and the ways in which treatment is used as a deterrent in determining whether an offender can maintain custody or remain in contact with the child or family.

### 5A-5: Criminal Prosecution of Child Abuse Offenders

The impact of criminal prosecution of child abuse on the protection of children has not been rigorously evaluated. The question of whether to criminally prosecute child maltreatment offenders is shaped by competing views of the role of the legal system in influencing behavior and responding to individuals, families, and community needs. Those who are opposed to criminal action believe that it hurts the family, that the criminal justice system is insensitive to families' and children's needs, and that district attorneys and police officers focus more on prosecution than on referrals for treatment and services. Those who favor criminal prosecution believe that it is an effective way to enforce the laws, deter future abuse, discourage unacceptable behavior, and coerce individuals into treatment. This perspective reflects a belief that, as a matter of policy, one should not selectively forgo prosecution of criminal behavior for the sole reason that the victim is related to the offender.

There are no evaluations in this area that meet the committee's criteria for inclusion. The research cited in this section is either descriptive or lacks control groups.

In most states, reports of maltreatment are made to a designated child protection agency (see discussion in section 5A-1 above). After investigating, the agency may report serious cases to law enforcement officials (some states require child protective services to report all cases of abuse and neglect to the district attorney). Once a case is referred to law enforcement, prosecutors have broad discretion in whether or not to file charges and whether to drop or accept the case.

Research focusing on the decision making of prosecutors has examined variables that play a role in the acceptance and rejection of cases; decisions to prosecute vary widely, with many factors determining whether a prosecutor decides to proceed (Whitcomb, 1992). In a federally sponsored 3-year study in four cities, prosecutors were influenced by mandatory reporting requirements, statutes regarding procedural and evidentiary practices, and the availability of alternatives to prosecution, such as counseling (Office of Juvenile Justice and Delinquency Prevention, 1994). Another study found three primary characteristics related to prosecutors' decisions to file charges: age and maturity of the victim, the relationship between the victim and the perpetrator, and the evidence of abuse (Borland and Brady, 1985).

Younger children may be less competent to testify and lack credibility, so their cases may be screened out. The relationship of the offender to the child poses questions regarding safety and the likelihood that the abuse will occur again. A study of initial decisions by prosecutors in sexual abuse cases found that offenders who were fathers, stepfathers, and uncles were more likely to be prosecuted than brothers, child care workers, or babysitters (MacMurray, 1989). This study also found that cases involving male victims were more likely to be prosecuted than those involving female victims.

Because of the hidden nature of child abuse, prosecutors may feel there is not enough physical or medical evidence to successfully prosecute a case. The nature of the abuse itself may also determine whether prosecution is pursued. A 1993 American Bar Association survey of 600 prosecutors found that they reported prosecuting fewer physical than sexual abuse cases (Smith and Elstein, 1993), despite the fact that there is a high attrition rate in sexual abuse cases (Finkelhor, 1984). Overall, few child abuse and neglect cases go to trial; those that do raise questions concerning the ability and role of children as witnesses in the court system.

## 5A-6: Improving Child Witnessing

Children have not usually been considered believable witnesses in a court of law (Myers, 1994). Although an extensive body of literature has focused on their ability to adequately serve as witnesses, no evaluations in this area have been conducted that involve the use of comparison or control groups. The discussion that follows is based on other types of research.

In a criminal justice system designed for adults, issues such as children's competence to testify, their ability to distinguish fact and fiction, and the possible harm that their testifying presents pose special challenges. Researchers have explored children's memory, suggestibility, and ability to distinguish truth from fantasy (Goodman, 1984; Goodman et al., 1987). Their credibility rests on the knowledge that they are able to recall and report events reliably. In general, laboratory studies involving eyewitness accounts indicate that children as young as four years of age can present testimony that is as reliable as that of adults (Melton, 1985). Interestingly, children are no more likely to lie than adults (Myers, 1994). Errors in their testimony are primarily those of omission (Goodman et al., 1987). When questioned through free recall about what they have experienced, children may be less forthcoming than adults but are nonetheless accurate in their descriptions (Melton, 1985). However, retrospective studies of children demonstrate that traumatic events are often vividly remembered (Terr, 1981, 1983). The threat of injury and degree of trauma may also result in children's attempting to control their fear by reconstructing events to make them seem less threatening (Eth and Pynoos, 1985).

The need to question children in a detailed manner raises concerns about their suggestibility and the extent to which their developmental level allows them to be influenced by others. Myers (1994) notes that researchers studying children's susceptibility to suggestion can be separated into two groups. One emphasizes children's susceptibility when being tested in artificially and sometimes extremely stressful situations. The second group acknowledges children's limitations but offers evidence that they can resist suggestion. Identifying children's strengths and weaknesses, these researchers concentrate on methods to improve testimony (Goodman et al., 1987).

Research comparing children and adults in simulated situations has shown that younger children (age 3 and below) consistently recall less information and answer objective questions less accurately (Goodman et al., 1987), although other results reveal that adults and 6-year-olds differed little in their ability to answer objective questions (Goodman and Reed, 1986). Younger children, like adults, have proven to be more suggestible when the interviewer is seen as an authoritative figure (Ceci et al., 1987). Although children may have difficulty distinguishing between their own thoughts and actions, they are able to separate *another* person's actions from their own thoughts (Johnson and Foley, 1984). The potential suggestibility of children necessitates careful interviewing techniques by professionals involved in legal investigation and prosecution of child maltreatment.

Given that most research is conducted in artificial circumstances that often bear little resemblance to the courtroom or the judicial process, the strength of laboratory research findings is uncertain when applied to real-life situations. The courtroom presents children with a mystifying and stressful environment. Cross-examination, facing the defendant, and testifying for long periods of time may affect children's ability to testify competently and accurately.

The impact of testifying can be harmful or beneficial for children; there is evidence for both. Some researchers believe that testifying in the courtroom can further traumatize children (Office of Juvenile Justice and Delinquency Prevention, 1994). Others believe that testifying can be beneficial, if children are provided with an opportunity to tell their story and to be believed (Runyan et al., 1988).

### 5A-7: Evidentiary Reforms

Increased recognition of the need to assist and protect child witnesses in court has led to the development of innovative procedural and evidentiary approaches, many of which raise issues of constitutionality, due process, and fairness. Reforms have involved system changes, such as modifications in the rules of evidence, exceptions to the restricted use of hearsay testimony, and the use of child advocates in the courtroom. A primary concern has been to shield children from having to confront the defendant in person. The use of videotaping and closed circuit television, which allows for a live transmission to the courtroom from a nearby location, is currently allowed in some states. The impacts of these reforms on children, adolescents, adults, and legal procedures remain unknown.

Although evidentiary reforms are the subject of intense debate, there are no evaluations in this area that meet the committee's criteria for use of a comparison or control group. Research to determine the efficacy of various reforms is limited, and knowledge of their actual impact on children is anecdotal. Innovations that enhance a child's ability to recall and relate with accuracy may improve the prosecution of child maltreatment cases that involve criminal acts. But given that the court must choose among the rights of the defendant, standards of evidence, and the potential harm to the child, further investigation of the reforms under consideration is warranted.

### 5A-8: Procedural Reforms

Recognizing that children often need support when they testify in the courtroom, provisions to allow for victim advocates and guardians ad litem have increased. Victim advocates are often part of a community-based program not officially affiliated with the criminal justice system. Guardians ad litem ("for the suit") are appointed by the court to represent the best interests of the child in a legal proceeding. Statutes vary with regard to the types of hearings and proceedings that advocates can attend, but usually one person, such as a parent, relative, or friend, is permitted to stay with the child and may even hold the child's hand (Whitcomb, 1992). Legal issues surrounding guardians ad litem include questions regarding their legal status, their proper function and responsibility, and their right to privileged communication with the child (Whitcomb, 1992).

In this area no evaluations meet the committee's criteria for inclusion. One study that did not include a comparison group found that children testifying in criminal court were better able to answer questions and appeared less frightened when a parent or loved one was allowed to remain with them (Goodman et al., 1987). Additional efforts to streamline the judicial process have been made but remain unevaluated in the research literature. Recent innovations include the development of specialized child advocacy teams, multidisciplinary teams to coordinate investigations, and specialized police investigative units.

## DOMESTIC VIOLENCE INTERVENTIONS

Before the 1970s, legal institutions responded with ambivalence to violence toward wives and intimate partners. The convergence of the interests of feminists, victim advocates, and legislators led to a series of reforms beginning in the late 1970s to strengthen criminal justice responses to wife beating (Lerman, 1981; Dutton, 1988). By 1980, 47 states had passed domestic violence legislation mandating changes in protective orders, enabling warrantless arrest for misdemeanor assaults, and recognizing a history of abuse and threat as part of a legal defense for battered women who kill their abusive husbands.[1]  Police response and arrest procedures changed not only in response to these pressures, but also pursuant to successful litigation by women against police departments for their failure to enforce criminal laws and protect them from violent partners (see, for example, *Scott v. Hart*, U.S. District Court for the Northern District of California, C76-2395; *Bruno v. Codd*, 47 N.Y. 2d 582, 393 N.E. 2d 976, 419 NYS 2d 901, 1979; and *Thurman v. City of Torrington*, 595 F. Supp. 1521, 1984).

The array of statutory, procedural, and organizational reforms has covered nearly every aspect of the legal system.  Police departments have adopted pro-arrest or mandatory arrest policies.  Domestic violence units were formed in prosecutor's offices, and treatment programs for abusive husbands were launched in probation departments and by community-based groups.  Reforms in protective and restraining order legislation enabled emergency, ex parte relief that included no-contact provisions as well as economic and other tangible assistance to battered women.  These forms of relief, as well as the application of criminal laws, were extended to women in unmarried cohabiting couples and to divorced and separated women.  A small number of jurisdictions have developed coordinated, systemic responses that bring to bear the full range of social controls and victim supports for battered women.

Interventions to control violence against adult intimate partners reflect three separate but related policy goals: criminal punishment and deterrence of batterers, rehabilitation of batterers, and protective interventions designed to ensure the safety and empowerment of victims.  Legal institutions have been used to advance each of these goals, but the evaluations of interventions are complicated by the lack of common measures that could assess whether progress in one area helps or impedes the achievement of other policy goals.  In addition, the research literature does not include evaluations of general deterrent efforts of these reforms (the extent to which legal interventions reduced the level of domestic violence in a community).  The literature examines the effects of legal interventions only on the identified cases to which they apply.

Eight interventions are reviewed in the sections that follow:  (1) reporting requirements, (2) protective orders, (3) arrest procedures, (4) treatment for domestic violence offenders, (5) criminal prosecution, (6) specialized courts, (7) systemic approaches, and (8) training for criminal justice personnel.  The sections are keyed to the appendix tables that appear at the end of the chapter.

### 5B-1:  Reporting Requirements

Unlike the reporting of child maltreatment, which is mandatory by law in all states, the reporting of domestic violence is often part of the state's injury report-

---

[1]The "battered woman's defense" was applied not only in cases in which the woman killed the man during an attack, but also in cases in which the man was not actively threatening or abusing the woman at the time of the incident (Schneider, 1980).

ing requirements and varies by state jurisdiction. As of August 1996, 45 states and the District of Columbia had laws that require health professionals to report, usually to law enforcement officials, certain injuries suspected of being caused by domestic violence (Hyman et al., 1995); 41 states require reporting by health care practitioners when a patient presents an injury that appears to have been caused by a gun, knife, firearm, or other deadly weapon. In 18 states and the District of Columbia, a report is required when the patient's injuries are suspected of having resulted from an illegal act; since battering—the physical or sexual assault of an intimate partner—is considered criminal in all states, this requirement is tantamount to requiring reports for injuries caused by domestic violence. In only five states do the reporting laws specifically and narrowly require the reporting of injuries when domestic violence is suspected.

In 1994, California enacted the first state legislation requiring health care professionals to report domestic violence to legal agencies. More uniform reporting could provide datasets similar to those available for child maltreatment, thereby allowing better tracking of prevalence trends. However, the disadvantages of mandatory reporting discussed above (5A-1) may be even more serious for domestic violence than for child maltreatment. Those who work with battered women argue that mandatory reporting could undermine the autonomy of adult women, prevent them from seeking necessary services, and in some cases put them at increased risk of serious harm.

There have been no evaluations of reporting requirements for domestic violence. In light of the potential dangers to victims, careful evaluation of the new mandatory reporting law in California seems warranted before other states pass similar requirements.

### 5B-2: Protective Orders

Beginning with the passage of the Pennsylvania Protection from Abuse Act in 1976, every state now provides for protective orders in cases of domestic violence (Klein, undated). Protective orders are civil injunctions that establish restraints against a person accused of threatening or harassing the individual who requests the order. Civil orders of protection (also known as restraining orders) are issued by the courts upon request by a victim of domestic violence; they state that the offender (the "respondent") may not assault her, enter her home, approach her, or have any communication with her for a specified period of time. States typically allow for temporary and permanent protective orders; temporary orders are in effect for a short period of time, often several weeks, and may be issued on an emergency basis without a hearing. A permanent order may be awarded after a hearing; permanent protective orders are often good for one to three years (Klein and Orloff, 1996).

The advantages of protective orders are that they are victim-initiated and timely. They allow a relaxed standard of proof, focus on the victim's protection, and can prescribe a wide range of specific interventions that address safety and economic well-being. However, only a few studies have examined their effectiveness in reducing domestic violence; the extent to which protective orders are used in conjunction with criminal prosecution and the types of errors that are avoided as well as associated with relaxed evidentiary standards are generally unknown. There are no evaluations in this area that meet the committee's criteria for inclusion.

In the absence of controlled studies, it is not possible to determine the role that protective orders play in discouraging the recurrence of violence. It has been suggested that temporary protective orders are frequently violated and that few sanctions exist for violations (Harrell et al., 1993). Protective orders can be issued by civil or criminal courts, but the large majority are handled by civil courts. The police have a long-standing ambivalence about the priority of enforcing civil remedies in the criminal justice system, and poor coordination of information between the civil and criminal systems may make it difficult for police to know who has a protective order when a "domestic" call is received. One study indicates that protective orders against respondents with a criminal history are likely to be less effective in deterring future violence than those obtained against respondents without such a history (Keilitz et al., 1996), but this study lacks a comparison or control group. Although protective orders are not designed to deter violent behavior, they may play a role in providing security to and building self-esteem for victims (Keilitz et al., 1996). It is uncertain whether protective orders can help deter future violence when combined with criminal prosecution or social interventions, highlighting the need for research experimentation to compare the relative impact of comprehensive legal reform efforts and single law enforcement strategies. Weak enforcement and limited punishment for violations may undermine the utility of the protective order.

The use of electronic devices to monitor compliance with protective orders is a recent innovation in a number of communities. These systems include alarm systems in victims' homes, portable panic buttons that victims can activate when offenders approach, and bracelets worn by the offender that set off alarms if he comes within a specified distance of the victim's home. Electronic systems have the potential to generate a swift response from police in the event of the violation of a protective order. Whether or not these systems increase victim safety has not yet been determined; however, both technical and operation problems have hindered the performance of electronic monitoring in home confinement programs for other crimes.

### 5B-3:  Arrest Procedures

Arrest for domestic violence is perhaps the best-studied intervention for family violence. Many evaluations employ experimental designs, random assignment groups, common measures, and replication studies that represent exemplary methods of evaluation. Table 5B-3 lists eight evaluations of arrest that meet the committee's criteria for inclusion.

The Minneapolis Domestic Violence Experiment is one of the first and most widely cited and influential criminal justice experiments in the area of family violence research (Sherman and Berk, 1984a). In that study, street-level police officers' responses to misdemeanor spouse assault were determined by random assignment to one of three treatments: (1) arresting the suspect, (2) ordering one of the parties out of the residence, and (3) advising the couple. Using victim interviews and official records of subsequent police contact, the researchers reported that the prevalence of subsequent offending—including assault, attempted assault, and property damage—was reduced by nearly 50 percent when the suspect was arrested (Sherman and Berk, 1984a:267). It is important to emphasize that only misdemeanor cases were included in the experiment, an eligibility criterion that reduces the generalizability of the experiments to felony cases involving serious assault or rape.

The study findings were widely publicized (Sherman and Cohn, 1989). The U.S. Attorney General's Task Force on Family Violence endorsed the study's findings and recommended that state and local agencies adopt a policy toward spouse assault (U.S. Attorney General, 1984). Following the attention given to this single study's results, a dramatic change in formal policy consistent with the study's findings was reported by police departments in both large and small U.S. cities (Sherman and Cohn, 1989).

The Minneapolis experiment was a critical event in changing public and scholarly perceptions of nonfelony spouse assault from a family problem amenable to mediation and other informal, nonlegal interventions (Bard and Zacker, 1971) to a violation of the law requiring a formal criminal justice sanction. However, the initial reports of deterrent effects in the Minneapolis experiment were tempered by later criticisms of limitations in the design and claims of the overreach of its conclusions (Binder and Meeker, 1992). Replications of the Minneapolis experiment were conducted in five jurisdictions (see Table 5B-3): Omaha, Nebraska (Dunford et al., 1990); Charlotte, North Carolina (Hirschel and Hutchison, 1992); Milwaukee, Wisconsin (Sherman et al., 1992a); Dade County, Florida (Pate and Hamilton, 1992); and Colorado Springs, Colorado (Berk et al., 1992a). Known collectively as SARP (the Spouse Assault Replication Program), these five studies were designed with features that were intentionally similar: arrest as the selected treatment intervention; common eligibility criteria (misdemeanor cases of domestic violence); the use of victim reports and police reports as measures of outcome; and the use of random assignment. Although execution of each study varied among the five sites, some of which was necessitated by local law, the shared design format and common measures allowed general insights to be drawn from the five jurisdictions.

None of the five replication experiments show that arrest per se works in general to reduce subsequent violence. The findings on the specific deterrent effect of arrest on the prevalence of reoffending—the central finding of the Minneapolis experiment—differ by data source and by site (Garner et al., 1995; Fagan and Browne, 1994). The policy implication of these findings is that arrest of all misdemeanor cases will not on average produce a discernible effect on recidivism. Although it is important to acknowledge a distribution of effects across the five sites, it is not clear whether this distribution is significant.

Conclusions about the ineffectiveness of deterrence based on the police experiments may be limited by the weak "dosage" of punishment in the arrest group—that is, in most cases arrest was the only sanction imposed. Most offenders were not prosecuted once arrested. Few were handcuffed, most spent only a few hours in custody, and only a few were jailed overnight (Sherman, 1992a). In some cases, however, augmentations were included—the Milwaukee group included an arrest-and-hold treatment (regarded as a higher dose than just arrest). The Omaha experiment included an "offender-absent" group: arrests were not made, but warrants were issued for batterers who had fled the scene prior to the arrival of police (Dunford et al., 1990). Felony cases were included in the Omaha offender-absent experiment, which had consistent evidence of deterrence.

The implications of these replication experiments do not imply that arrest is unnecessary. Apart from its effect on recidivism, arrest may serve the public's interest that justice be done, or it may serve as a general deterrent for others in the community—an impact that was not examined in the SARP studies. Furthermore, arrest may have an important effect on certain kinds of people. For example, most of the five SARP studies demonstrated a finding of "conditional deterrence"—that is, arrest and overnight incarceration awaiting arraignment appeared to deter batterers with strong informal social control, but not those who lack such controls. Tests of this hypothesis with data from four of the replications conducted by three independent teams of investigators (Sherman et al., 1992a; Pate and Hamilton, 1992; Berk et al., 1992b) all concluded that employed suspects were deterrable by arrest, whereas unemployed suspects were either less deterred or became more violent after randomly assigned arrest.

The interactions between employment status and arrest are limited by the fact that arrest was not randomly assigned to the employed and unemployed groups; they are also limited by the use of somewhat different measures of repeat offending across sites (Garner et al., 1995). But they were given further support by a reanalysis of the Milwaukee experiment that examined the amount of informal control in the community (Marciniak, 1994). Suspects randomly assigned to arrest in census tracts with low unemployment were deterred by arrest, independent of their individual employment status; suspects in high unemployment areas were more violent following arrest than after a warning.

The conclusion that the deterrent effect of arrest for misdemeanor violence depends on the level of informal social control led to recommendations against mandatory arrest laws that apply to misdemeanors in concentrated poverty areas (Sherman, 1992a), and in favor of community policing policies reached in collaboration with local leaders. Such a proposal, however, does not address the potential general deterrent effects of mandatory arrest policies.

No rigorous tests of the general deterrent effects of arrest, let alone prosecution or sentencing, are available for either misdemeanor or felony domestic violence. Low prosecution rates for misdemeanor arrest—as low as 5 percent in Milwaukee (Sherman, 1992a)—suggest that major increases in prosecution will require a shift in the priorities and resources of local jurisdictions. Whether more court-imposed sanctions in combination with arrest could create general or specific deterrence of domestic violence remains unknown. Most research in this area generally does not examine the effects of different sentences on different types of batterers once domestic violence cases are prosecuted.

Further research on deterrent effects of legal interventions, both general and individual, should be a high priority. The Omaha offender-absent experiment, which remains unreplicated almost a decade after it was first reported, suggests that the use of warrants achieved a deterrent effect for suspects who were absent by the time police arrived, even though deterrence was not indicated by arresting offenders who were still present at the scene (Dunford et al., 1990). The deterrent effects of police intervention were clearer and more consistent across different outcome measures in this experiment than in any of the other conditions, indicating that the continuing threat of legal sanctions may have a stronger deterrent effect than the actual imposition of a sanction through the arrest process. Since almost half of all domestic violence suspects leave the scene before police arrive (Sherman, 1992b), offender-absent policy deserves far more attention. So does the finding that arrest backfires in urban poverty areas, where requests for police responses to domestic violence are heavily concentrated. Domestic violence policies are a critical part of the larger research agenda for such areas, where other kinds of violence are also highly concentrated (Wilson, 1996).

The difficulty of comparing results across different study designs illustrates several major challenges for family violence research evaluations: (1) maintaining experimental controls in service settings can involve substantial resource commitments by both the research team and the service agency; (2) the vast array and complexity of potential interventions necessitate careful identification of the critical components that warrant experimental analysis; (3) critical components often vary between experimental sites (for example, the length and severity of confinement practices may differ within and between jurisdictions); (4) certain interventions may stimulate different types of follow-up actions (such as the loss of a job or parole violation) that can interact with the arrest event; and (5) variations in the reporting and analysis procedures of individual studies can result in inconsistent reports of program effectiveness (Garner et al., 1995).

Attention to identification of critical components in interventions, common measures, and consistent program and research definitions in study design will improve the ability of the research community to provide more explicit guidance to the policy makers and service providers in designing law enforcement interventions for family violence. The selection of outcomes of interest beyond recidivism rates can provide insights into other dimensions of behavior or service system characteristics that may be directly influenced by arrest policies and practices. Other outcomes that merit consideration in future evaluation studies are the impact of arrest on interactions between victim and offender, the impacts of arrest on others in the household (including children) and in the community, and the cost and unintended consequences of arrest policies. The latter category includes consideration of improper or unwarranted arrests and the likelihood of disproportionate arrests of certain groups of offenders (minority, low-income, unemployed).

### 5B-4: Court-Mandated Treatment for Domestic Violence Offenders

Mandating batterers to a treatment program in conjunction with other criminal justice sanctions, as a condition of probation or as an alternative to other sanctions, is gaining increasing popularity in courts across the country. Treatment interventions for batterers vary in several respects. They are administered by different service sectors, including probation departments, social service agencies, mental health settings, private agencies, battered women's shelters, and self-help groups. Treatment interventions and settings vary in their underlying assumptions about the causes of intimate violence and their operational characteristics, including the duration, frequency of contacts, skills of the service provider, and the objectives of treatment. Many interventions address anger management or the relationship of power and control to the use of violence; victim safety is often linked to offender's behavioral changes as central components of program development.

The courts generally do not recognize different types of batterers or make efforts to match batterer profiles to specific treatment types (Saunders and Azar, 1989), yet there may be considerable need to address these issues (Andrews et al., 1990). For example, violence toward intimates may be more intractable to treatment interventions for men with longer and more serious histories of intimate violence, men with criminal histories for stranger violence, and men with histories of traumatic exposure to violence as children (Fagan et al., 1984; Hamberger and Hastings, 1989).

There is little experimental or quasi-experimental evidence to evaluate the effectiveness of batterer interventions. Edleson and Tolman (1992) reviewed 19 studies published between 1981 and 1990 and found only one that used an untreated control group. Most studies have no comparison group and, of those that do, most rely on comparisons of program completers with noncompleters, a selection bias that presents serious obstacles to the assessment of treatment effectiveness. Two studies now under way will address the shortcomings of the research; one includes a randomized trial (Davis and Smith, 1995; Gondolf, 1995).

Table 5B-4 lists eight evaluations of treatment interventions that meet the committee's criteria for inclusion. In only one study were subjects randomly assigned to treatment or control conditions, but the sample size was very small (Palmer et al., 1992).

Two of the studies compare program completers to program dropouts (Edleson and Grusznski, 1989; Hamberger and Hastings, 1988) and four compare treated groups to nontreated groups (Chen et al., 1989; Dutton, 1986; Harrell, 1992; Palmer et al., 1992). Four of these six studies found significant differences in the rates of repeat domestic violence between those who completed treatment and those who either dropped out or did not receive treatment (Dutton, 1986; Edleson and Grusznski, 1989; Hamberger and Hastings, 1988; Palmer et al., 1992). In the other two, although there were no significant differences, the trend was for a lower rate of repeat domestic violence among treated batterers. Chen et al. (1989) also looked at the rate of being charged for any crime. Although they did not find a significant difference for domestic violence charges, men who were treated had significantly lower rates of being charged for any crime than those who were not treated.

Variations exist in the measurement of recidivism. Of the two studies that found no significant differences due to treatment, one relied solely on police data and the other solely on interview data; there does not appear to be a clear-cut difference between them. However, all the studies cautioned that using only offender self-reports was likely to underestimate the amount and severity of violence.

Several studies looked not only at repeat physical violence, but also at verbal and emotional abuse after treatment. Two found that verbal and emotional abuse continued even though physical violence rates were reduced (Edleson and Grusznski, 1989; Hamberger and Hastings, 1988). In contrast, another study found no significant difference in the reduction of physical violence between batterers in treatment and the control group, but it did find a significant decrease in verbal and emotional abuse by the treatment group (Harrell, 1992).

Because most of the studies did not use a random assignment design, the differences in outcome cannot be definitively attributed to the treatment. Although most of the studies statistically controlled for group differences, there may have been unidentified personality, motivational, or other traits that influenced the rates of repeat domestic violence.

Four studies dealt specifically with groups who had been mandated to treatment by the courts. Two found court-mandated treatment to significantly reduce recidivism rates, and two found no significant difference between treated and nontreated offenders. However, the high dropout rates among those in court-mandated treatment were striking. Between 25 and 37 percent of the offenders mandated to treatment in these studies either never showed up at all or dropped out fairly early in treatment. This rate of attrition is similar to that for batterer treatment in general (33 to 50 percent drop out after the first session) (Feazell et al., 1984). Several of the researchers noted that the criminal justice system imposed few or no sanctions on those who did not fulfill their treatment obligation. This omission of sanctions for noncompleters raises serious questions about victim safety, since battered women are more likely to remain with a batterer who goes to treatment (Gondolf and Fisher, 1988). Court-mandated treatment may give these women a false sense of security.

Concern about the high attrition rates in these programs has fostered interest in examining whether pregroup preparation influences completion rates (Tolman and Bhosley, 1989). There was no significant difference in the percentage of men who went on to join the treatment group by type of pregroup preparation. Furthermore, the attrition rates do not appear to be much different from those achieved by programs with no preparation sessions.

As court-mandated treatment for batterers has become more pervasive, a number of states have set standards for programs, including length of treatment and type of program. Little empirical evidence currently exists to guide this standard setting (Edleson and Syers, 1990). The absence of quasi-experimental studies that can examine the comparative effects of different therapeutic approaches (psychopathology, cognitive-behavioral, and power control) and different types of treatment settings (individual, group, couples) with different types of batterers is a striking omission in the family violence research literature. Although a variety of treatment approaches appear to have positive effects for some batterers, dropout rates remain high and court mandates do not appear to facilitate completion rates for the typical offender. The absence of sanctions for failure to complete treatment is an area that warrants further attention to determine whether the positive effects of treatment are enhanced or restricted when penalties exist for dropping out.

## 5B-5:  Criminal Prosecution

Historically, prosecutors, like the police, have been accused of disinterest in family violence cases, failing to file cases presented by the police and discouraging willing victims from pursuing criminal complaints. With the advent of special prosecution units in the early 1980s, an atmosphere and organizational context developed in prosecutors' offices in which spouse assault cases had high status. This created incentives for vigorous prosecution of domestic violence cases and reduced competition with other high-visibility cases in other units for scarce trial and investigative resources (Forst and Hernon, 1985). In addition, some prosecutors adopted no-drop policies that avoided the last-minute withdrawal of charges by victims, practices that frustrated both police and judges. Critics suggested, however, that no-drop policies discouraged some women from use of the legal system to end the violence. Furthermore, the costs associated with no-drop policies and more aggressive discretionary decisions to bring charges remain uncertain.

Few studies have documented the effects of prosecution on spouse or partner assault. Most studies of prosecution of partner violence have focused on prosecutorial decision making regarding the sorting and selecting of cases for prosecution (e.g., Schmidt and Steury, 1989). One study found subgroup differences similar to those reported by Sherman et al. (1991) for arrests (Fagan, 1989). Men with prior arrest records or lengthy histories of severe violence toward their partners were more likely to reoffend if prosecuted, compared with men who were not prosecuted. Again, evidence of counterdeterrent effects raises serious questions not only about the extent to which legal sanctions could achieve deterrent effects, but also about the interactions of violent men with legal institutions that may produce this effect. The consistent absence of research on the effects of different sentences makes it difficult to assess the impact of court actions on diverse subgroups.

Table 5B-5 lists the only study on prosecution that meets the committee's criteria for inclusion. In the Indianapolis Domestic Violence Prosecution Experiment, the most comprehensive study of prosecution, 678 cases were randomly assigned to one of three recommended prosecution goals representing the judges' traditional response to these cases: diversion to counseling, probation with counseling, and other sentencing such as fines, probation, jail time (Ford and Regoli, 1993). No differences in repeat violence were found for any of the three case disposition practices. The only combination of policy and practice affecting new violence was permitting victims to drop charges and whether or not they did so. Victims who were permitted to drop charges but did not do so were significantly less likely to experience revictimization within 6 months after case closure.

The results of this study suggest small marginal gains in deterrence from the use of the threat of prosecution. However, the results are difficult to interpret due to the small sample sizes. Furthermore, as in the arrest studies, the most serious offenders—those with previous felony convictions or prior convictions of violence against the same victim—were not included. The Indianapolis study, however, does raise the hypothesis that the threat of prosecution, placed in the hands of the victim to use in her efforts to end her partner's violence, may have deterrent effects (Ford, 1991; Ford and Regoli, 1993). When coupled with informal sources of social control, the threat of prosecution may have greater deterrent salience compared with the more typical deterrence model, in which threats are contingent on the dynamics and processes of legal institutions.

## 5B-6: Specialized Courts

The creation of specialized courts for spouse and partner assault cases is a response to the devaluation of these cases in regular courts. The "stream of cases" argument suggests that cases are prioritized for processing and the allocation of punishment resources according to their relative severity compared with other cases in the same context (Emerson, 1983; Jacob, 1983). In this view, domestic violence cases may be assigned a lower priority for prosecution and punishment when placed alongside cases of violence involving strangers.

In the specialized court, intimate violence does not compete with other violence cases. This type of court seeks to reduce the large number of domestic violence cases that are dropped from the legal system because of prosecution difficulties and the reluctance of many complaining witnesses to testify or provide evidence. It also seeks to assign substantive punishment—such as fines, supervised probation, and imprisonment—and broaden the range of sanctions beyond the narrow band of arrest-only cases.

There are no evaluations of specialized courts that meet the committee's criteria for inclusion. The use of the experimental protocols in court evaluations is rare, often because of the legal and ethical complications as well as problems in design and methodology (Fagan, 1990). What follows is based on the descriptive literature.

The Dade County (FL) Domestic Violence Court represents an interdisciplinary and integrated system-wide approach in which members of the court, led by the judiciary, work together as a team toward a shared goal of reducing family violence. It is a criminal court with a civil component that can serve as a coordinated, systemic response to the treatment of domestic violence cases in the courts, dealing with misdemeanor cases, civil orders of protection, and violation of civil protection orders. The Dade County Domestic Violence Court has been evaluated using an experimental design; most of the analysis is focused on the role of substance abuse in domestic violence and the effect of a treatment approach that integrates batterer and substance abuse treatment (Goldkamp, 1996).

### 5B-7: Systemic Approaches

Systemic responses that coordinate criminal justice, social service, and community-based programs have been developed in a few jurisdictions, notably Duluth, Minnesota; Quincy, Massachusetts; and San Francisco. Although these efforts may take many forms, at a minimum they involve efforts to establish communication among criminal justice and social service agencies, the establishment of advocacy services to meet victims' needs, and policies aimed toward more aggressive apprehension and sanctioning of offenders (Worden, 1995). Coordinated community approaches frequently emphasize batterer intervention programs as the appropriate destination for offenders: the criminal justice system's role is to apprehend, supervise, and punish offenders for failure to comply with treatment requirements.

Although there may be many benefits and impacts of coordinated responses, these programs are very difficult to evaluate (see the discussion in Chapter 7). Establishing comparison conditions internally or across communities requires examining the separate components that contribute to the intensity of social control in a community. In this type of analysis, the effects of prosecution or advocacy need to be distinguished from the effects of treatment design or content to identify the critical components that contribute to change in individuals and law enforcement systems.

A broader discussion of service integration and community-charge interventions is included in Chapter 7. In this discussion we review systemic approaches that are focused on and administered by law enforcement agencies.

Table 5B-7 lists two evaluations of coordinated efforts that meet the committee's criteria for inclusion. One study looked primarily at process variables—that is, the impact of coordinated efforts on arrest rates, prosecution rates, and rates of mandated counseling (Gamache et al., 1988). The study found a statistically significant increase in the percentage of calls that resulted in arrest and the percentage of arrests that resulted in prosecution following establishment of a community intervention project in each of three communities. There was also a significant increase in the percentage of men mandated to counseling in each of the communities, indicating that coordination among various parts of the criminal justice and social service systems may increase criminal justice responses to domestic violence. However, as discussed in other sections of this chapter, arrest, prosecution, and treatment do not necessarily ensure a reduction in future violence.

The other study examined the impact of public education and joint police/social worker home visits on recidivism and the use of services (Davis and Taylor, 1995). Residents of public housing projects in three police districts were randomly assigned to receive public education about domestic violence services or to a control group. At 6-month follow-up, no significant differences were observed in the number or severity of victim-reported incidents of repeat violence between the experimental and control groups; however, both of the experimental groups were significantly more likely to call the police for the repeat violence than were control groups.

Systemic approaches designed to increase social controls that will lead to reductions in domestic violence in a community have yet to be tested rigorously in the evaluation literature. Some preliminary but promising evidence suggests that these comprehensive approaches increase law enforcement activity in the area of arrests and prosecutions, but their long-term effects on community safety, recidivism, and deterrence are not yet known.

## 5B-8: Training for Criminal Justice Personnel

Because the criminal justice and legal systems have tended to avoid involvement in family matters, some interventions have been aimed primarily at mobilizing these systems and overcoming their resistance to involvement in domestic violence. These efforts include legal reforms that allow (or mandate) warrantless arrest (see section 5B-3; Dunford et al., 1990); the training of police, prosecutors, and judges (see Chapter 8); and mandatory reporting laws (see section 5B-1).

New laws and policies are likely to have little impact on practice unless police officers, prosecutors, judges, and other criminal justice personnel are aware of them and are trained to implement them. Many jurisdictions have instituted some form of training on domestic violence for certain professionals. Training frequently includes information on the prevalence of family violence, on the dynamics of family violence (such as why women stay with an abusive spouse), and on local policies and resources.

There are no evaluations of the effectiveness of different training programs (Worden, 1995).

## ELDER ABUSE INTERVENTIONS

Legal responses to elder abuse have developed more slowly and are narrower in scope than responses to other forms of family violence. Laws that provide specific penalties for elder abuse and neglect that are separate from laws prohibiting their underlying crimes (such as assault) have only recently been enacted (Tatara, 1995). These statutes generally either follow the model of a state's child abuse statute and apply it to the elderly, or simply provide for an enhanced penalty if a crime is committed against an elderly person.

Jurisprudential reforms similar to those developed for spouse assault (e.g., warrantless arrests for misdemeanor assaults) and child abuse (e.g., procedures for child testimony) have not been forthcoming in the area of elder abuse. Moreover, there has been no pressure of increased caseloads to generate these reforms, and limited advocacy compared with the aggressive lobbying by feminist groups on behalf of battered women and child welfare advocates for abused children. Similar to the situation with regard to domestic violence cases over two decades ago, only the most serious cases are brought to the attention of criminal justice agencies, despite the modification of reporting laws to provide notice to law enforcement when cases of elder abuse are substantiated by adult protective services workers. Elder abuse cases remain the most hidden of all family violence, at least in terms of their presence in criminal court dockets. Their presence in civil court dockets is also limited to cases involving guardianship or court-ordered services in which abuse is alleged.

The role of the legal system in dealing with elder abuse increased during the 1980s (Anetzberger, 1995). Following the pattern set by responses to child abuse, mandatory reporting laws were passed in some states to bring abused elders and their abusers to the attention of appropriate authorities, often adult protective services agencies. In addition, some states have passed laws that increase the penalties for crimes against the elderly. However, criminal prosecution of elder abuse remains rare (Korbin et al., 1991).

Unlike child abuse, elder abuse often includes financial exploitation, which can include outright theft of an elderly person's property, coerced or involuntary transfer of property, and improper use of joint tenancies, powers of attorney, or joint signatories on bank accounts. Some interventions specifically pertain to financial abuse and others to all types of elder abuse.

Five legal interventions for elder abuse are discussed in the sections below: (1) reporting requirements, (2) protective orders, (3) education and legal counseling, (4) guardians and conservators, and (5) arrest, prosecution, and other litigation. The committee found no evaluations of interventions for elder abuse that meet its criteria for inclusion. The sections that follow are based on descriptive literature.

## 5C-1:  Reporting Requirements

Mandatory or voluntary reporting of elder abuse is specified in 42 states and the District of Columbia (Wolf, 1996).  Studies in this area have examined variations in reporting practices and compared the effectiveness of voluntary and mandatory reporting systems (Alliance Elder Abuse Project, 1981; Wolf et al., 1984; U.S. General Accounting Office, 1991b). A study by the General Accounting Office reported the view of supporters of mandatory reporting that legal requirements are necessary to encourage reporting practices and to remove impediments, such as fear of lawsuits, that might deter reports of elder abuse. The report also reported the view of proponents of voluntary reporting that legal requirements are not necessary because other factors, such as public education, prevention efforts, and caregiver relationships, will promote reporting practices. The General Accounting Office concluded that reporting laws, whether mandatory or voluntary, are not considered as effective as a high level of public and professional awareness in identifying, preventing, and treating elder abuse.

The states of Illinois and Pennsylvania have adopted voluntary reporting practices combined with emphasis on public and professional education (Illinois Department on Aging, 1990; Pennsylvania Attorney General's Task Force, 1988). One researcher observed that increasing the knowledge and undertstanding of providers of human services for the aging who are at risk of abuse or neglect, rather than reporting requirements, would contribute more effectively to the identification, treatment, and prevention of elder abuse (Wolf, 1996).

## 5C-2:  Protective Orders

Most states have civil processes for separating older persons who are victims of physical abuse from abusers other than spouses (Eisenberg, 1991). In cases of physical abuse by a spouse, orders of protection are available to elderly victims under domestic violence provisions (see section 5B-2). Some states have adapted protective orders to also cover cases of financial abuse.  For example, Illinois amended its Domestic Violence Act to allow prompt intervention in cases involving financial abuse of an elderly person in the same manner as physical abuse has been dealt with.

There have been no studies evaluating the effectiveness of orders of protection in ensuring the safety of victims of elder abuse. Findings from the limited research on orders of protection in cases of domestic violence are not encouraging. Victims of elder abuse also face additional difficulties that may make them reluctant to seek an order of protection (Eisenberg, 1991). First, if the elderly victim is physically dependent on the abuser, removing the abuser from the home or ordering no contact with the victim may result in the need for the elderly victim to be placed in a long-term care facility. Second, if the victim does not own the home, such as when an elderly person resides with a son or daughter, questions may arise about whether the elderly victim has a right to stay in that home.

### 5C-3: Education and Legal Counseling

Educating older people about their legal rights to privacy, autonomy, control of assets, medical and personal decision making, and freedom from abuse is thought to be one important means of preventing elder abuse. For competent elderly persons, the provision of information about their legal rights and the possible consequences of such actions as property transfers and granting powers of attorney may be sufficient to prevent financial abuse by a family member or caregiver. Anecdotal evidence from a legal clinic in Illinois suggests that legal counseling may help the elderly person make informed decisions independent of the influence of family members or caregivers who are trying to exploit them (Eisenberg, 1991). Legal assistance can also help the elderly person to place assets outside the reach of third parties. For example, signatories on bank accounts can be changed, accounts can be consolidated under the elderly person's name, and existing powers of attorney can be revoked. An attorney may also provide referrals to appropriate social services that can provide support to the elderly person.

The situation becomes more complicated if the elderly abused person is not competent to make decisions regarding personal care and property and did not make previous arrangements through a durable power of attorney or living trust. In such cases, a substitute decision maker must be appointed before any informal or formal legal remedies can be pursued.

Although anecdotal evidence suggests that legal counseling and other legal remedies may prevent abuse and improve the lot of the elderly victim of financial abuse, there have been no rigorous evaluations of these interventions.

### 5C-4: Guardians and Conservators

In order to protect the person or property of an incapacitated elderly person, it is common for the court to appoint a substitute decision maker. Although the term varies from state to state, *guardian* often refers to someone authorized to make decisions about personal care, such as housing or health care; *conservator* often refers to someone authorized to make decisions about property.

Traditionally, the assignment of a guardian for an elderly person was tantamount to declaring that person incompetent and leaving him or her no right to make decisions about personal or property matters. Although there are those for whom this level of guardianship is necessary, many elderly persons have difficulties in handling only specific areas of their lives. Guardianship and conservatorship policies have been criticized for lack of due process provisions, unnecessary and inappropriate loss of basic civil liberties, and inadequate standards, regulation, and oversight of surrogate decision makers (Wilber, 1991). To overcome some of these criticisms, states have moved toward the availability of limited guardians or conservators with authority to make decisions only on matters beyond the elderly person's ability to decide. In many states, the elderly person retains all rights not specifically removed by the court and given to the guardian (Legal Counsel for the Elderly, Inc., 1987).

It seems logical to assume that the appointment of a guardian or conservator is a useful remedy in instances of abuse or neglect of an incompetent elderly person. However, there is also the potential for abuse by the guardian or conservator. There have been no evaluations of the impact on elder abuse of appointing guardians or conservators. Nor have there been evaluations comparing the impact of general guardianship or conservatorship to that of more limited forms of surrogate decision-making power.

## 5C-5: Arrest, Prosecution, and Other Litigations

Most states do not keep arrest statistics for elder abuse, and very few such offenders are prosecuted (Tatara, 1995). There have been no studies of arrest or prosecution of elder abuse. Recent training programs have emerged for police, prosecutors, and bank employees to enhance their ability to detect and respond appropriately to elder abuse and exploitation.

Litigation to redress financial abuse is often a measure of last resort. An abused elderly person may be reluctant to pursue litigation against a family member. Courts, lawyers, and litigation can be intimidating and may frighten an elderly abused person. Court costs and legal fees can be prohibitively expensive. Finally, remedies to undo financial abuse are not straightforward and, in most states, must be borrowed from other areas of law that may not be familiar to many lawyers and judges (Eisenberg, 1991). In the early 1990s, states began passing legislation specifically aimed at remedies for financial abuse of the elderly, which may make it easier to successfully bring suit against a perpetrator of financial abuse.

## CONCLUSIONS

The most extensive area of study in evaluation of law enforcement interventions for family violence is the field of domestic violence. The most rigorous evaluation studies in this area focus on arrest policies and practices. Although arrest remains the most common and most studied form of law enforcement intervention in family violence cases (especially in the area of domestic violence), it is important to note that few arrests are made for any form of family violence given the reported prevalence. Prosecution remains the exception, and only a few cases receive substantive punishment. The broad array of existing interventions—including the use of mandatory reporting systems, protective orders, prosecution, specialized procedural and broad-based systemic reforms in the juvenile and domestic violence courts—has not received rigorous attention in the research literature and the effects are generally unknown.

Evaluations of legal interventions for family violence generally focus on the impact of the intervention on recidivism. Important outcomes in other domains, such as victim and community safety, offender health or well-being, level of family functioning, and the rights of those charged are generally unexamined. Local variations in reporting and law enforcement practices often inhibit the use of common measures in cross-site research studies, and rigorous efforts to impose systematic data collection practices can inhibit collaborative efforts between researchers and law enforcement officials. Even in such areas as the evaluation of spouse assault arrest policies, in which a number of replication studies have been conducted, consistent findings remain elusive because of significant variation in study design and outcome measures. The impact of these interventions on family violence remains poorly understood.

Despite these limitations, some tentative conclusions can be drawn from the research reviewed in this chapter:

- State reporting systems constitute an intervention that affects the largest number of children and families in the area of family violence. The passage of mandatory reporting laws for child and elder abuse has been followed by increased reports of abuse and neglect. However, mandatory reporting systems have not been studied rigorously to determine whether the costs associated with administering a large investigative process have improved access to services or increased the safety and well-being of children or the elderly and their families. The comparative rate of errors in mandatory and voluntary reporting systems, in terms of both false positives and false negatives, remains uncertain.
- None of the five spouse arrest replication experiments reviewed show that arrest in the absence of other sanctions works *in general* to reduce subsequent violence by the offender. Some research studies suggest that arrest may be a deterrent for employed and married individuals (people who have a stake in social conformity) and may lead to an escalation of violence among those who do

not, but this hypothesis has not been tested by specifically examining the impact of arrest on groups that differ in social and economic status.

• The continuing threat of legal sanctions may have a stronger deterrent effect in the area of domestic violence than the actual imposition of a sanction through the arrest process. This finding deserves further attention in future research studies and offender-absent policies, since almost half of all domestic violence suspects leave the scene before police arrive. The interaction of arrest policies with individual and community factors is another intriguing area of research that warrants further investigation not only in family violence studies, but also in studies of the effectiveness of criminal justice interventions in family interactions in different types of neighborhoods.

• Anecdotal evidence suggests that specialized units and comprehensive reforms in police departments, prosecutors' offices, and specialized courts have improved the experiences of abused children and women. Some research suggests that protective orders may be an effective deterrent of future domestic violence when they are combined with the prosecution of violations, suggesting that comprehensive legal reforms are needed rather than relying on a single strategy.

• Court-mandated treatment is becoming increasingly prevalent in the area of domestic violence, but the effectiveness of batterer treatment has not been examined in rigorous scientific studies. Batterer treatment programs may be helpful but require further effort to enforce referrals, to establish penalties for failure to comply with program requirements, to develop program components that can address the needs of different types of batterers, and to consider the unintended results that may be a consequence of the treatment program.

• The absence of strong theory and common measures to guide the development of family violence treatment regimens, the heterogeneity of offenders (including patterns of offending and readiness to change) who are the subjects of protective orders or treatment, and low rates of attendance, completion, and enforcement are persistent problems that affect both the evaluation of the batterer treatment interventions and efforts to reduce the violence. A few studies suggest that court oversight does appear to increase treatment completion rates, which may enhance victim safety in the area of domestic violence, but it has not yet led to a discernible effect on recidivism rates in general.

• Evaluations of legal interventions for elder abuse are virtually nonexistent. Many have been modeled on experiences with child abuse that may not be applicable to adults. Building evaluation components into elder abuse interventions as they are established could greatly improve the knowledge base in this area.

TABLE 5A-3   Quasi-Experimental Evaluations of Court-Mandated Treatment
for Child Abuse Offenders

| Intervention | Citation | Initial/Final Sample Size<br>Duration of Intervention<br>Follow-up |
|---|---|---|
| Court-mandated treatment for child abuse offenders. | Irueste-Montes and Montes, 1988 | N(X) = 35/24<br>N(O) = 30/18<br><br>3 years |
| Court-mandated family treatment program emphasizing child management skills. | Wolfe et al., 1980 | N(X) = 25<br>N(O) = 46 |

SOURCE:  Committee on the Assessment of Family Violence Interventions, National
Research Council and Institute of Medicine, 1998.

| Data Collection | Results |
|---|---|
| Behavioral observations of parent-child dyads | Treated families in both mandatory and voluntary participation groups significantly increased their use of praise and descriptive praise with their children and significantly reduced their use of criticism. All subjects continued to attend to their children's annoying behaviors. Results of this comparison indicate that court-mandated treatment does not necessarily render abusive and neglectful parents less amenable to treatment. |
| Completion of treatment | Court-ordered participants were five times more likely to complete treatment than voluntary participants. |

TABLE 5A-4    Quasi-Experimental Evaluations of Treatment for Sexual Abuse
Offenders

| Intervention | Citation | Initial/Final Sample Size Duration of Intervention Follow-up |
|---|---|---|
| In-patient, multimodal treatment for incest offenders and pedophiliacs consisting of group psychotherapy, social skills training, anger management, human sexuality education, psychodrama, films discussing victims, and stress inoculation. | Lang et al., 1988 | N(incest offenders) = 29 N(pedophiles) = 22 Minimum of 6 months 3-year follow-up |
| Modification of sexual preference through electrical aversion, masturbatory reconditioning, and self-administration of smelling salts contingent on sexual thoughts about children. | Marshall and Barbaree, 1988 | N(X) = 68 N(O) = 58 Treatment group includes incest offenders as well as nonfamilial molesters; recidivism data reported separately for incest offenders |

SOURCE: Committee on the Assessment of Family Violence Interventions, National
Research Council and Institute of Medicine, 1998.

| Data Collection | Results |
| --- | --- |
| Phallometric monitoring of sexual arousal patterns, recidivism data from law enforcement and clinics, psychometric assessments of mood states (anger, suspicion, anxiety, etc.) | Incest offenders showed improvement on 16 of 19 measures and showed more significant improvements on 5 measures compared with pedophiles. After a 3-year follow-up, two (7%) incest offenders and four (18%) pedophilic men reoffended according to law enforcement reports and community and outpatient clinic intake data. |
| Sexual preference as measured by plethysmography, official recidivism data | Treated patients had lower recidivism rates than untreated patients, although recidivism for all patients increased over longer follow-up periods. Younger offenders and offenders who had engaged in genital-genital contact were most likely to reoffend. |

TABLE 5B-3  Quasi-Experimental Evaluations of Arrest Procedures

| Intervention | Citation | Initial/Final Sample Size<br><br>Duration of Intervention<br><br>Follow-up |
|---|---|---|
| One of four police dispositions: arrest coupled with protective order, protective order with crisis counseling of offender, protective order only; mediation. | Berk et al., 1992a | N = 1,658 randomly assigned to one of four treatments<br><br>Follow-up at 6 months after entering study |
| One of three police dispositions: mediation, separation, or arrest. | Dunford et al., 1990 | N(mediation) = 91/85<br>N(separation) = 89/80<br>N(arrest) = 83/77<br><br>Victims interviewed 6 months postintervention |
| On-scene warrantless arrest. | Ford and Regoli, 1993 | N = 188/106<br><br>Victims interviewed 6 months postintervention |
| One of three police responses: advising/ separation, citation to the offender, arrest. | Hirschel and Hutchinson, 1992 | N = 573 |
| Arrest or nonarrest. | Pate and Hamilton, 1992 | N = 815<br><br>Victims interviewed 6 months postintervention |

| Data Collection | Results |
| --- | --- |
| Police records and victim interviews | Results support evidence for a deterrent effect of arrest among "good risk" offenders who presumably have more to lose from being arrested. The balance of evidence is more equivocal for a "labeling effect" in which arrest increases the likelihood of new violence. |
| Police records, including court appearances and convictions, Conflict Tactics Scales completed by husbands and wives | No differences by disposition were found in prevalence or frequency of repeat offending. |
| Recidivism rates: characteristics of violent incidents (severity, frequency, and length of time between the old and new incidents); all data gathered from victim interviews, official records, police records, complaints to court | Policy alternatives to traditional sentencing do not appear more effective in protecting victims 6 months following case settlement. When defendants are arrested under a warrant and their victims are permitted to drop charges and choose not to, those women are significantly more likely to be safe from continuing violence. |
| Arrest recidivism, self-report of subsequent violence by victim | Arrest of misdemeanor spouse abusers does not appear to be a more effective deterrent to repeat abuse than other police responses. |
| Interviews with victims conducted immediately after the presenting incident and again 6 months afterward. | Overall, formal arrest has no effect on occurrence of a subsequent assault. Arrest does have a statistically significant deterrent effect among employed suspects, whereas arrest leads to a significant increase in subsequent assaults among unemployed suspects. |

TABLE 5B-3   *(Continued)*

| Intervention | Citation | Initial/Final Sample Size Duration of Intervention Follow-up |
|---|---|---|
| Mediation or arrest. | Sherman and Berk, 1984a | N = 314/161<br><br>Victims interviewed 6 months postintervention |
| One of three police responses: short arrest, full arrest, and mediation. | Sherman et al., 1992b | N = 1,200/563<br><br>Victims interviewed 6 months postintervention |
| One of three police responses: arrest, citation, or no action. | Steinman 1988, 1990 | N(X) = 49/48<br>N(O) = 168/156<br><br>12- to 24-month follow-up |

SOURCE: Committee on the Assessment of Family Violence and Interventions, National Research Council and Institute of Medicine, 1998.

| Data Collection | Results |
| --- | --- |
| Police reports of subsequent violence, interviews with victims | Arrested suspects manifested significantly less subsequent violence than those who were ordered to leave. The victim report data show that the arrested subjects manifested significantly less subsequent violence than those who were advised. |
| "Hotline" reports called in to local battered women's shelter by police encountering a case of domestic battery, arrests for repeat violence, offense reports of repeat violence, two interviews conducted with victim | Results show no evidence of an overall long-term deterrent effect of arrest. The initial deterrent effects observed for up to 30 days disappear. By 1 year later, short arrest alone, and short and full arrest combined, produce an escalation effect. Arrest has different effects on different types of offenders. |
| Conflict Tactics Scales, victim interviews, police and court records of repeat violence | Compared with no action, arresting and citing offenders produced more abuse in baseline cases and less when tied to other sanctions. Court sanctions coordinated with arrest policies did not lower abuse directly, but they transformed arrest and, to a smaller effect, citations into deterrents. |

TABLE 5B-4    Quasi-Experimental Evaluations of Court-Mandated Treatment
for Domestic Violence Offenders

| Intervention | Citation | Initial/Final Sample Size<br>Duration of Intervention<br>Follow-up |
|---|---|---|
| Court-mandated batterer treatment. | Chen et al., 1989 | N(court-referred abuses) = 120 (12% attended no sessions, 63% attended more than three-fourths of the sessions) N(nonreferred abuses) = 101<br><br>8 2-hour sessions |
| Court-mandated batterer treatment. | Dutton, 1986 | N(X) = 50 N(O) = 50<br><br>3 hours per week for 16 weeks<br><br>Follow-up ranged between 6 months and 3 years postintervention |
| Orientation groups, therapeutic treatment groups, and follow-up self-help group for batterers. | Edleson and Grusznski, 1989 | Study One N(program completers) = 32; 27 of their female partners were interviewed N(noncompleters) = 31; 30 of their female partners were interviewed<br><br>Study Three: N(program completers) = 112; 84 of their female partners were interviewed N(noncompleters) = 47; 37 of their female partners were interviewed |

| Data Collection | Results |
|---|---|
| Recidivism reports and a weighted offense scale to measure recharging on any offense, with violent offenses given more weight | Results indicate that the relationship between attendance and recidivism is not linear. Clients who attended 75% of the treatment sessions or more showed decreased recidivism; others showed no impact. |
| Police records, including court appearances and convictions; Conflict Tactics Scales completed by husbands and wives | Program completers had a 4% recidivism rate 3 years posttreatment according to police records. Conflict Tactics Scales scores reported by both treated husbands and wives showed significant posttreatment decreases from pretreatment levels. Rates of verbal aggression also decreased posttreatment. |
| Interview with female partners, modified Conflict Tactics Scales | Approximately two-thirds of the men who completed treatment were found to be nonviolent 6-10 months postintervention. Slightly more than one-half of the men who received some treatment but did not complete the program were reported as nonviolent postintervention. |

TABLE 5B-4   (*Continued*)

| Intervention | Citation | Initial/Final Sample Size Duration of Intervention Follow-up |
|---|---|---|
|  | Edleson and Grusznski, 1989 (*continued*) | Therapy groups met 2.5 hours twice a week for 8 weeks. Self-help follow-up groups met 2.5 hours per week for an indefinite period. |
|  |  | Follow-up interviews about 1 year after intake. |
| Three treatment modalities were explored: a self-help model, an education model, and a combined model of group work; each was offered in 12 and 32 sessions to batterers. | Edleson and Syers, 1990 | N(X) = 283/70 12 weeks of one 2.25-hour session per week; or 16 weeks of two 2.25-hour sessions per week |
|  |  | 6- and 18-month follow-up |
| Cognitive behavioral skills training program for male spouse abusers with three components: cognitive restructuring, communication/assertiveness, and active-coping relaxation. | Hamberger and Hastings, 1988 | N(X) = 71/32 N(noncompleters) = 36 |
|  |  | 3 weeks of psychometric evaluation and 12 weeks of 2.5 hours of weekly group therapy |
|  |  | 1-year follow-up |

| Data Collection | Results |
|---|---|
| Reports of repeat partner violence, incidence and severity, use of threats of violence as reported by partner or batterer if partner not available | Two-thirds of the men who completed the intervention programs who could be located at follow-up were found to be nonviolent. Short-term, relatively structured group treatment tended to produce the most successful results. Men's involvement with the courts and lack of prior mental health treatment predicted lower levels of violence at the 18-month follow-up. |
| Physical violence recidivism as reported by batterer or partner on Conflict Tactics Scales, and official police records of calls and arrests | Results showed significant decreases in occurrence of violent behaviors after treatment and up to 1-year follow-up in subjects (32) completing the intervention. Compared with program dropouts (36), completers showed a lower rate of physical violence recidivism over the 1-year follow-up period. There was evidence of continued psychological abuse among completers in some cases. |

TABLE 5B-4   *(Continued)*

| Intervention | Citation | Initial/Final Sample Size Duration of Intervention Follow-up |
|---|---|---|
| Court-mandated, cognitive-behavioral batterer treatment offered by three organizations: a nonprofit association, a church sponsored agency, and a feminist organization. | Harrell, 1992 | N(nonprofit) = 43<br>N(church) = 51<br>N(feminist) = 13<br>25% did not complete assigned treatment<br>N(0) = 86<br><br>Nonprofit: 12 weekly group sessions of 1 to 1.5 hours<br>Church: individual intake session followed by eight group sessions of 1 to 1.5 hours<br>Feminist: minimum of 12 weekly group sessions of 1.5 hours<br>4- to 6-month postintervention follow-up |
| Court-managed batterer treatment in a psychoeducational, unstructured group. | Palmer et al., 1992 | N(X) = 30/17<br>N(O) = 28/15<br><br>10 weekly 1.5 hour sessions<br><br>1-year follow-up |
| Group preparation for men about to enter batterer treatment group. | Tolman and Bhosley, 1989 | N(Tx1) = 44/16<br>N(Tx2) = 68/34<br><br>Tx1 = maximum of four group sessions, 1 hour each<br>Tx2 = intensive pre-groupworkshop, 12 hours over 2 days |

SOURCE: Committee on the Assessment of Family Violence and Interventions, National Research Council and Institute of Medicine, 1998.

| Data Collection | Results |
| --- | --- |
| Data gathered from victim and offender interviews: reports of severe violence, physical aggression, threats of violence, psychological abuse | Treatment did not appear to reduce the prevalence or incidence of abuse. There were no significant differences between treated offenders and those not ordered to treatment in the cessation of severe violence or threats of violence. In both groups, 80-85% abstained from severe violence during the treatment period. A significantly smaller proportion of offenders in treatment abstained from physical aggression: 57% for treated offenders versus 88% for nontreated offenders. |
| Subject and partner reports and police reports of repeated violence against partners, Basic Personality Inventory | Recidivism rates based on police reports were found to be lower for the treatment group than for the control group. They were also found to be lower for men initially exhibiting greater depression. Short, unstructured treatment intervention seemed to have long-term benefits. |
| Rate of joining the treatment group after completing the orientation; rate of attendance at batterer treatment group after completing the orientation. | The intensive workshop format resulted in significantly fewer dropouts from the ongoing group prior to completion of four sessions. The impact of the intensive workshop may diminish over time. |

TABLE 5B-5    Quasi-Experimental Evaluations of Criminal Prosecution

| Intervention | Citation | Initial/Final Sample Size Duration of Intervention Follow-up |
|---|---|---|
| Prosecution options: diversion to counseling, probation with counseling, other sentencing, drop permitted. | Ford and Regoli, 1993 | N(diversion) = 112/84 N(probation) = 116/74 N(other) = 112/83 N(drop permitted) = 112 Follow-up 6 months after settlement of case |

SOURCE: Committee on the Assessment of Family Violence Interventions, National Research Council and Institute of Medicine, 1998.

TABLE 5B-7    Quasi-Experimental Evaluations of Systemic Approaches

| Intervention | Citation | Initial/Final Sample Size Duration of Intervention Follow-up |
|---|---|---|
| Home follow-up visits by social workers and police; public education. | Davis and Taylor, 1995 | N(X) = 436/414 72% of victims were interviewed at 6 months postintervention |
| Implementation of coordinated police, judicial, and social service response. | Gamache et al., 1988 | Three communities |

SOURCE: Committee on the Assessment of Family Violence Interventions, National Research Council and Institute of Medicine, 1998.

| Data Collection | Results |
| --- | --- |
| Repeat violence, severity and frequency of violence, time to reoffense, data collected from victim interviews, offender interviews, and police records | Policy alternatives to traditional sentencing do not appear more effective in protecting victims 6 months following case settlement. When defendants are arrested under a warrant and their victims are permitted to drop charges and choose not to, those women are significantly more likely to experience less violence. |

| Data Collection | Results |
| --- | --- |
| Victims' self-reports of violence (modification of Straus' weighing system), police records, awareness and use of domestic violence services | Results indicate no effects of home visits or public education on the number or severity of violent incidents as reported by victims. Data did indicate significant increases in reports of violence to the police as a function of both home visit and public education interventions. |
| Arrest data, rate of prosecution, number of convicted batterers mandated to counseling | Community intervention projects had a significant impact on both police and judicial responses to woman battering. |

# 6

# Health Care Interventions

In the last three decades, knowledge about the short- and long-term health effects associated with abuse and neglect, combined with the advocacy efforts on behalf of victims of family violence, have stimulated health professionals to focus attention on its causes, consequences, treatment, and prevention (Alexander, 1990; Chadwick, 1994). This enhanced interest has been accompanied by an increase in the number and variety of health intervention programs (Kolko, 1996a; Infante-Rivard et al., 1989). Although individual clinicians may respond to the needs of individual patients, clinical settings and public health agencies often do not address family violence as a health and social problem (*Journal of the American Medical Association*, 1990; Hamberger and Saunders, 1991; Kurz, 1987; McLeer et al., 1989). Several professional associations have recommended diagnostic and treatment guidelines for family violence, but health care interventions for family violence are generally not incorporated into standard medical care, health data reporting systems, or health care reimbursement practices.

In their direct contact with individual patients, who may include past, present, and future victims of family violence, health care providers have daily opportunities to screen for, diagnose, treat, and prevent individual cases of child abuse and neglect, domestic violence, and elder abuse. Estimates of the impact of family violence on the public health and the health care system indicate that family violence accounts for 39,000 physician visits each year; 28,700 emergency room visits, 21,000 hospitalizations, and 99,800 hospital days Rosenberg and Mercy, 1991). They can provide important linkages between individual health services, social support networks, community resources, and more comprehensive preventive efforts; in their roles as researchers and advocates, they can integrate their

*206*

expertise in direct patient care with efforts to expand the range of health and social services available to their patients and the general population. Health care professionals interact with the legal system and the social service system as mandated reporters, forensic examiners, and expert witnesses.

The health care system consists of two broad sectors: the medical care sector is focused on services for individuals, and the public health sector is concerned with community-based efforts to improve the quality of care for special groups, including the poor and persons with infectious diseases and chronic or debilitating health problems. The interventions described in this chapter are primarily medical interventions; they focus on individuals and the treatment of patients for injuries or illnesses, including mental illnesses, that may or may not be reported as consequences of family violence. The medical model includes interventions such as screening, diagnostic and therapeutic services, referrals for specialized services, and follow-up care to maintain the patient's health and prevent the recurrence of health disorders.

Current violence prevention efforts in the medical care system generally focus on particular populations defined by gender, age group, or type of violence. Some efforts involve system-wide approaches that include interactions between health care providers and representatives of community agencies, advocacy groups, and the media to address family violence in the general population. Prevention efforts have usually targeted individuals rather than the family unit, with the exception of services based in family practice and some mental health settings.

In contrast, prevention efforts in the public health system include programs and interventions to improve the health of the public or special populations within a community. In the last decade, the field has embraced violence as a subject within its mandate, and proponents have contributed new tools and perspectives to changing abusive and violent behavior and preventing its injurious consequences (Mercy et al., 1993). The formulation of violence as a public health issue dates to the 1985 surgeon general's Workshop on Violence and Public Health, convened by Surgeon General C. Everett Koop to encourage health professionals to begin to respond to the consequences of interpersonal violence (U.S. Department of Health and Human Services, 1986). Modeled on historical successes in controlling infectious diseases, the public health approach aims to reveal underlying patterns of violence in communities, to identify individuals and groups at risk, and to highlight and control the risk factors and behaviors that are associated with child abuse, domestic violence, and elder abuse (Rosenberg and Fenley, 1992) (Figure 6-1, Table 6-1).

Oriented toward communities and prevention rather than the treatment of individuals and consequences, the public health perspective is not prominent in most of the interventions described in this book. The emphasis on proactive responses to social problems that have major health consequences has the potential to engage the public health system and individual health care providers in a

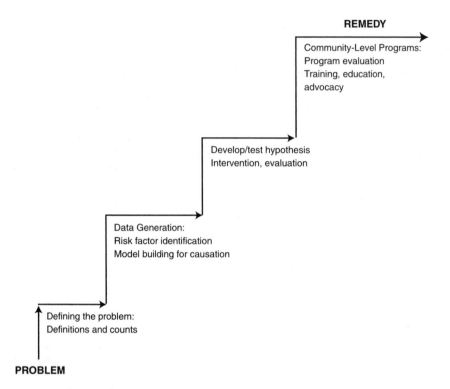

FIGURE 6-1  Public health scientific method and its role in family violence research. SOURCE: Mercy et al. (1993). Copyright 1993, The People-to-People Health Foundation, Inc., Project HOPE, http://www.projhope.org/HA/. Reprinted by permission of *Health Affairs*.

broad network designed to provide not only health care services but also referrals to others who can address the legal and social dimensions of family violence before harmful effects have occurred. The public health perspective also promotes the use of scientific knowledge and quality assurance and performance measures to achieve community health goals (see Box 6.A). The committee sees real value in a strong commitment to public health approaches to the prevention of family violence, although work in this area has a long way to go to establish viable prevention strategies and demonstrate evidence of their effectiveness.

The existing research on health care interventions focuses primarily on the incidence and prevalence of abuse in specific populations, the characteristics of victims and perpetrators, and the health consequences of victimization. Although attention is most often given to the immediate impact of family violence on victim use of health services and resources, the health impact of family violence can affect different stages of development over the life course, including pregnancy outcomes and fetal development, infancy, early and middle childhood,

TABLE 6-1  Public Health Strategies for Preventing Violence and Its Consequences

| Strategy | Description | Intervention Examples |
|---|---|---|
| Change individual knowledge, skills, or attitudes | Deliver information to individuals to:<br>—Develop prosocial attitudes and beliefs<br>—Increase knowledge<br>—Impart social, marketable, or professional skills<br>—Deter criminal actions | —Conflict resolution education<br>—Social skills training<br>—Job skills training<br>—Public information and education campaigns<br>—Training of health care professionals in identification and referral of family violence victims<br>—Parenting education<br>—Home visitation programs for young, poor, single mothers<br>—Family therapy |
| Change social environment | Alter the way people interact by improving their social or economic circumstances | —Adult mentoring of youth<br>—Job creation programs<br>—Respite day care<br>—Battered women's shelters<br>—Economic incentives for family stability |
| Change physical environment | Modify the design, use, or availability of:<br>—Dangerous commodities<br>—Structures or space | —Control of alcohol sales at local events<br>—Gun laws and restrictions (e.g., in schools) |

SOURCE: Modified from Mercy et al. (1993). Copyright 1993, The People-to-People Health Foundation, Inc., Project HOPE, http://www.projhope.org/HA/. Reprinted by permission of *Health Affairs*.

adolescence, adult stages, and the latter stages of life. Family violence has been identified as a contributing factor for a broad array of fatal and nonfatal injuries and health disorders, including pregnancy and birth complications, sudden infant death syndrome, brain trauma, fractures, sexually transmitted diseases, HIV infection, depression, dissociation, psychosis, and other stress-related physical and mental disorders (*Journal of the American Medical Association*, 1990). Family violence has also been associated with numerous major social problems, including aggressive, violent, self-injurious, and suicidal behavior; teen pregnancy; runaway and homeless youth and adults; substance abuse; and delinquency and crime (Malinosky-Rummell and Hansen, 1993; National Research Council, 1993a; Widom, 1989a,b,c). Family violence has been identified as the causal

## BOX 6.A

In 1991, one of the priority areas identified in the Public Health Service report *Healthy People 2000* is the need for information to guide public health policy at the state, local, and national levels and to develop common health goals that can help change social norms that may contribute toward a health problem. Among its 300 goals, *Healthy People 2000*, in its revised form (U.S. Department of Health and Human Services, 1995), includes the following objectives related to family violence:

• Reverse to less than 22.6 per 1,000 children the rising incidence of maltreatment of children younger than age 18 (Baseline: 22.6 per 1,000 in 1986).
• Reduce rape and attempted rape of women age 12 and older to no more than 108 per 100,000 women (Baseline: 120 per 100,000 in 1986).
• Reduce physical abuse directed at women by male partners to no more than 27 per 1,000 couples (Baseline: 30 per 1,000 couples in 1985).
• Extend protocols for routinely identifying, treating, and properly referring suicide attempters, victims of sexual assault, and victims of spouse, elder, and child abuse to at least 90 percent of hospital emergency departments (Baseline data unavailable).
• Extend to at least 45 states implementation of unexplained child death review systems (Baseline: 33 states in 1991).
• Increase to at least 30 the number of states in which at least 50 percent of children identified as physically or sexually abused receive physical and mental evaluation with appropriate follow-up as a means of breaking the intergenerational cycle of abuse (Baseline data unavailable).
• Reduce to less than 10 percent the proportion of battered women and their children turned away from emergency housing due to the lack of space (Baseline: 40 percent in 1987).
• Increase to at least 50 percent the proportion of elementary and secondary schools that teach nonviolent conflict resolution skills, preferably as a part of comprehensive school health education (Baseline data unavailable).
• Extend coordinated, comprehensive violence prevention programs to at least 80 percent of local jurisdictions with populations over 100,000 (Baseline data unavailable).

As with many of the national objectives, however, baseline and follow-up data were not available at the national level and data constraints were even more severe at state and local levels (Stoto, 1992; U.S. Department of Health and Human Services, 1995).

An Institute of Medicine report has recently proposed a community health improvement process to integrate various perspectives on the determinants of health and performance monitoring and to marshal collective resources in a community to improve the health of its members (Institute of Medicine, 1997). The process includes 12 recommended prototype indicators, including the prevalence of physical abuse of women by male partners; the number of confirmed child abuse cases reported to authorities and the percentage receiving child protective services and appropriate medical care; and the existence of protocols for health care professionals to identify, treat, and properly refer suicide attempts, victims of sexual assault, and victims of spouse, elder, and child abuse.

link in some health and social problems resulting from cases that involve physical injuries, withholding medication, complications of forced sex, or inability to use barrier protection. Although linkages in many other areas are uncertain and often highly individualistic, the presence of family violence as a risk factor in such an expansive range of health disorders has created strong interest in identifying medical interventions to address family violence.

Evaluations of family violence treatment and prevention interventions in health care settings are not well developed in the research literature. Child maltreatment interventions are the most commonly studied services, especially mental health services and home visitation programs. Evaluations of health care provider training, identification, and screening programs are extremely rare in all three areas of family violence. Documentation of histories or reports of family violence, for either children and adults, are generally not part of medical practice. As a result, the impact of interventions on an individual's health history or on the general health of a community often is unknown.

As in social service and the legal interventions, progress in evaluating the effectiveness of health care interventions is hampered by numerous methodological and design constraints. There are very few quasi-experimental or experimental studies; those that exist do not use control groups or other hallmarks of rigorous design. Rather, they are essentially individual program descriptions, with information about patient demographics and characteristics and caseload and process measures. One important exception to this observation is the set of studies that have been conducted on home visitation interventions, which are usually based in a community public health agency. These studies are some of the few evaluations of family violence interventions to use randomized assignment, rigorous assessment measures for maternal and child well-being, and lengthy follow-up periods (15 years in one study).

This chapter reviews health care interventions and the available evaluations of them, first for child maltreatment, then for domestic violence, and finally for elder abuse. As discussed in Chapter 1, our decision to treat interventions according to their institutional settings necessitated somewhat arbitrary categorizations. The discussion of certain interventions would be equally appropriate in the chapters on social services or the legal system, but we have categorized as health related all interventions that occur primarily in a health care setting. The chapter includes brief descriptions of some interventions of great interest in the field that are in the early stages of development but have not been evaluated.

## CHILD MALTREATMENT INTERVENTIONS

Evidence of child maltreatment appears to health care providers as multiple and recurrent injuries, injury histories inconsistent with physical findings, and injuries inconsistent with children's developmental capability to sustain them on their own (examples of the latter are a 2-month-old infant with a fractured arm and a prepubertal child with a sexually transmitted disease). Health care providers are required under state law to report suspicions of child maltreatment to child protective service officials.

The response of the health care system to child abuse and neglect involves identification of maltreatment and referral of victims and perpetrators for associated health care, social, and legal services; treatment for the immediate and long-term medical and psychological consequences; and the reporting of abuse and neglect to the appropriate investigatory authorities in order to initiate protective intervention on behalf of the child. Although all children who come to the attention of the health care system and who require medical care are treated, identification and reporting of maltreatment are inconsistent and are influenced by health care providers' awareness, training, and judgment (see the discussion of mandatory reporting in Chapter 5). As a result, some (possibly many) children do not receive appropriate services and may not be viewed as at risk for future maltreatment.

Six interventions are reviewed in this section: (1) identification and screening, including the use of hospital multidisciplinary teams and the role of health care professionals as expert witnesses, (2) mental health services for child victims of physical abuse and neglect, (3) mental health services for child victims of sexual abuse, (4) mental health services for children who witness domestic violence, (5) mental health services for adult survivors of child abuse, and (6) home visitation and family support programs. The sections are keyed to the appendix tables that appear at the end of the chapter.

## 6A-1: Identification and Screening of Child Maltreatment[1]

Organizations for health care professionals have initiated training programs designed to increase knowledge for recognizing, diagnosing, documenting, and treating child abuse. The range of efforts includes integrating health care professionals into interdisciplinary multiagency teams and interventions (American Academy of Pediatrics, 1991; American Medical Association, 1992a,b, 1995); issuing guidelines for interview techniques, behavior observations, and physical examinations; and providing health care providers with information about reporting requirements and community resources for social and legal assistance to patients. Physician guides and visual diagnosis kits have been designed to assist health professionals in establishing the causes of injuries in both obvious and obscure cases of child maltreatment.

Local community-based programs that unite public health and clinical settings also serve an educational and awareness-raising role. The Preventing Abuse and Neglect Through Dental Awareness (PANDA) Coalition in Missouri, for

---

[1]See also the discussion of mandatory reporting procedures in Chapter 5.

example, includes state medical, public health, and social service representatives committed to educating dental professionals about how to identify and report child abuse and neglect (Missouri Department of Health, 1995).

Although evaluations have examined the impact of training about child maltreatment on the knowledge and behavior of health care providers, they have not examined links between training experiences, provider practices, service referrals, and patient outcomes. Nor have they examined the possibility that increased detection may provide diminishing returns for both child and adult victims if additional remedies are not available. As a result, the ability of health care providers and institutions to recommend appropriate care for recognized victims of family violence, monitor treatment implementation and success, and influence eventual health outcomes for children and families has yet to be adequately documented.

Table 6A-1 lists the only evaluation of an identification and screening program that meets the committee's criteria for inclusion. It compared child health and rates of reported maltreatment outcomes for two groups of high-risk mothers using a screening device and a comprehensive health services program for one group and routine services for the other (Brayden et al., 1993). Although infant health improved in the treatment intervention, the comprehensive program did not alter the rates of reported abuse for high-risk mothers and was associated with an increased number of neglect reports, possibly a result of surveillance bias.

The authors attribute the failure of this intervention to demonstrate reduced rates of maltreatment in part to the possibility that the psychosocial treatment of the mothers may not have been intensive enough to offset past adverse environmental influences, even though the medical aspect of the intervention improved infant health. The authors also observe that group discussions for high-risk mothers may have been a poor choice, since it may have unintentionally facilitated poor parenting practices. This evaluation suggests that improving health care provider knowledge or behavior alone may not be sufficient to influence maltreatment outcomes if the availability and efficacy of other intervention services are not considered.

## Hospital Multidisciplinary Teams

Many health care facilities use multidisciplinary teams to improve identification and case management for victims of child maltreatment identified in hospitals. These teams are generally composed of hospital administrators, social workers, physicians, nurses, and mental health professionals who perform several roles: providing medical consultation on individual cases; assisting with the psychosocial management of the family while in crisis; initiating and coordinating outpatient care and follow-up; conducting integrated case reviews with representatives from social services and legal agencies; and educating other health care providers.

The use of multidisciplinary teams has not been evaluated to assess child health outcomes. Several hospitals have now disbanded their teams because of lack of resources and smaller populations of pediatric patients.

## The Health Professional as Expert Witness

In cases of physical or sexual abuse, the medical record that documents the history and physical examination of the victim may be the most important piece of evidence heard by the court. Physician statements and medical records can justify important exceptions to hearsay rules (which vary from state to state), thereby allowing the child to speak about the nature of the event, the circumstances, and the identities of the persons involved (see also the discussion of improving child witnessing in Chapter 5). The health professional can collect, document, and present evidence of abuse; discuss the likelihood of maltreatment and possible perpetrators; and if necessary advocate for the child's safety and best interests.

In theory, the preparation and training of health care professionals regarding expert testimony can improve their effectiveness and willingness to appear in court on behalf of patients and enhance the use of the victim's medical records as evidence (Stern, 1997). Such training may also make them better witnesses for the defense as well as better prosecution witnesses. No studies have evaluated the impact of such training programs, however, and uncertainty exists as to whether they improve collaborative efforts between health professionals and the law enforcement officials, improve the prosecution of offenders and the protection of victims, or alter long-term health outcomes for children. In addition, the absence of compensation for the time and diagnostic tests that may be involved in preparing such testimony may discourage many health professionals from participating in law enforcement actions.

## 6A-2: Mental Health Services for Child Victims of Physical Abuse and Neglect

No consistent set of mental health consequences has been identified for children who have been maltreated (Goldson, 1987; Malinosky-Rummell and Hansen, 1993; Kolko, 1996a), although they have been reported to be developmentally delayed, have behavior disorders, and be recognizably different from their age peers in ways than cannot be attributed to physical injuries alone (Cicchetti and Carlson, 1989; Wolfe, 1987). (Note that victims of child sexual abuse are discussed in the next section.) Some children show many symptoms immediately; some show symptoms some time after the abuse; and some seem to show no visible effects of their experiences at all. Different factors may account for this variation in the emotional and mental health impact of maltreatment, including the level of parental support, cognitive-attributional perspectives, and the presence or absence of other stressful factors in the child's environment. More research is required to investigate the variability in children's responses to their experiences in order to develop effective intervention programs (Salzinger et al., 1993).

Children who have been maltreated are typically referred to psychotherapy or counseling for a range of problems, including hyperactivity, impulsiveness, delinquency, aggressive or undisciplined behavior, noncompliance, social withdrawal, isolation, anxiety, phobias, and depression. They may receive any one or a combination of services (individual/group/family therapy and psychodynamic/ cognitive-behavioral/psychoanalytic).

Table 6A-2 lists five evaluations in this area that meet the committee's criteria for inclusion. Two of the studies involved evaluations of the impact of treating social withdrawal in preschool children who had experienced or were assessed to be at high risk for physical abuse or neglect (Fantuzzo et al., 1987, 1988). The interventions were designed to enhance positive peer social interactions in a community-based day treatment center for maltreated children that integrates comprehensive counseling and education services for parents (the Mt. Hope Family Center in Rochester, New York, provided the site for each of the studies). The evaluations indicated that the treatment group in each study achieved developmental gains, enhancement of self-concept, and positive oral and motor skills that enhanced the social behavior of the maltreated children. Although the studies included a small number of participants (in one case, only four children each in the treatment and comparison groups), they are noteworthy in their assessment of the impact of the intervention across multiple domains of child functioning and their efforts to isolate critical components of the intervention strategy (for example, experimenting with adult versus peer-initiated social interactions).

Two studies by Kolko (1996a,b) involved a comparison of treatment conditions for children who had experienced physical abuse. In a comparison of two primary treatment conditions (cognitive-behavioral therapy and family therapy), both treatments appeared to reduce parental anger and force, but cognitive-behavioral therapy showed a significantly larger reduction than family therapy on these measures (Kolko, 1996a). An important observation in this study indicated that one-fifth of the cases showed heightened parental force in both the early and the late phases of treatment, suggesting a subgroup of families who were less responsive to services.

In a second study, 55 cases of physically abused, school-age children were randomly assigned to one of three groups: (1) individual child and parent cognitive-behavioral therapy, (2) family therapy, or (3) routine community services (Kolko, 1996b). Relative to routine community services, both individual cognitive-behavioral and family therapy were associated with greater reductions in child-to-parent violence and children's externalizing behavior, parental distress and risk of abuse, and family conflict and cohesion, although the three conditions reported improvements across time on several of these measures. Although not statistically different, abuse recidivism rates in the three intervention conditions for children in this study were 10 percent (cognitive-behavioral therapy), 12 percent (family therapy), and 30 percent (routine community services); the rates for the participating adult caretakers were 5 percent (cognitive-behavioral therapy), 6 percent (family therapy), and 30 percent (routine community services). No significant differences between cognitive-behavioral and family therapy were observed on consumer satisfaction or maltreatment risk ratings at termination.

### 6A-3: Mental Health Services for Child Victims of Sexual Abuse

In 1994, McCurdy and Daro estimated that 150,000 sexual abuse cases were substantiated by child protective services. Interventions in these cases include counseling programs for the child victims, treatment programs for the offenders (discussed in Chapter 5), and family therapy programs (often comparable to those discussed in section 4A-1 in Chapter 4). Prior studies indicate that between 44 and 73 percent of children who are reported as victims of sexual abuse receive some form of counseling or psychotherapy related to their victimization (Finkelhor and Berliner, 1995; Chapman and Smith, 1987; Finkelhor, 1983; Lynn et al., 1988). Other studies show that between 20 and 50 percent of victims are asymptomatic at the time of disclosure (Kendall-Tackett et al., 1993). Some children remain symptom free, others develop problems at a later developmental stage (Gomes-Schwartz et al., 1990). Furthermore, for those children who do develop symptoms, the effects vary widely (Kendall-Tackett et al., 1993).

Traditional treatment of sexually abused children includes three service approaches: the lay or paraprofessional approach, which utilizes peer counseling and support groups; the group approach, which emphasizes group therapy and education; and individual counseling, which may be provided by social workers or mental health professionals (Keller et al., 1989). Treatment types include individual, family, and group interventions and what is offered depends on the child's age, level of functioning, gender, type of victimization, availability of resources in a geographic area, and the orientation of the treatment provider (Pogge and Stone, 1990; Lanyon, 1986; Keller et al., 1989). Treatment programs reflect a variety of intervention goals: to address a child's response to the abuse, to destigmatize the experience, to increase the child's self-esteem, to prevent the onset of short or long-term adverse effects, and to prevent future abuse (Kolko, 1987; James and Masjleti, 1983; Calhoun and Atkenson, 1991; Beutler et al., 1994; O'Donohue and Elliott, 1992).

Outcome measures are typically comparative measures of the victim's mental health or externalizing behaviors (sexual play with other children, self-stimulation) relative to untreated victims. Several behavioral inventories and checklists are available, although other methods, such as observations of the child at home and at school, are also used (e.g., Downing et al., 1988). Interventions may not only address effects of past abuse but also teach children skills to avoid further abuse. Recognizing that sexual victimization can have profound effects on family dynamics and other family members, therapeutic interventions may address the nonoffending parent as well as the child victim (Deblinger et al., 1996; Oates et al., 1994).

Table 6A-3 lists seven evaluations of interventions in this area that meet the committee's criteria for inclusion. Six of these evaluations examined therapeutic interventions. Three studies compared treatment groups with no-treatment control groups (Deblinger et al., 1996; Oates et al., 1994; Verleur et al., 1986); the others compared competing treatment formats (Berliner and Saunders, 1996; Cohen and Mannarino, 1996; Downing et al., 1988). All six showed improvements in victim mental health following a variety of therapeutic interventions. The efficacy of abuse-specific treatment has been demonstrated in three studies (Cohen and Mannarino, 1996; Deblinger et al., 1996; Verleur et al., 1986).

In a seventh study, an experimental group of female adolescent incest victims who received sex education therapy in group treatment showed significant increase in positive self-esteem and increased knowledge of human sexuality, birth control, and venereal disease compared with the control group (Verleur et al., 1986). The latter finding is significant because less rigorous studies have shown that child sexual abuse victims are likely to be more sexually active than other children and therefore may have greater need for such knowledge.

A review of 29 nonexperimental studies of therapeutic interventions for child victims of sexual abuse found only 5 that demonstrated beneficial outcomes attributable to the intervention as opposed to the passage of time or some other factor outside therapy (Finkelhor and Berliner, 1995). In a similar review of the literature, the researchers were unable to assess the effectiveness of any mental health interventions for sexually abused children because of the limited numbers of studies and methodological problems (O'Donohue and Elliott, 1992). Consistent benefits of treatment for child victims of sexual abuse have been reported in clinical pre-post studies, although no specific type of therapeutic intervention has been shown to have significant impact when compared with others in experimental studies.

## 6A-4: Mental Health Services for Children Who Witness Domestic Violence

Whether or not they are also the victims of abuse themselves, some children who witness violence in their home or their community not only are more disturbed in their interpersonal relationships than other children, but also are at significant risk of repeating dysfunctional relationship patterns, which can contribute to a cyclic pattern of family violence (Bell and Jenkins, 1991; Zuckerman et al., 1995; Jaffe et al., 1986a,b). Some of these children show psychological or behavioral reactions to witnessing violence similar to those of children who have been abused themselves (Fantuzzo et al., 1991; Hurley and Jaffe, 1990; Kashani et al., 1992; Osofsky, 1995a,b).

In reviewing the literature on the effects of witnessing violence in the home, retrospective studies suggest that boys who witness domestic violence are more likely to use violence against their own dating partners and wives (Hotaling and Sugarman, 1990). Girls who witness domestic violence may also be more violent in dating relationships, but such exposure does not appear to be a significant risk factor for adult victimization. Many gaps and inadequacies exist in this research area, including the absence of longitudinal studies that inhibit understanding of the interactions and pathways involved. A recent secondary analysis of a domestic violence database from the Spouse Assault Replication Program (SARP) (discussed in Chapter 5) provides valuable insights in examining the prevalence and situational characteristics of children exposed to substantiated cases of adult female abuse and additional developmental risk factors (Fantuzzo et al., 1997). The authors report that children are often involved in multiple and intricate ways in domestic disputes, beyond simply witnessing physical or sexual assaults. A sizable number of children in such households are the ones who call for help, are identified as a precipitant cause of the dispute that led to violence, or are physically abused themselves by the perpetrator.

Mental health services for children who witness domestic violence are a relatively new intervention strategy, but several preventive intervention and treatment programs have emerged as a secondary prevention strategy—one targeted to families who meet certain case criteria (Osofsky, 1997). One such program is Boston City Hospital's Child Witness to Violence Project (Groves et al., 1993; Zuckerman et al., 1995; Groves and Zuckerman, 1997). The goals of the intervention are to increase stability and safety in a child's environment, to treat psychological and developmental problems related to witnessing violence, to educate and support parents in managing marital conflict and eliminating violence, and to stimulate discussion by families about the role of violence. This program has not been evaluated.

Table 6A-4 lists two evaluations of one type of group treatment program for child witnesses that meet the committee's criteria for inclusion. These evaluations suggest that interventions for children who witness violence at home have beneficial effects, but they offer contradictory evidence as to which variables are most likely to be affected.

Following a 10-week group counseling intervention focused on a number of outcomes, interview data indicated significant gain in two areas: the children were able to report more safety skills and strategies and had more positive perceptions of their mothers and fathers (Jaffe et al., 1986b). No differences were found on their perception of their responsibility for the violence between their parents.

In contrast, a replication of the same treatment program found no significant differences between treatment and control groups in knowledge of safety and support skills (Wagar and Rodway, 1995). Significant improvement was noted in the treated children's attitudes and responses toward anger and sense of responsibility for parents and violence in the family. The real contribution of these interventions for children who witness domestic violence remains unclear; it is also uncertain whether such interventions influence the incidence of domestic violence between adult partners.

The evaluation of future interventions of children exposed to violence is complicated by the interaction of multiple risk factors, including the violence that the child witnesses, the general home atmosphere, violence in the community, and violence that involves the child as victim. Since family violence usually operates in concert with other pathogenic influences, effective interventions require recognition of the broader context of the child's family and neighborhood environments.

Another issue for research is emerging evidence suggesting that, although some children may be profoundly affected by exposure to violence, many do not develop marked problems (King et al., 1995). Considerable literature on protective factors or resilience examines how many children exposed to extreme circumstances manage not only to survive, but also to thrive in the face of such adversity (Garmezy, 1985, 1993; Rutter, 1990). In order to develop effective prevention and intervention strategies, it is crucial to understand the processes by which some individuals remain confident and develop supportive relationships despite difficult circumstances. Future study designs, preferably longitudinal, should give equal attention to variables that may protect children and be associated with more positive outcomes (Osofsky, 1995a). Existing services (such as Head Start programs) can provide natural opportunities for collaborative partnerships between family violence researchers and service providers (including child care workers, early childhood educators, parents, and community leaders) that examine not only the problems that arise in situations in which children are exposed to domestic violence but also the family, community, and cultural strengths that provide important compensatory mechanisms in addressing the impact of such exposure (Fantuzzo et al., 1997). These opportunities can assist with the development of tools to address the hard-to-count and the hard-to-measure dimensions of family violence, child development, and family functioning, especially in high-risk environments in which young children may be disproportionately vulnerable to familial stress factors.

### 6A-5:  Mental Health Services for Adult Survivors of Child Abuse

A positive correlation has been shown between childhood sexual abuse and mental health problems in adult life. The effects of abuse on victims may manifest themselves at different phases of the life cycle; some victims may not require, or may not have access to, mental health services until they reach adulthood. Therapeutic interventions for adult survivors of child abuse may be delivered through individual or group therapy. Few evaluations of either approach have been done. Studies of adult victims are rare and are characterized by the same methodological problems as research on child victims.

Table 6A-5 lists the only evaluation in this area that meets the committee's criteria for inclusion. Using a randomized clinical trial design, it tested the hypothesis that different kinds of group therapy can recreate the experience of family, and in this setting adults can relearn healthy interpersonal skills (Alexander et al., 1989, 1991). Group therapy was more effective than a wait-list condition in reducing depression and alleviating distress, with differences maintained at the 6-month follow-up. Fearfulness and social adjustment were also affected differentially by the two types of group therapy used.

### 6A-6: Home Visitation and Family Support Programs

Home visitation and family support programs, which are usually administered by public health agencies, constitute major preventive interventions that show important promise in addressing the problem of child maltreatment. In contrast to the parenting practices and family support services discussed in Chapter 4, home visitation is offered to families at risk of child maltreatment but who have not been reported for it; home visitation seeks to influence parenting practices during critical transitions in family life.

Home visitation is a health care strategy to improve child health and development outcomes in families determined to be at risk for poor infant and child outcomes, based on risk factors of low birthweight, prematurity, young age of mother, primiparity, maternal education, poverty or low socioeconomic status, lack of maternal social support, and substance abuse (Brayden et al., 1993; Infante-Rivard et al., 1989; Seitz et al., 1985; Bennett, 1987; Brooks-Gunn, 1990; National Research Council, 1993a; Institute of Medicine, 1994). In traditional practice, home visiting programs generally begin with prenatal care for the mother and then extend through the first or second years of her child's life. Home visitors attempt to improve bonding by educating parents about children's physical, cognitive, and social development, by teaching parents more effective parenting and child management techniques, and helping them develop access to family support services and community resources. Although the primary focus is on the mother and her role as the primary caregiver, family functioning, individualized family and child needs, and the role of community are also considered. Although there are few evaluations in this area, it is one of the few interventions that have included long-term (15-year) follow-up studies (Olds et al., 1997), suggesting that home visitation can provide an important contribution to widespread strategy for reducing family violence.

Table 6A-6 lists the nine evaluations in this area that meet the committee's criteria for inclusion, five of which are follow-up studies of one intervention, the

Prenatal/Early Infancy Study in Elmira, New York (Olds, 1992; Olds et al., 1986, 1988, 1994, 1995). These studies reported a significant impact on certain family health-related outcomes, including: improved prenatal health behaviors, such as improved maternal diet, reduced smoking, and greater social support; increased infant birthweight and mother's length of pregnancy, including a 75 percent reduction in preterm delivery (Olds et al., 1988). The study also reported improvements in maternal personal development by stimulating continued efforts at school or in the workforce and by postponing the birth of a second child.

Evaluation indicates that the intervention also affected child health and safety. It improved the safety of the home environment, reduced the number of emergency department visits for child injuries and ingestions, and had some effect on reports of abuse and neglect. In the highest-risk group—poor unmarried teenagers—home visitation reduced the number of subsequent child maltreatment reports during the first two years of their infant's life to 4 percent for the treatment group compared with 19 percent for the control group. This decrease during the first two years of their infant's life is linked by the researchers to improvement in parent's knowledge, parenting skills, and bonding with infants.

Four years after the completion of the intervention, however, no difference existed between the treatment and control groups in their behavioral and developmental outcomes or the rates of child abuse and neglect (Olds et al., 1994). This finding has been attributed to selection bias in the original sample—home visitors and other service personnel who continued to have contact with the mothers in the treatment groups may have been more sensitive to and more likely to report signs of child maltreatment that would otherwise not come to the attention of child protection agencies. A 15-year follow-up study of the long-term effects of the original intervention indicated that the prenatal and early childhood home visitation program showed positive results, including a reduction in the number of subsequent pregnancies, the use of welfare, child abuse and neglect rates, and criminal behavior on the part of low-income, unmarried mothers (Olds et al., 1997).

During the time between the first and second evaluations, the program evolved from a high-intensity demonstration and research study into a community services program administered by local governmental offices. During this transition, changes occurred in the program definition, target audience, educational training of the provider, extent and coordination of services, and caseload per home visitor (Institute of Medicine, 1994), which may have diluted the overall impact of the original design of the intervention (U.S. General Accounting Office, 1990).

The Elmira project was replicated in Memphis, Tennessee, in a largely low-income African American population (Olds et al., 1995). After two years of project implementation, positive outcomes were reported in interim measures associated with child maltreatment, but the children were still too young to provide any significant data on rates of reports of abuse or neglect. In the Memphis study, women reported fewer attitudes associated with child abuse (lack of empa-

thy for children, a belief in physical punishment to discipline infants and toddlers). At 12 and 24 months of the project, the homes of nurse-visited women
were rated as more conducive to healthy families than those of the control group.

The Healthy Start program, administered by the Hawaii Department of Maternal and Child Health, is a second model of home visitation; it began in 1985 as
a 3-year demonstration project and became a state program in 1988. The Hawaii
program offers parent education and support as well as counseling and support in
gaining access to such community resources as housing, financial assistance,
medical aid, nutrition, respite care, employment, and transportation.

Initial data on the effects of the Hawaii Healthy Start program suggest that it
has a positive impact on reducing child abuse and neglect; two evaluations of the
program are under way but have not yet been completed. The National Committee for Prevention of Child Abuse is conducting a clinical trial with high- and
low-risk families randomly receiving home visits or no treatment, but the evaluation study has not yet been published. Outcomes to be monitored include
parental functioning, child physical and cognitive development, parent-child interactions, use of formal and informal community supports, and child abuse rates
as measured using standardized psychometric instruments. This evaluation will
examine program features such as the use of paraprofessionals as home visitors,
methods for determining service intensity and duration, and methods for identifying target populations and delivering the most effective home care. The study
will provide recommendations to over 25 states that have demonstrated an interest in replicating the program. A second evaluation of Healthy Start is being
conducted at Johns Hopkins University but has not yet been published.

In response to early reports that home visitation may improve family functioning and child health, some researchers have concluded that the statistical
evidence is not sufficient to support the efficacy of nurse visitation programs on
child abuse events or child development and well-being for all children (Infante-
Rivard et al., 1989). Variations in the levels of service provision and family
compliance, difficulties in the measurement of abuse, and broader intervening
psychosocial and socioeconomic factors that affect families make the current
research difficult to interpret. Reliance on official reports as measures of child
abuse and neglect may underestimate the true incidence or prevalence of such
events. Surveillance bias is another methodological problem, since the homes to
which health professionals have routine access may be more likely to be reported
for abuse or neglect than homes that are never visited.

Despite the methodological difficulties and uncertainties about the duration
of program impact on preventing child maltreatment, home visitation remains
one of the most promising interventions for prevention of child abuse or neglect;
there is some indication of its success with families at risk, and it would be useful
to compare its benefits as a secondary (targeted) or a primary (provided to all)
strategy. An important consideration is the issue of cost, since the provision of

health and social services to a large number of families in their homes over a lengthy period can be expensive.

We describe below a number of projects that have not yet been evaluated.

*Healthy Families America.* A new initiative for abuse prevention, called Healthy Families America, is based on the Hawaii Healthy Start program. At present, it exists as a consultation service to communities that are planning state or local home visitation programs. Its goal is to encourage the development of a universal system for parent education and support, including home visitation services for families who request additional support (Bond, 1995). Although Healthy Families America has not yet been evaluated, the program has established a research network to assess the implementation of the intervention.

*Bright Beginnings.* In 1995 the state of Colorado initiated the Bright Beginnings program to provide universal, voluntary home visitation by community volunteers from birth through age 3 weeks. The intervention is designed to foster positive child social and health outcomes, to reduce the incidence of child maltreatment, and to provide prenatal care for every pregnant woman in the state by 1998. The program has not been evaluated.

*Anticipatory guidance at well-baby visits.* Most families do not have access to home visitor services. Most new babies and their mothers are seen in the health care setting for a prescribed routine of well-care visits, which may provide many opportunities to offer the same kinds of prevention strategies as home visitation. This strategy has not yet been evaluated, and its comparative strength relative to home visitation or other community family support services is not known.

## DOMESTIC VIOLENCE INTERVENTIONS

The consequences of domestic violence may be one of some women's most significant health problems. Entry into the health care system serves as a common point of intervention for battered women (Parsons et al., 1995; Commonwealth Fund, 1996; American Medical Association, 1992c). Battered women seek extensive medical care over the life course; domestic violence is one of the most powerful predictors of increased health care utilization (Bergman and Brismar, 1991; Koss et al., 1991; Felitti, 1991). Recent studies indicate that between 2 and 14 percent of women seeking medical services had experienced domestic violence in the past 1-12 months; a quarter of these cases had experienced severe abuse involving more than four incidents over the last 12 months (Abbott et al., 1995; McCauley et al., 1995; Gin et al., 1991). The lifetime prevalence of domestic violence reported in one study was over 50 percent; 16.9 percent of the women seeking health services were still with the partner who had abused them (Abbott et al., 1995).

The physical consequences of domestic violence include acute injuries as well as chronic injury, chronic stress and fear, intimidation, entrapment, and lack of control over health care or support systems. These consequences include a range of medical, obstetric, gynecological, and mental health problems, including chronic or psychogenic pain, chronic irritable bowel, pelvic inflammatory disease, chronic headaches, atypical chest pains, abdominal and gastrointestinal complaints, gynecologic problems, and sexually transmitted disease (American Medical Association, 1992c). The mental health consequences include post-traumatic stress disorder, depression, suicide attempts, and nonspecific disorders, such as headaches, insomnia, and anxiety (Bergman and Brismar, 1991; American Medical Association, 1992c).

Although a broad array of negative health outcomes is associated with domestic violence, a significant number of women who seek health services as a result of violent experience do not identify themselves as victims. Inadequate screening and identification of battered victims is thought to be linked to providers' lack of knowledge and awareness of battering as a significant women's health problem; lack of time, privacy, and social services resources; and frustration about victims who return to violent partners (Sugg and Inui, 1992; Warshaw, 1989, 1993; Friedman et al., 1992).

The current health care response to domestic violence is a blend of medical care, public health, and advocacy approaches. The efforts of the domestic violence advocacy community, individual clinicians, and a growing number of professional societies have generated standards of care and major initiatives to increase provider awareness, to establish and distribute clinical guidelines, and to offer strategies for improving institutional responses to domestic violence. Many professional societies, including the American Medical Association, the American Nurses Association, the American College of Obstetricians and Gynecologists, the Association of American Medical Colleges, the Joint Commission on Accreditation of Healthcare Organizations, the American College of Emergency Physicians, the American College of Physicians, the American Academy of Family Physicians, and the American College of Nurse-Midwives have generated standards of care relevant to domestic violence. Innovative hospital-based advocacy programs are increasing in number, and medical and nursing programs are beginning to integrate family violence materials into their standard curriculum (Warshaw, 1996).

In the sections that follow we review two types of interventions for battered women: (1) screening, identification, and medical care responses and (2) mental health services. The sections are keyed to the appendix tables that appear at the end of the chapter.

## 6B-1: Domestic Violence Screening, Identification, and Medical Care Responses[2]

Much of the health care system's response to domestic violence focuses on screening and identification. Despite widespread recognition of domestic violence as a public health problem in the 1990s, many clinicians have difficulty integrating routine inquiry about domestic violence into their day-to-day practice. The reluctance of health professionals to ask questions about domestic violence is associated with several factors, including close identification of the practitioner with the patient, especially among female clinicians who have personal histories of abuse; fear of offending patients; lack of training and knowledge about appropriate interventions; inability to control the situation or cure the problem; lack of time to deal appropriately with abuse; and lack of coverage or reimbursement for referral or recommended services (Tilden et al., 1994; Sugg and Inui, 1992). Training and institutional reform efforts are now under way to address these factors and to develop strategies for social change that can integrate public health and advocacy-based principles into traditional medical care to enhance the prevention of domestic violence (Warshaw, 1993, 1996). Integrating principles of prevention, safety, empowerment, advocacy, accountability, and social change into clinical care practices, however, requires attention to structural components of the health care system that inhibit optimal care as well as attention to the philosophy and process of clinical training (Warshaw, 1996). The enhancement of domestic violence training programs in health care settings also raises issues about the quality and verifiability of the added identifications and the points at which such increased case detection provides diminishing returns for both victims and health care providers.

Pregnancy is an important opportunity for abuse assessment and intervention. Screening for abuse prior to or during pregnancy may be effective in identifying patterns of family violence, due to the frequency and pattern of prenatal visits. Screening for domestic violence is usually included in outpatient clinic care rather than in private care settings, but the latter are also beginning to change. Recent studies have shown that the incidence of abuse during pregnancy is equal to or greater than other health complications for which women are routinely screened (such as gestational diabetes and preeclampsia), and that abuse has the potential for lethality for both mother and fetus (Gazmararian et al., 1996). Abuse during pregnancy has been linked to low-birthweight outcomes for infants (Parker et al., 1994; Bullock et al., 1989; Schei et al., 1991), an increased rate of miscarriage (Gielen et al., 1994), and maternal postpartum depression (associated with lack of support from a partner). It is not certain if abuse increases during pregnancy, but studies have indicated that 7.4 to 20 percent of

---

[2]See also the discussion of mandatory procedures in Chapter 5.

women experience abuse in the 12 months prior to their pregnancy (Campbell and Parker, 1992; Gazmararian et al., 1996; McFarlane et al., 1992). The timing and overlap between wife abuse and child abuse are cause for concern and warrant research (Straus and Gelles, 1990).

Effective and efficient use of screening in health care settings requires several key factors: awareness among health care professionals of the possibility for domestic violence in both general and clinical populations, especially in obstetrics, family practice, primary care, and mental health settings; the existence of sensitive and specific screening tools that can integrate questions about domestic violence into routine health histories; adequate training to overcome discomfort in asking and responding when patients reveal abuse experiences; and resources to facilitate referral once victims are identified.

As in the area of child maltreatment, organizations for health care professionals have initiated efforts to assist physicians in identifying and treating battered patients. In 1989 the American College of Obstetricians and Gynecologists joined Surgeon General Everett Koop to launch a public awareness campaign. In 1992, the American Medical Association (1992a) published diagnostic and treatment guidelines for interview techniques, behavior observations, and physical examinations. In addition, health care organizations provide information to health care providers about state and federal reporting requirements, community resources to which patients may be referred for social services and legal assistance, emergency temporary custody arrangements, guidelines for testimony on abuse findings in legal proceedings, and risk management regarding legal liability.

Also in 1992, the Joint Commission on Accreditation of Healthcare Organizations required emergency departments and hospital ambulatory care services to have written procedures and staff training for the identification and referral of victims of violence. For the first time, hospital accreditation was directly linked to compliance with standards for the care of patients who were battered by their partners. Since then, many state medical societies and public health departments have adopted these published standards.

Table 6B-1 lists four evaluations in this area that meet the committee's criteria for inclusion. These studies assessed the effectiveness of training programs and emergency department protocols in identifying battered women. The studies use times-series designs to examine outcome data before and after the implementation of an intervention. Using rates of identification of abused women as the outcome measure, the studies show that appropriate protocols can be developed and implemented that are specific to enhancing identification of battered women.

A study done at the emergency department of the Medical College of Pennsylvania, which serves a predominately low-income, inner-city population (McLeer and Anwar, 1989), concluded that staff training and protocols increased recognition of abused women, although the enhanced identification process was not maintained in the absence of institutionalized policies and procedures for diagnosing and treating victims of domestic violence (McLeer et al., 1989). Using the same study design and outcome measure to evaluate an identification protocol implemented among nursing staff at a university hospital in the Northwest, a second study concluded that enhancing the knowledge and interview skills of nurses can increase the identification of battered women (Tilden and Shepard, 1987).

Another study used a prospective design for screening domestic violence victims in the emergency room setting (Olson et al., 1996). They screened all women ages 15-70 who came to a Level I trauma center using a chart modification method, adding the question, "Is the patient a victim of domestic violence?" to the emergency department record. Two percent of women were identified as victims of domestic violence at baseline; 3.4 percent were identified during the chart modification month; and 3.6 percent were identified when an educational component involving training about the causes and impacts of domestic violence was added to the chart modification. The relative rate for identifying victims of domestic violence was 1.8 times higher when the question was asked than during the control month; the educational component did not appear to enhance identification.

These identification studies must be considered cautiously, since time-series study designs have well-known limitations, including the inability to control all variables that could influence the outcome (Campbell and Stanley, 1966). The limitation that is most significant to emergency department research is the frequent turnover in staff, which alters the proportion of staff who have undergone training during the study period. Changes in the socioeconomic and cultural environments used in these studies did not appear to alter or seem likely to influence the findings, according to the authors. However, the Olson study also highlights the importance of recognizing the limits of training and screening questions as isolated interventions. These approaches may have greater impact if they are part of a comprehensive approach designed to address domestic violence that provides ongoing reinforcement and changes in institutional cultures that can improve the quality of health care for victims of abuse.

Although they have not been completed, evaluations are currently under way for a number of other programs designed to enhance health provider responses to domestic violence. The Health Resource Center, administered by the Family Violence Prevention Fund in San Francisco, has developed a manual and a training model for teams of health care providers and advocates to improve hospital, clinic, and community responses to domestic violence. This model evolved from a growing recognition that traditional training was not sufficient to change individual provider behavior or to generate the kinds of system changes necessary to respond appropriately to victims of domestic violence. In 1994, a 3-year evaluation of it was undertaken by the Johns Hopkins School of Nursing in collaboration with the Trauma Foundation/San Francisco Injury Center and the University of Pittsburgh's Center for Injury Research and Control. A randomized trial will evaluate the program's impact on staff attitudes, infrastructure changes and responses to victims needs, effectiveness of screening instruments, and patient satisfaction. The evaluation component of the training program, funded by the Centers for Disease Control and Prevention, involves 12 hospitals in Pennsylvania and California.

Another evaluation study under way and funded by the Centers for Disease Control and Prevention compares three hospitals in which the WomanKind program is already in place with three control hospitals in the Minneapolis area. WomanKind is a hospital-based program combining education and training with a network system for health professionals, social workers, and advocates involved in caring for domestic violence patients. The study will measure changes in knowledge, attitudes, and skills among health care providers and advocates; frequency of diagnosis and referral; patient satisfaction with services; number of repeat contacts with the program; and utilization of community services.

The Agency for Health Care Policy and Research has funded a 3-year study that is designed to help primary care providers in a managed care setting identify and treat victims of domestic violence. Health care providers will be educated about both acute and chronic presentations and consequences of domestic violence, and protocols for enhanced case management techniques will be initiated. Program effects on detecting battering and on preventing recurrences will be assessed, along with a critical analysis of program costs (Agency for Health Care Policy and Research, 1996). A unique aspect of this study is its ability to follow a specific patient population over an extended period of time.

Staff training programs and protocols, by themselves, do not ensure that patients will receive the services they need. Regardless of the training of medical staff, ensuring victim access to services depends on availability and accessibility of local resources, insurance coverage and financial strategies for reimbursement of medical services, and assurances of confidentiality and safety. Establishing an appropriate therapeutic plan depends not only on characteristics of providers but also on an institutional culture and community resources that support services for female victims by addressing such structural barriers as cost, reimbursement, and accessibility (Flitcraft, 1993; Warshaw, 1993).

For yet another set of interventions in this area, no evaluations are either scheduled or completed. They are, however, of interest to the field and are described briefly below.

*St. Luke's-Roosevelt Hospital.* St. Luke's-Roosevelt Hospital in New York City is developing a comprehensive intervention to obtain a statistical assessment of domestic violence related to medical visits; to provide victim advocates for emergency department patients; to provide referrals for counseling; and to foster cooperation among the law enforcement, criminal justice, and health care systems. This intervention has initiated universal screening of all women over 17 years of age in two emergency department facilities, using a structured protocol and form to document domestic violence. Project outcomes have not been tested in the medical, social service, or legal settings.

*AWAKE.* The Advocacy for Women and Kids in Emergencies (AWAKE) program at Children's Hospital in Boston screens mothers of abused children for domestic violence in order to improve the welfare of the mothers and prevent future incidents of child abuse (Robertson, 1995). The program offers immediate risk assessment and safety planning, counseling services, support groups, and an educational program; it provides access to housing as well as legal and medical providers. AWAKE attempts, whenever possible, to keep mothers and children together and maintain the family. Multigenerational programs like this are good examples of how coordination of care and interagency cooperation can maximize resources available for patient care. They need to be evaluated to understand what components of these teams are most effective for securing services for abuse victims and improving health outcomes for both adult and child victims.

### 6B-2: Mental Health Services for Domestic Violence Victims[3]

Mental health consequences of domestic violence are significant and prompt women to seek services as frequently as do physical problems. In controlled studies, battered women are consistently found to be more depressed than other women on various instruments (Bland and Orn, 1986; Jaffe et al., 1986a). In other studies, depression was the strongest indicator of domestic violence among women seeking medical care at a family practice medical center (Saunders et al., 1993); a significantly higher prevalence of major depression existed among battered women than in the larger population under study (Gleason, 1993). Significant predictors of depression in battered women include the frequency and severity of abuse, other life stressors, and their ability to care for themselves; these were stronger than prior history of mental illness or demographic, cultural, and childhood characteristics (Campbell et al., 1997; Cascardi and O'Leary, 1992).

In mental health care settings, post-traumatic stress syndrome is widely recognized as a frequent consequence of violent victimization (Koss et al., 1994). Higher rates have been documented among battered women in shelters than in other groups of women (Gleason, 1993; Woods and Campbell, 1993). Many of the symptoms that emerge following domestic violence are included among the criteria for a diagnosis of post-traumatic stress syndrome: reexperiencing the traumatic event (nightmares and flashbacks), avoidance and numbing (avoidance of thoughts and reminders of the trauma), and increased arousal (problems in sleeping and concentrating, exaggerated startle reactions) (American Psychiatric Association, 1994). There is a strong possibility that post-traumatic stress syn-

---

[3]Mental health services programs for batterers are discussed in Chapter 5, since most clients are referred to these treatment programs by legal authorities following an arrest.

drome is underdiagnosed by primary care providers, who tend to focus only on the obvious symptoms of sleep disorder and stress reactions.

Surprisingly few studies have investigated substance abuse among battered women. Two studies of medical emergency departments, neither of which was controlled, show an association between alcoholism and being assaulted by a partner (Stark and Flitcraft, 1988; Bergman and Brismar, 1991).

Other studies have found an association between abuse and illicit drug use (Plichta, 1996) and increased alcohol problems (Jaffe et al., 1986a; Miller et al., 1989). Studies of abuse during pregnancy have also reported an association with substance abuse (Amaro et al., 1990; Campbell and Parker, 1992; Parker et al., 1994). A key question that has not been well studied is the extent of mental health symptoms, including substance abuse, that may have existed prior to the family violence compared with problems that develop as a consequence of the violence.

Table 6B-2 lists four evaluations of mental health services for domestic violence that meet the committee's criteria for inclusion (see also the discussion of evaluations of advocacy services for battered women in section 4B-3, which include mental health measures in their assessments of the intervention). Bergman and Brismar (1991) studied whether a screening and supportive counseling intervention would decrease battered women's use of hospital services for somatic or psychiatric care. Several limitations, such as sampling bias, inadequate proxy or indicator measures, inadequate power to detect effect, and lack of information regarding other potentially confounding factors, make it difficult to draw conclusions.

Cox and Stoltenberg (1991) report significant improvement from pre- to post-test in assertiveness and self-esteem for a group of 9 women in a battered women's shelter who volunteered to participate in a group counseling program. The program had been developed to improve the skills needed to end violent relationships, but it did not report how many women returned to their abusers when they left the shelter.

Since a high percentage of women seen in mental health settings are unidentified battered women, the effects of different types of treatment formats (individual, group, couples) and protocols deserve rigorous evaluation to examine their impact on women who have experienced domestic violence (see also the discussion of peer support groups for battered women in Chapter 4).

The merits and advisability of couples counseling, a common form of family therapy for domestic violence offenders and victims, have received significant attention and debate (Walker, 1994; O'Leary et al., 1994). Many victim advocates believe that couples counseling programs fail to address issues of power, control, and violence used by the batterer and issues of safety, empowerment, and increased options for the victim. Although couples counseling treatment programs may be effective in some situations (when violence is stimulated by alcohol, for example, or when it occurs at a low level), there is need for caution so that the danger to women is not increased by the therapy.

Harris et al. (1988) report as the most important result of their study that offender-victim couples are more likely to complete a group treatment program than a couples counseling program. In treatment groups, participants in the couples counseling format were four times more likely to drop out than those in the group program. All participants showed positive changes in psychological well-being, regardless of treatment group. The goal of ending violence in the relationship was achieved for 23 of 28 women who could be located for follow-up interviews, but this figure (82 percent) is suspect since the women who dropped out of treatment could not be located and may have dropped out because of an increase in violence. No difference was noted for level of violence between treatment groups. The evidence about the advisability of couples counseling as a whole is inconclusive.

In the past, research on victims of domestic violence has focused on identifying victims and the psychological consequences of battering. Efforts are now under way to shift the focus from clinical treatment to a broader set of health and safety goals designed to reduce the impact of violence and ultimately prevent its occurrence. Tensions between clinicians and victim advocates have been fostered, in part, by the lack of an integrated framework that could address both the social and psychological needs of battered women. Careful attention to project design will encourage scientific evaluation of different treatment models to assess their outcomes and relative effectiveness while ensuring appropriate delivery of needed services.

## ELDER ABUSE INTERVENTIONS

Very few programs offer interventions for elder abuse in health care settings; most that do adapt models used to prevent child abuse and neglect and domestic violence. Research in this field is in an early stage of development, and observers have noted that, as long as elder abuse is seen as tangential to geriatrics and gerontology, research on elder abuse interventions will remain undeveloped (U.S. House Select Committee on Aging, 1981). No rigorous evaluations of such programs have been published.

As noted in the discussions of child maltreatment and domestic violence, provider awareness of family violence and mandated reporting requirements do not necessarily translate into effective treatment and prevention services. Ehrlich and Anetzberger (1991) found that, although state departments of health were aware of elder abuse reporting laws, very few had implemented abuse identification and reporting practices. Particular problems arise in the field of elder abuse because the victims have the right to self-determination unless there is reason to doubt their competence to make decisions concerning their own welfare. In extreme circumstances, a hospital can authorize a protective service admission if it decides that the elderly person, upon discharge, would not be safe back in his or her home setting; this option, although viable, can be difficult to achieve when hospitals seek to reduce economic costs or do not regard patient safety as part of their concern. Another option is to keep the elderly person in an emergency unit overnight until an intervention can be put in place in collaboration with social service or law enforcement officials, so that she or he can go home to a safe environment (Carr et al., 1986; Fulmer et al., 1992).

In this section we review three interventions for abused elders: (1) identification and screening programs, (2) hospital multidisciplinary teams, and (3) hospital-based support groups. There are no evaluations in this area that meet the committee's criteria for inclusion; the sections that follow are based on descriptive literature.

## 6C-1:  Identification and Screening

Guidelines for the detection and treatment of suspected elder abuse have been published by the American Medical Association (1992d).  Although 42 states now have reporting requirements for elder abuse, few hospitals have established adult protective teams.

In Seattle, Harborview Medical Center has developed an elder abuse detection and referral protocol for all geriatric disciplines (Tomita, 1982).  The protocol includes medical history, presentation of signs and symptoms, functional assessment, physical exam, caregiver interview, collateral contacts, and case plans.  Program services include client or caregiver service intervention, staff training, referrals to community services, and case follow-up (Quinn and Tomita, 1986).

## 6C-2:  Hospital Multidisciplinary Teams

Hospital multidisciplinary teams are also used in elder abuse cases.  The San Francisco Consortium for Elder Abuse Prevention, for example, consists of representatives from a variety of professions and settings, including case management, family counseling, mental health, geriatric medicine, civil law, law enforcement, financial management, and adult protective services.  The team meets monthly to review and assess multiproblem, multiagency cases of elder abuse (Wolf and Pillemer, 1994).

Regulations for protective services in Illinois require that any protective services program serving an area that includes 7,500 or more people age 60 and older have a multidisciplinary team that represents protective services, medical care, law enforcement, mental health, financial planning, and religious institutions.  Special training programs regarding elder abuse are also available in many communities for those who must respond to the needs of the elderly as health professionals, social service personnel, or caregivers.

## 6C-3: Hospital-Based Support Groups

Following the model of existing hospital-based support groups for families affected by diseases of the aged such as Alzheimer's, for the caregivers of elderly relatives, and for abused elders themselves (Wolf and Pillemer, 1994), support groups are intended to provide information and social support to minimize frustrations and tensions that may lead to abusive or neglectful behavior. Although descriptive data are available for many support group efforts, they often lack standards or outcomes against which to measure their effectiveness, and they do not assess the effects on the community.

The integration of elder abuse health interventions into the broad network of support services for the elderly sponsored by the Older Americans' Act and the federal Administration on Aging represents a promising approach that deserves further consideration in the treatment and prevention of elder abuse. An integrated approach allows health professionals to become part of a community effort focused on early recognition and responses that can be sustained in the absence of a crisis. Yet such initiatives, whether specific to elder abuse or to generally improve the lives of older people, are notable for their lack of measured effectiveness.

## CONCLUSIONS

Three key areas have received significant research attention in the development of health care interventions for family violence: (1) identification and screening practices for all forms of family violence, (2) mental health services for victims of child maltreatment and domestic violence as well as children who witness domestic violence in their homes, and (3) home visitation services for families at risk of child maltreatment. Although the research base in the first two of these three areas is still in an early stage of development, some significant observations are clear:

• Efforts to encourage health care providers to ask their patients routine questions about the source and nature of their injuries and to inquire about experiences with abuse are only a first step in addressing in health settings the broader dimensions of family violence. Chart modification practices and training to raise provider awareness of the characteristics and consequences of child maltreatment, domestic violence, and elder abuse appear to be successful strategies for improving the rate of identification of current and potential victims of family violence. However, isolated interventions in these areas do not guarantee that health or mental health services will be available for identified victims or offenders, or that they will be referred or will receive treatment and services.

• Advocacy efforts focused on safety and enhanced options for the protection of women and children have stimulated numerous reforms in health care services in addressing family violence. These efforts are now encouraging comprehensive approaches in health care system reforms that seek to integrate awareness of and familiarity with family violence by health professionals, the development of sensitive and specific screening tools that can be used in routine inquiries, and resources to facilitate client referral once victims are identified. What remains uncertain is the extent to which these approaches will affect the documentation of incidents and histories of experience with family violence in individual and group health records, and the impact of such documentation on health care provider referral and reimbursement practices.

Whereas the efforts of social service and law enforcement agencies may be of primary importance in investigating and intervening in violent home situations involving child maltreatment and elder abuse, in cases of domestic violence and child maltreatment involving adolescents, health care providers can help increase options for victims as well as hold batterers accountable for their actions. Exploratory programs are examining whether health care providers can work with social service, legal, and community organizations to provide direct services to victims as well as perpetrators and also join community efforts to change conditions that foster family violence. The evaluation of this diverse range of efforts will require creative approaches that focus on institutional processes, economic costs and benefits, and professional behavior as well as individual case characteristics and health outcomes.

• Evaluations of different forms of mental health service interventions for maltreated children suggest that individual cognitive behavior therapy and family therapy offer comparative advantages, relative to routine community services, in addressing the impact of family violence on child outcomes, especially in self-esteem and the management of stress. A few small studies of therapeutic interventions designed to improve the social interactions of maltreated children with their peers have shown promise in reducing the withdrawn and other isolating behaviors that often characterize young children who have experienced abuse and neglect. In the area of child sexual abuse, consistent benefits of mental health services for victims have been reported. Although no specific type of therapeutic intervention has been shown to have significant impact when compared to others in experimental studies, abuse-specific treatments have been found more effective than nonspecific therapies in achieving positive changes on measures of traumatic effects and on self-esteem, anxiety and depression, and externalizing behavior.

• Interventions for children who witness domestic violence in their homes represent an important area of study that is just beginning to emerge in the research literature. Valuable partnership opportunities for researchers and service providers who are in regular contact with young children can assist with the development of tools to address the hard-to-count and the hard-to-measure risk and protective factors that may exist in communities where young children may experience multiple stresses in their families and neighborhoods; these may require greater emphasis on secondary prevention strategies.

• For women who have experienced domestic violence, the different types of treatment formats in mental health service interventions have not yet received sufficient research attention to make it possible to endorse a particular type of treatment. Careful scientific evaluation of different treatment models is needed to assess their outcomes and relative effectiveness with specific types of treatment groups.

• Home visitation represents one of the most carefully evaluated and promising opportunities for the prevention of child maltreatment. The documented benefits of early home visitation programs has stimulated the development of an array of models that reflect different service goals and vary in terms of their services, personnel, resources, length, and intensity. Rigorous evaluations of different models of home visitation services will be required to identify particular domains of parent and child behaviors that can be influenced through health and support services as well as critical components in client-practitioner and family interactions that foster effective collaborative relationships.

The public health sector, both in its proactive approach to addressing community health issues and its responsibility to ensure that at-risk populations receive essential health services, has sought to place violence prevention in the mainstream of public health (Foege, 1986). Yet making family violence prevention a priority in public health will require a delicate negotiation of difficult ethical and legal issues in an often volatile political environment. Strategies are needed to effect a balance between risk and protection factors in developing case detection and social support approaches and in establishing safeguards to protect the rights of privacy and confidentiality of individuals and families.

The implications for family violence interventions created by the restructuring of health care services in this country need far greater attention. Cost-containment models may impose new limits on the abilities of health care providers to ask about their client's experience with violence, to provide counseling services, to become a point of consistent interaction with their patients, and to engage in nonreimbursable collaborative ventures designed to improve the quality of care for the community. Managed care models may also encourage prevention efforts, however, especially if patient populations can be followed over extended periods and specific interventions are shown to reduce the total cost of health care services.

Most important in improving and expanding health care responses to family violence is resolving the question of whether the role of health interventions should be limited to reactive treatment of immediate injuries and crisis intervention or extended to include collaboration in developing community health promotion, improved treatment, and the prevention of violence. As professional organizations expand their role in alerting health care professionals about symptoms, consequences, and interventions for victims of child maltreatment, domestic violence, and elder abuse, they will need to educate their constituencies about alternative settings in which victims gain access to recommended services. Health care providers will also need to develop collaborative efforts with other private and public agencies to increase the availability of recommended services and to determine the appropriate balance between primary and secondary preventive interventions.

**APPENDIX TABLES BEGIN ON NEXT PAGE**

TABLE 6A-1  Quasi-Experimental Evaluations of Identification and Screening
of Child Maltreatment

| Intervention | Citation | Initial/Final Sample Size<br>Duration of Intervention<br>Follow-up |
|---|---|---|
| Identification protocol for high-risk expectant mothers followed by psychosocial support, education about self-care and healthy pregnancy behaviors, biweekly support group offered to primiparous women of low socioeconomic status in Nashville, Tennessee. | Brayden et al., 1993 | N(X) = 141<br>N(high-risk comparison group) = 122<br>N(low-risk comparison group) = 264 |

SOURCE: Committee on the Assessment of Family Violence Interventions, National
Research Council and Institute of Medicine, 1998.

| Data Collection | Results |
| --- | --- |
| Official, substantiated reports of child abuse and neglect | Physical abuse was found for 5.1% of the study population; neglect was substantiated for 5.9%. Prediction efforts were effective in identifying risk of physical abuse but not of neglect. Comprehensive health services did not alter the reported abuse rate for high-risk parents and was associated with an increased number of neglect reports. |

TABLE 6A-2    Quasi-Experimental Evaluations of Mental Health Services for Child Victims of Physical Abuse and Neglect

| Intervention | Citation | Initial/Final Sample Size<br><br>Duration of Intervention<br><br>Follow-up |
|---|---|---|
| Nine months of therapeutic day treatment program for physically abused and neglected children aged 3.9-5.9 years; also counseling and educational services for parents. | Culp et al., 1991 | N(X) = 17<br>N(O) = 17<br>Profile<br>Both groups tested at 0 and 9 months<br>6 hours per day, 5 days per week |
| Peer social initiation intervention at a community-based day treatment facility for maltreated preschool children. | Fantuzzo et al., 1987 | N(X) = 4<br><br>Two children reobserved at 4-week follow-up |
| Peer and adult social initiation intervention. | Fantuzzo et al., 1988 | Peer initiation N = 12/6<br>Adult initiation N = 12/7<br>N(O) = 12/6<br><br>2-month postintervention follow-up |
| Individual child and parent cognitive-behavioral therapy (CBT) and family therapy (FT) provided to 55 physically abused, school-aged children and their offending parents/families. | Kolko, 1996a,b | N(CBT) = 25<br>N(FT) = 18<br>N(O) = 12<br><br>Control group received routine community services<br><br>12 1-hour weekly clinic sessions within a 16-week period<br><br>1-year follow-up |

SOURCE: Committee on the Assessment of Family Violence Interventions, National Research Council and Institute of Medicine, 1998.

| Data Collection | Results |
|---|---|
| Perceived Competence and Social Acceptance Scale, Early Intervention Developmental Profile | The treatment group had significantly higher scores for cognitive competence, peer acceptance, and maternal acceptance. |
| Observation of play triads | The introduction of peer social initiation intervention preceded increases in the observed numbers of positive social interactions for the treatment children. Two children retested at 4 weeks maintained gains at follow-up. |
| Observation of play dyads, Preschool Behavior Questionnaire, Brigance Diagnostic Inventory of Early Development | The peer treatment condition resulted in greater improvements over time in positive social behaviors than adult initiation or control groups. |
| Conflict Tactics Scales, Weekly Report of Abuse Indicators, Child Abuse Potential Inventory, Severity Ratings of Individualized Treatment Problems, Sexual Abuse Fear Evaluation, Children's Attributions and Perceptions Scale, Youth Self-Report, Children's Hostility Inventory, Child Behavior Checklist, Child Conflict Index, Global Assessment Scale for Children, Brief Symptom Inventory, Beck Depression Inventory, Child Rearing Interview, Parenting Scale, Parent Opinion Questionnaire, Parent Perception Inventory, Family Environment Scale, Family Assessment Device, Conflict Behavior Questionnaire, official reports of abuse and neglect. | Overall levels of parental anger and physical discipline/force were lower in CBT than FT families, though each group showed a reduction on these items from the early to late treatment sessions. |

TABLE 6A-3    Quasi-Experimental Evaluations of Mental Health Services for
Child Victims of Sexual Abuse

| Intervention | Citation | Initial/Final Sample Size Duration of Intervention Follow-up |
|---|---|---|
| Conventional sex abuse specific group therapy (8 weeks) and same treatment with an added focus on stress inoculation and gradual exposure (10 weeks) provided to sexually abused children ages 4-13. | Berliner and Saunders, 1996 | $N(X1) = 48$ $N(X2) = 32$ 8 weeks and 10 weeks 1- and 2-year follow-up |
| Cognitive behavioral treatment (CBT) and nondirective supportive treatment (NST), provided in 12 1.5-hour sessions to parent and child. | Cohen and Mannarino, 1996 | $N(CBT) = 39$ $N(NST) = 28$ 12 1.5-hour sessions |
| Child-only therapeutic treatment, mother-only therapeutic treatment, mother and child therapeutic treatment offered to sexually abused children and their nonoffending parent. Provided in 12 weekly treatment sessions by mental health therapists trained in cognitive behavioral interventions. | Deblinger et al., 1996 | $N = 100/90$ $N(child) = 25$ $N(mother) = 25$ $N(child\ and\ mother) = 25$ $N(O) = 25$ Comparison group received only routine community services |
| Psychodynamic (P) group counseling, reinforcement therapy orientation counseling (RTO) offered to school-aged children who were confirmed victims of sexual abuse. | Downing et al., 1988 | $N(P) = 12$ $N(RTO) = 10$ Psychodynamic counseling offered on a weekly basis for 1 year; reinforcement theory counseling provided in 5-6 weekly sessions with monthly follow-up thereafter for 1 year |

| Data Collection | Results |
| --- | --- |
| Fear Survey Schedule for Children, Sexual Abuse Fear Evaluation Scales, Revised Children's Manifest Anxiety Scale, Child Behavior Checklist, Children's Depression Inventory, Child Sexual Behavior Inventory, Parent Information Form, Therapist Information Form | Both treatment groups improved significantly over time on most outcome measures. No significant differences were found between groups in improvement on fear and anxiety symptoms. |
| Preschool Symptom Self Report, Child Behavior Checklist, Child Sexual Behavior Inventory, Weekly Behavior Report | Within-group comparison of pretreatment and posttreatment outcome measures demonstrated that, although significant changes were not observed in the NST group, the CBT group had significant improvement on most outcome measures. |
| Schedule for Affective Disorders and Schizophrenia for School-Age Children, State-Trait Anxiety Inventory for Children, Child Depression Inventory, Child Behavior Checklist, Parenting Practices Questionnaire | Results indicated that mothers assigned to the experimental treatment condition described significant decreases in their child's externalizing behaviors and increases in effective parenting skills; their children reported significant reductions in depression. Children who were assigned to the experimental intervention exhibited greater reductions in post-traumatic stress disorder symptoms than children who were not. |
| Home observations, parental reports, school observations, teacher reports | Abused children's depression and self-esteem remained relatively stable over time; many of the problem behaviors observed by their parents abated over 18 months. The abused children improved slightly more than nonabused controls. |

TABLE 6A-3   (*Continued*)

| Intervention | Citation | Initial/Final Sample Size Duration of Intervention Follow-up |
|---|---|---|
| Selected therapeutic interventions. | Oates et al., 1994 | N(X) = 84/64<br><br>Treatment group was compared with age and sex-matched comparison group |
| Homogeneous group therapy and sex education with same-sex therapists and clients for 15 adolescent female incest victims in a residential treatment facility. | Verleur et al., 1986 | N(X) = 15<br>N(O) = 15<br><br>6 months |
| A communications training program for offending and nonoffending parents in sexually abusive families offered by the Hillsboro, Oregon, chapter of Parents United. | Wollert, 1988 | N(X) = 6 (3 couples, 3 singles)<br><br>Treatment group compared with a delayed training comparison group from the same Parents United chapter<br><br>Eight 90-minute weekly sessions<br><br>8-week follow-up |

SOURCE: Committee on the Assessment of Family Violence Interventions, National Research Council and Institute of Medicine, 1998.

| Data Collection | Results |
|---|---|
| Children's Depression Inventory, Achenbach Child Behavior Checklist, McMaster Family Assessment Device, General Health Questionnaire, Indices of Coping Responses, Newcastle Child and Family Life Events Schedule | Although the control children's self-esteem, depression, and behavior scores showed little change over time, the treatment children's scores were more likely to move toward the normal range although some remained dysfunctional. No relationship was found between therapy and outcome. |
| Coopersmith Self-Esteem Inventory, Anatomy/Physiology Sexual Awareness Scale, behavioral observations by resident professionals, daily behavior logs | Female incest victims in the experimental group showed significant increase in positive self-esteem as measured by the inventory and developed increased knowledge of human sexuality, birth control, and venereal disease when compared with the control group. |
| An 11-item self-assessment scale | Posttraining scores of experimental subjects were higher than controls. Experimental subjects maintained these scores upon follow-up; the scores of the control group increased when the program was administered by a student therapist. |

TABLE 6A-4   Quasi-Experimental Evaluations of Mental Health Services for Children Who Witness Domestic Violence

| Intervention | Citation | Initial/Final Sample Size / Duration of Intervention / Follow-up |
|---|---|---|
| Ten-week group treatment program for children ages 8-13 to treat the effects of witnessing spouse abuse at home. | Jaffe et al., 1986b | N(X) = 28 N(O) = 28 10 weeks |
| Ten-week group treatment program for children ages 8-13 to treat the effects of witnessing spouse abuse at home. | Wagar and Rodway, 1995 | N(X) = 16 N(O) = 22 10 weeks 6-month follow-up |

SOURCE:  Committee on the Assessment of Family Violence Interventions, National Research Council and Institute of Medicine, 1998.

TABLE 6A-5   Quasi-Experimental Evaluations of Interventions of Mental Health Services for Adult Survivors of Child Abuse

| Intervention | Citation | Initial/Final Sample Size / Duration of Intervention / Follow-up |
|---|---|---|
| Group therapy and Interpersonal Transaction (IT) group therapy modalities for women sexually abused as children by a family member. | Alexander et al., 1989, 1991 | N (X) = 65 N (O) = 58 1.5 hours per week for 10 weeks 6-month follow-up |

SOURCE:  Committee on the Assessment of Family Violence Interventions, National Research Council and Institute of Medicine, 1998.

| Data Collection | Results |
|---|---|
| Child Witness to Violence Interview, Parent Perception Inventory, Child Behavior Checklist | Preliminary results suggest immediate benefits in terms of safety skill development and positive perceptions of each parent. |
| Child Witness to Violence Questionnaire; Conflict Tactics Scales, Parent Interview Questionnaire | Significant improvements in pre- to posttest for the experimental group in attitudes and responses toward anger and sense of responsibility for parents' violence. The second variable, safety and support skills, showed no significant difference between groups. |

| Data Collection | Results |
|---|---|
| Beck Depression Inventory, Modified Fear Survey, Symptom Checklist, Revised, Social Adjustment Scale Interview, Locke-Wallace Marital Adjustment Scale, Group Climate Questionnaire, Group Leadership Behavior Inventory | Both groups proved to be effective relative to the wait-list control condition. Treatment gains were maintained at 16-month follow-up. The structure of the IT group appeared to reduce fearfulness for highly symptomatic women. Participants in the process condition improved over time in social functioning. |

TABLE 6A-6   Quasi-Experimental Evaluations of Home Visitation and Family Support Programs

| Intervention | Citation | Initial/Final Sample Size<br><br>Duration of Intervention<br><br>Follow-up |
|---|---|---|
| Home visitation program designed at the Royal Victoria Hospital in Montreal, Canada, to promote better child health and development for infants of working-class families. One group received home visits starting prenatally, group two received visits from 6 weeks postpartum, and group three received no visits. | Larson, 1980 | N(X1) = 35/26<br>N(X2 )= 40/27<br>N(O) = 40<br><br>N(X1) = 17 months<br>N(X2) = 15 months |
| A home visitation program for women at risk for out-of-home placement of their newborns. Biweekly home visits by trained community members from the baby's first postpartum check-up until first birthday, providing postpartum health and social services. | Marcenko and Spence, 1994 | N(X) = 125/110<br>N(O) = 100/77<br><br>Comparison group received standard agency services including prenatal, postpartum, family planning, and gynecological services, on-site HIV testing, and social services<br><br>Average 10 months |
| Hawaii's Healthy Start home visitation program for mothers judged to be at risk for child maltreatment. Mothers selected during postpartum hospital stay. | National Committee to Prevent Child Abuse, 1996 | N(X) = 181<br>N(O) = 191<br><br>1 year<br><br>12-, 18-, and 24-month follow-up for some clients |

| Data Collection | Results |
|---|---|
| Inventory of Home Stimulation, Maternal Behavior Scale, HOME Environment Scale, children's health status | Significant differences were found for mothers receiving prenatal and postnatal visits over other groups. These included a reduced accident rate, higher scores on assessment of home environment and maternal behavior, and a lower prevalence of mother-infant interaction problems. |
| Addiction Severity Index, history of Child Protective Services involvement, HOME Environment Scale, Norbeck Social Support Questionnaire, Brief Symptom Inventory, Rosenberg's Self-Esteem Scale | After an average of 10 months exposure, the experimental group reported significantly increased social support, greater access to services, and decreased psychological distress. |
| Child Abuse Potential Inventory, Michigan Screening Profile of Parenting; Maternal Social Support Index; Nursing Child Assessment Satellite Training | Early and intensive home visitation by paraprofessional produces measurable benefits for participants in the areas of parental attitudes toward children, parent-child interaction patterns, and type and quantity of child maltreatment. Mothers who received home visits showed significant reductions in Child Abuse Potential scores three times faster than nonvisited mothers. Six confirmed cases of maltreatment occurred in the visited families as compared with 13 involving the control counterparts. |

TABLE 6A-6    (*Continued*)

| Intervention | Citation | Initial/Final Sample Size Duration of Intervention Follow-up |
|---|---|---|
| Home visits by nurses providing education about child development and nutrition compared with a prenatal-only condition and a no-visit condition; free well-child visits and transportation to clinic were provided for single, primiparous mothers of low socioeconomic status in rural New York. | Olds, 1992 Olds et al., 1986, 1988, 1994, 1995 | N(transportation, well-child care) = 94 N(prenatal visits) = 100 N(pre/postnatal visits) = 94 N(O) = 90 N(high-risk nurse-visited infancy) = 18 N(comparison high-risk nurse-visited pregnancy) = 22 |
| Home visits biweekly during the 10-month school year for 2 years. The home visitor brings a gift of a toy or book to the family each week and demonstrates how verbal interaction between children and adults can be encouraged. Provided to parents of children aged 2 years in Bermuda. | Scarr and McCartney, 1988 | N(X) = 78 N(O) = 39 2 years |

SOURCE:  Committee on the Assessment of Family Violence Interventions, National Research Council and Institute of Medicine, 1998.

| Data Collection | Results |
|---|---|
| Interviews, infant assessment, medical records, Bayley Scales, Cattel Scales, Infant Temperament Q-Sort procedure, Caldwell and Bradley Home Environment Scales, records of abuse and neglect reports | Nurse-visited children lived in homes with fewer hazards for children, had 40% fewer injuries and ingestions, 45% fewer behavioral and parental coping problems noted in the physician record, and 35% fewer visits to the emergency room than the nonvisited children. Beneficial effects for visited mothers were noted in their efforts to pursue their education, employment, and reductions in subsequent unintended pregnancies. High-risk mothers (described as young, adolescent, and poor) visited during their child's infancy were less likely to be reported for child abuse and neglect (0.04) than high-risk mothers who received visits only during pregnancy (0.18). Treatment contrasts for groups at lower risk did not reach statistical significance. |
| Stanford-Binet Test of Intelligence, Bayley Scale of Mental Development, achievement test designed to assess the curriculum of the program, delay of gratification test, Infant Behavior Record, Cain-Levine Social Competence Scale, Childhood Personality Scale, parent report, Parent as Educator review, discipline techniques interview, maternal teaching test | The program had few demonstrable effects on any segment of the sample, even for the socioeconomically disadvantaged. |

TABLE 6B-1    Quasi-Experimental Evaluations of Domestic Violence
Screening, Identification, and Medical Care Responses

| Intervention | Citation | Initial/Final Sample Size / Duration of Intervention / Follow-up |
|---|---|---|
| Emergency room protocol for obtaining trauma history. | McLeer et al., 1989 | N (female trauma patients identified as being battered preprotocol) = 5.6% |
| | McLeer and Anwar, 1989 | N (female trauma patients identified as being battered immediately after protocol introduction) = 30% |
| | | N (female trauma patients identified as being battered 8 years after the protocol was introduced, with no formal effort to continue its use in the emergency department) = 7.7% |
| | | 8-year follow-up to measure rates of identification |
| Emergency department protocol to identify battered women. | Olson et al., 1996 | N (female trauma patients identified as battered preprotocol) = 2.0% |
| | | N (female trauma patients identified as battered after emergency department chart was modified to ask questions about domestic violence) = 3.4% |
| | | N (female trauma patients identified as being battered after 30-day domestic violence education for emergency department staff) = 3.6% |

| Data Collection | Results |
| --- | --- |
| Review of hospital records to measure number of women identified as battered | The percentage of women identified positive for battering increased from 5.6% to 30% following staff training and institution of the protocol in the emergency room. |
| Review of hospital records to measure number of women identified as battered | Twenty-five (2%) cases were identified as domestic violence in the baseline month, 49 (3.4%) in the chart modification month, and 49 (3.6%) in the education month. |

TABLE 6B-1    (*Continued*)

|                                   | Citation            | Initial/Final Sample Size<br>Duration of Intervention<br>Follow-up |
|-----------------------------------|---------------------|--------------------------------------------------------------------|
| Intervention                      |                     |                                                                    |
| Emergency department protocol to identify battered women. | Tilden and Shepherd, 1987 | N (female trauma patients identified as being battered preprotocol) = 9.72%<br><br>N (female trauma patients identified as being battered postprotocol) = 22.97% |

SOURCE: Committee on the Assessment of Family Violence Interventions, National Research Council and Institute of Medicine, 1998.

| Data Collection | Results |
| --- | --- |
| Hospital records | Enhanced knowledge and interviewing skills of nurses can lead to increased identification of battered women. |

TABLE 6B-2   Quasi-Experimental Evaluations of Mental Health Services for Domestic Violence Victims

| Intervention | Citation | Initial/Final Sample Size / Duration of Intervention / Follow-up |
| --- | --- | --- |
| Emergency room counseling by a social worker, overnight hospital stay even if not warranted by injuries, counseling after release, referrals to social services, legal services offered to women self-identified as battered. | Bergman and Brismar, 1991 | N(X) = 58<br>N(O) = 59<br><br>5-year follow-up |
| Personal and vocational counseling provided to abused women in a shelter. Second treatment group received same counseling and also used a personality factors instrument. | Cox and Stoltenberg, 1991 | N (counseling only) = 9<br>N (counseling + personality instrument) = 7<br>N(O) = 6<br><br>Five 2-hour modules over 2 weeks |
| Group counseling (partly single sex and partly coed) and couples counseling formats for battered women and their spouses. | Harris et al., 1988 | N(group) = 23<br>N(couples) = 35<br>N(O) = 10<br><br>Includes group counseling, couples counseling, and no-treatment control group<br><br>Ten weekly 3-hour sessions for groups; length of couples counseling determined by therapist on an individual basis<br><br>6-month to 1-year posttreatment follow-up |

| Data Collection | Results |
| --- | --- |
| Use of somatic and psychiatric hospital care during 10 years before to 5 years after presentation in the emergency room | The use of somatic hospital care was dramatically higher among the battered women than among the control women. No decrease in use of care by the women who entered the program during the 5-year follow-up period. |
| Rosenberg Scale, Rotter Internal-External Locus of Control Scale, Adult Self-Expression Scale, Multiple Affect Adjective Checklist, Career Maturity Inventory | The group with the personality factors instrument administration and interpretation showed significant improvement in measures of anxiety, depression, hostility, assertiveness, and self-esteem. The group with the COPS System Interest Inventory and Sixteen Personality Factors Questionnaire utilization showed no significant improvement on any of the measures. |
| Profile of Mood States, Texas Social Behavior Inventory, Social Support Questionnaire, Reid-Ware Three Factor Locus of Control Scale, Conflict Tactics Scales | The group program was not significantly more effective than individual couple counseling in reducing physical violence or improving the participants' level of psychological well-being. Those who received couple counseling were four times more likely to drop out of treatment than those who participated in the group program. |

TABLE 6B-2    (*Continued*)

| Intervention | Citation | Initial/Final Sample Size / Duration of Intervention / Follow-up |
|---|---|---|
| Therapy groups for violent couples and for battering men and abused women separately, provided to couples in which the man had used violence at least two times within the past year, but where the violence did not result in injuries for which the wife sought medical attention. | O'Leary et al., 1994 | N = 70/37<br><br>14 weeks<br><br>1-year follow-up |

SOURCE: Committee on the Assessment of Family Violence Interventions, National Research Council and Institute of Medicine, 1998.

| Data Collection | Results |
| --- | --- |
| Modified Conflict Tactics Scales, Psychological Maltreatment of Women Scale, Dyadic Adjustment Scale, Positive Feelings Questionnaire, Beck Depression Inventory, fear of husband scale, attribution of responsibility scale | Participants in both forms of treatment for wife abuse reported a significant reduction in both psychological and physical aggression at posttreatment and at 1-year follow-up. No significant differences between treatments on any dependent variable. Both treatments evidenced improvement in marital quality at both posttreatment and 1-year follow-up. |

# 7

# Comprehensive and Collaborative Interventions

Social service, law enforcement, and health care professionals have consistently noted that family violence is often only one aspect of the troubled lives of individuals and families who come to their attention. Family violence often occurs in a social context that includes substance abuse, homelessness, poverty, discrimination, other forms of violence, and mental disorders. Researchers and service providers have also recognized that protective factors are often in place in these same communities that mitigate problems for the majority of residents. The presence of multiple risk and protective factors in the physical and social environments of those who experience family violence is receiving increased attention in the design of treatment and preventive interventions (National Research Council, 1993a,b, 1996). Recent theories have emphasized the importance of interactions among family violence, neighborhood environments, and the broader social culture on a range of factors, such as poverty, unemployment, discrimination, and community violence, that may contribute to, or inhibit, family violence.

Three separate but complementary initiatives have emerged to address the complex interactions of risk and protective factors, multiple problems, and environmental effects on family violence: (1) service integration, (2) comprehensive services focused on separate problems that share common risk factors (also called cross-problem interventions), and (3) community-change interventions that target social attitudes, behaviors, and networks. Although the overall goals and characteristics of these three initiatives are similar, they use different strategies in seeking to accomplish change and to improve the quality and range of family violence prevention, treatment, and support services in community settings. The first focuses primarily on using existing services more effectively within a community; the second responds to the needs and strengths of the whole person or family; and the third addresses the community or society itself as the subject of the intervention.

Experience with these initiatives is relatively recent, and research in this area is still largely descriptive. This early works indicates that

- the array of models that has emerged in the last decade are characterized by innovative and experimental approaches to service delivery;
- the emphasis on comprehensive (cross-problem) and collaborative (cross-sector or multiagency) approaches has attracted substantial interest and enthusiasm by community leaders and public and private agencies that sponsor family violence treatment and prevention programs;
- service integration efforts that go beyond agency coordination into the realm of collaboration and resource-sharing require extensive time, resources, leadership, and commitment by the participating agencies; and
- the creation of new organizational units, service strategies, and communication, information, and decision-making systems may be required to implement these initiatives.

Few evaluation studies exist to demonstrate whether comprehensive or collaborative approaches are more effective than traditional forms of service delivery in improving the outcomes of clients and communities. In many communities, the experimental initiatives often complement or extend traditional agency services rather than replace them, making it difficult to isolate the effects of the new approaches. The committee found no evaluations of any interventions discussed in this chapter that meet its criteria for inclusion; we do, however, raise key issues about the methods that should be used in studies of their effectiveness.

In this chapter, we describe what is known about service integration and cross-problem interventions that go beyond individual agencies and take the form of coordinating councils, task forces, multiagency programs, resource centers, and wraparound services. We also discuss community-change initiatives that are designed to shift the balance of power between service providers and community representatives and to foster new approaches that respond to particular needs or objectives as defined by a local community.

## TYPES OF INTERVENTIONS

### Service Integration Initiatives

The hallmark of service integration is collaboration within or between health, law enforcement, and social service agencies. Tremendous diversity characterizes the structure, style of operation, funding sources, and settings in which service integration interventions operate. They do, however, share the goal of enhancing the quality and design of services focused on discrete aspects of child maltreatment, domestic violence, and elder abuse by

- increasing service provider awareness of the multiple needs and complex histories of victims and offenders;
- identifying opportunities for integrating service plans to reduce duplication and inefficiency; and
- enhancing victim safety and diminishing the frustration and harm that can occur when victims are asked to describe a traumatic incident or relationship on multiple occasions in various institutional settings.

Some authors have characterized service integration as an evolutionary and hierarchical process (Swan and Morgan, 1993). The first level consists of informal cooperation, the second level involves interagency coordination and more formal utilization of existing resources, and the third level involves collaboration in which the participating agencies share common goals, mutual commitments, resources, decision making, and evaluation responsibilities. In some communities, for example, existing agencies are not prepared to embrace a true partnership but may share organizational resources with other programs through task force or coordinating committee efforts. Other communities have established a separate agency that provides a central physical location and organizational system supported by borrowed personnel from cooperating agencies and programs. Examples of the latter are the child advocacy centers that have emerged in numerous localities to assist with the identification, treatment, and documentation of child maltreatment, particularly child sexual abuse. Movement across the different levels of service integration is often uneven and is vulnerable to political and administrative factors that influence the integration effort and resource base of the participating agencies.

New programs can emerge that combine services across different types of violence or across institutional domains (Figure 7-1). But separate programs are not always necessary. Depending on the resources available in a particular program, victim advocates can provide their clients with legal assistance and social service referrals to counseling programs, emergency shelter, and child care regardless of their institutional setting.

## Comprehensive Services for Multiple Problems

Comprehensive services seek to improve the quality and impact of service delivery by responding to the multiple problems faced by troubled families in a single service setting. Such problems include violence in the home, substance abuse, inadequate housing, juvenile crime, school dropout, physical and mental health disorders, and unemployment. These efforts have been characterized as dealing with the whole victim or the whole family.

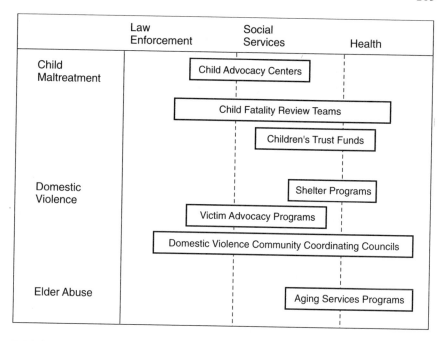

FIGURE 7-1   Examples of service integration initiatives. SOURCE: Committee on the Assessment of Family Violence Interventions, National Research Council and Institute of Medicine, 1998.

In some cases, a specialized unit is created to coordinate and administer a broad range of services; in others, an existing agency assumes a lead role. The administrative style and setting of a comprehensive services program may affect its acceptability to affected parties as well as its overall effectiveness. Comprehensive services are not often designed to significantly change the menu of services available to victims in a given community, but rather to improve client access to existing services and to enhance agency awareness of client needs, case histories with different service systems, and community resources and expectations. In some cases, especially in the area of violence prevention, these initiatives also seek to influence individual behavior and community attitudes about violence through outreach and public education.

## Community-Change Interventions

Community-change interventions involve shifting the locus of power and authority from centralized structures to the level of neighborhoods and community task forces; in achieving this goal, they often synthesize fragmented and categorized service systems (Connell et al., 1995; Kahn and Kamerman, 1996).

They attempt to create social networks in deprived communities that will enable local residents to exercise more power or autonomy in choosing or influencing the types of services available to them (Connell and Kubisch, 1996). Reform of political and social institutions is the primary focus of these interventions.

Community-change interventions are not the same as community outreach, although such efforts may overlap. The latter reflects a concern for community representation, local participation, and cultural diversity in order to improve service delivery, but it does not seek to achieve social change through political and social reforms.

The emphasis on community approaches as a general social strategy to support families and protect children has historical roots that span at least a century. The settlement houses that characterized the liberal reform movements of the nineteenth century, such as Hull House in Chicago, sought to serve a wide range of family needs in a neighborhood context (Halpern, 1990). Staff who lived in the settlement houses worked to establish a center that could spread the culture, values, and resources of mainstream middle-class America among poor and immigrant populations (Garbarino and Kostelny, 1994). These early efforts can be seen as precursors of modern victim advocacy programs, parent education programs, home visitation, battered women's shelters, and other family support services that seek to develop a national prevention strategy for family violence.

Other precursors to comprehensive community services include neighborhood-based projects to combat juvenile delinquency in the 1930s and the 1950s and the community action and model cities programs established during the war on poverty of the 1960s. Perhaps the most familiar examples of community-change interventions are the community development corporations of more recent decades (O'Connor, 1995; Halpern, 1994).

Interventions associated with this approach seek to create changes in social structures and networks on the assumption that these will lead to more responsive institutional and individual behaviors, as well as the creation of new resources that will improve the outcomes of residents and families in the community. Community-change interventions are often viewed as an instrument of progressive social reform, designed to engage multiple community resources in common efforts to foster social well-being rather than dividing the community into separate groups that focus on particular problems. This type of intervention also seeks to empower clients to gain access to services that may be scarce or located in inconvenient locations.

## EXAMPLES OF COMPREHENSIVE AND COLLABORATIVE INTERVENTIONS

The three types of community-based interventions discussed above include fatality review teams, child advocacy centers, coordinated community responses to domestic violence, family support resource centers, substance abuse and domestic violence treatment programs, community interventions for injury control, settlement houses, and shelters.

It is important to reiterate that these interventions have not been evaluated using control groups, and thus their effects on family violence remain undocumented. The committee presents brief summaries of innovative efforts in order to highlight insights into the potential benefits, as well as the challenges, of these approaches. Many of these interventions contain elements of service integration, comprehensive services, and community change as described in the earlier sections of this chapter. The variation in each type of program and the lack of in-depth case studies that could describe their basic goals and methods of operation make it difficult to characterize them in more precise terms at this stage of their development.

## Fatality Review Teams

It is estimated that 2,000 children die each year as a result of abuse or neglect by caregivers (Durfee, 1994). Half the fatalities identified as "fatal child abuse" or "homicide by caregiver" involve children less than 1 year old (Christoffel, 1990). Child fatality review teams are intended to provide a systemic, multi-disciplinary means by which several agencies can integrate information about child deaths in order to identify discrepancies between policy and practice, deficiencies in risk assessment or training practices, and gaps in communication systems that require attention. Since their inception in Los Angeles in 1978, child fatality review teams have emerged in 21 states to address the issue of severe violence against children and infants.

Some jurisdictions regard the most important outcome of child fatality review teams as the protection of siblings in the violent family; others emphasize the improvement of child protection efforts through better coordination and long-term collection of information. Emphasis is placed on the accurate classification of child deaths as homicides to decrease the number of homicides misidentified as accidental death, death by unknown cause, and sudden infant death syndrome (Lundstrom and Sharpe, 1991; Durfee et al., 1992). Improvements in the classification of child deaths are also thought to contribute to the collection of evidence to improve the prosecution of abusers.

Child fatality review teams are generally composed of representatives of the coroner or medical examiner's office, law enforcement agencies, prosecuting attorneys (from municipal, district, or state courts), child protective services agencies, and pediatricians and other health care professionals with expertise about child abuse. Some teams include representatives of mental health agencies, fire department or emergency personnel, probation and parole supervisors, educators and child care professionals, state or local child advocates, and sudden infant death syndrome experts (Granik et al., 1992). In some states, child fatality review teams review every child death; in others, they examine only suspicious deaths.

Investigation of child deaths requires special training in pediatric forensics, pathology, child abuse, and forensic investigation. Researchers have concluded that the specialized review team is more likely to identify the indicators of child abuse and neglect than coroners or physicians who do not have special training (Lundstrom and Sharpe, 1991).

The model of fatality review teams is now being adopted by some cities and states (such as Florida) to investigate domestic violence fatalities as well, but this experience has not yet been described in the research literature.

## Child Advocacy Centers

Community child advocacy centers have emerged to coordinate services to child victims of nonfatal abuse and neglect, especially in the area of child sexual abuse. The National Network of Children's Advocacy Centers estimates that there are 243 operational centers in 47 states in the United States.

An important goal of child advocacy centers is to reduce the redundancy, anxiety, and inconvenience that the child and family may experience as a result of family violence (especially sexual abuse). They seek to improve the handling of a maltreatment case during the stages of investigation, prosecution, and treatment by coordinating social services, health care, and law enforcement efforts. Typically, a child advocacy center is located in a facility that houses representatives of the jurisdiction's law enforcement, child protective services, prosecutors, child advocate, and mental health professionals. This model seeks to enhance interagency efficiency and effectiveness through the physical proximity of the center's multiagency staff, the designation of a child advocate who monitors the case through the various agency systems, and opportunity for formal and informal communication on a regular basis.

## Coordinated Community Responses to Domestic Violence

A variety of approaches have been developed to create safe environments for women who have experienced domestic violence: community partnering, community intervention, task forces or coordinating councils, training and technical assistance projects, and community organizing. Designated as "coordinated community responses," these interventions are examples of multiple forms of service integration (Hart, 1995).

*Community partnering* relies on grass roots organizations to develop various initiatives identified in a strategic plan for community action. *Community-wide intervention* programs represent a broader scope of effort and provide direct services to batterers as well as victims. The intervention projects generally focus on the criminal justice system to achieve greater accountability in the response to battered women and the deterrence of batterers. A well-known example of community-wide intervention is the Domestic Abuse Intervention Project in Duluth, Minnesota.

*Task forces or coordinating councils* are designed to coordinate and improve practices among key political leaders, public safety and emergency personnel, law enforcement officers, health care professionals, social service providers, and victim advocates to end violence against women. Task forces, often comprised of representatives of state and local government agencies and nonprofit organizations, may promulgate protocols or guidelines for practice, support training and technical assistance programs, identify areas in need of systemic reform, establish informal systems of communication, and facilitate conflict resolution and policy formation among diverse groups. In Seattle, for example, the Domestic Violence Coordinating Council includes several committees whose goal is to create and implement a five-year strategic plan to prevent domestic violence in the city.

### Family Support Resource Centers

In its 1995 annual report, the U.S. Advisory Board on Child Abuse and Neglect urged the development of a "comprehensive, child-centered, family focused, and neighborhood-based system of services" to help prevent child maltreatment and reduce its negative consequences among those who have already been victimized. Such a system would include informal family and neighborhood support, assistance with difficult parenting issues via community-based programs, and crisis intervention services. Many of these services are discussed in Chapter 4—the advisory board's emphasis is on blending them and providing them in a local residential setting. The advisory board recommended that such a system should be the principal component of a primary prevention strategy aimed at families with infants and toddlers to reduce fatalities from abuse and neglect, to increase child safety, and to improve the functioning of all families.

A proliferation of efforts designed to establish social support for families at risk for child abuse or neglect has been described in the research literature (see, for example, the discussion of parenting practices and family support interventions in section 4A-1, also Garbarino and Kostelny, 1994). Family support resource centers differ from traditional social service interventions focused on parenting because they are proactive and are available on a universal basis to all families in the community rather than embedded in a treatment program provided only to families who have been reported for child abuse or neglect. Examples of such programs are family support, such as the Family Focus program (Weissbourd and Kagan, 1994); social support networks, such as Homemakers (Belle, 1989); parent education projects, such as the New Parents as Teachers Program (Pfannenstiel and Seltzer, 1989); and home health visitor programs, such as the

Elmira project described in Chapter 6 (Olds et al., 1986; Olds and Henderson, 1990).

Family support resource centers seek to establish and strengthen social support systems that can link social nurturance and social control during formative periods of child and family development (Garbarino, 1987; Weiss and Halpern, 1991). This strategy is designed to enhance community resources that can alter parenting styles acquired and reinforced through a lifetime of experience in a sometimes dysfunctional familial and social world (Garbarino and Kostelny, 1994). Two questions pervade analyses of family support programs: Can family support be a short-term "treatment" strategy, or must it be a condition of life? Can family support succeed amid conditions of chronic poverty or very high risk? These questions pose limiting factors that may influence the effects of neighborhood support programs, including those focused on child maltreatment (Garbarino and Kostelny, 1994).

For parents who lack basic educational skills and experience with positive disciplinary practices, family support resource centers and parent support groups may help reduce the risks of maltreatment associated with corporal punishment and impulsive behaviors. However, these interventions may be ill-equipped to protect children in families with such problems as substance abuse, long-term health or mental health disorders, inadequate housing or homelessness, chronic unemployment, or other dysfunction that threatens the basic stability and integrity of family life. The length and intensity of effort necessary to support good parenting practices in these types of social settings may require extensive resources that can address the developmental stages of children and families and respond to shifting needs over time.

### Substance Abuse and Domestic Violence Treatment

It is beyond the scope of this report to review all community interventions that attempt to reduce family violence by addressing environmental and situational risk factors, such as poverty, unemployment, substance abuse, teenage and single parenting, and social isolation. We did, however, examine community intervention programs that seek to create opportunities for behavioral change in multiple dimensions, for example altering the link between substance abuse and violence against women.

Some communities have taken steps to integrate components of substance abuse treatment into domestic violence prevention programs and vice versa. These efforts take a variety of forms, including joint training on the two problems—an integrated approach—and the addition of a separate curriculum or speaker on a related topic—an additive approach. The relative effects of integrated and additive programs, compared with each other and with more traditional single-topic prevention programs, have not been evaluated.

One study of agency services in Illinois, indicated that, although service providers from both substance abuse and domestic violence programs wanted to collaborate with each other, their conceptual frameworks about causal factors and theories of change contained fundamental differences (Bennett and Lawson, 1994:286):

> Battered-women's advocates, in general, believe that abuse is a deliberate and volitional act. The batterer must accept full responsibility for his violence and must learn both self-control and respect for women. Addictions counselors generally believe that a disease process, beyond the control of the addict, causes dysfunctional behaviors.

These differences in beliefs may militate against service integration and comprehensive service initiatives. One study suggested as much by observing that data on the referral experience in substance abuse/domestic violence cross-problem interventions indicates a pattern of weak linkage and low referral rates (Bennett and Lawson, 1994). For example, 23 percent of the substance abuse staff surveyed stated that they never referred their clients to domestic violence programs. The authors concluded that service provider differences in beliefs about the role of self-control in substance abuse and domestic violence was the most significant factor that impeded collaboration.

## Community Interventions for Injury Control and Violence Prevention

Community interventions to address injury control and violence prevention are based on two assumptions: that multiple interventions aimed at one or more forms of injury will be more effective in reducing risk factors than a single intervention, and that an injury or violence prevention campaign that is oriented to the community will be more successful than one that is oriented to individuals. The community approach often involves public education campaigns in a particular community, highlighting the need for and ways to prevent all forms of injury or violence. More recently, public health efforts have been used to influence behavioral changes in the community with respect to risk factors and health outcomes, especially in preventing cardiovascular disease and smoking.

Youth violence prevention is one area of community interventions designed to integrate public health approaches with local crime control. A recent review of 15 evaluation studies of youth violence prevention programs identified several evaluation issues that require attention (Powell and Hawkins, 1996): the presence of multiple collaborating organizations; scientific and programmatic tension; the enrollment of control groups; subject mobility; the paucity of established and practical measurement instruments; complex relationships between interventions and outcomes; analytic complexities; unexpected and disruptive events; replicability; and the relative ease of research on individuals as opposed to groups. Many of these issues characterize evaluation research on other types of family violence interventions, suggesting the need for opportunities to exchange knowledge and expertise between these fields.

In 1992 and 1993, the Centers for Disease Control and Prevention launched a series of evaluations of 15 youth violence prevention projects in 12 U.S. cities and one county. Although these projects include different types of violence prevention strategies, they are all based on theoretical models that draw on scientific research (for a review see Powell and Hawkins, 1996). The strategies used to implement community-based youth violence prevention programs also may be valuable in planning family violence interventions because the youth violence programs often consist of multiple interventions implemented as a unit for a highly diverse population.

## Battered Women's Shelters

As mentioned in Chapter 4, the emergence in the 1980s of shelters for battered women as a major intervention focused on community change had its roots in the feminist and anti-rape movements of the 1970s (Schechter, 1982). These movements exposed ways in which existing health, legal, and social service systems were not responsive to the needs of women and stimulated institutional reforms to create alternative approaches to providing emotional and legal support in confronting male violence. Reforms were often stimulated by knowledge gained both from professionals involved in rape crisis centers and by the experiences and insights of rape crisis service providers, who were often suspicious of those who sought to blame women for male violence (Schechter, 1982).

Shelter providers often worked to connect individual victims and their supporters with political and economic resources that could break down the institutional and psychological barriers that isolated the experience of rape victims and battered women. Battered women's shelters thus became a catalyst for community service reforms as well as a direct service provider. This role fostered reforms that expanded professional service resources for battered women in a variety of institutional settings, including hospitals, emergency shelters, and women's health programs. Evaluations of the role and impact of battered women's shelters have often missed these effects because of their emphasis on direct service outcomes.

## Community Partnerships for Substance Abuse Prevention

In the early 1990s, the federal government initiated the Community Partnership Demonstration Program. Described as a "macro-strategy" by Cook et al. (1994), this intervention is designed to prevent abuse of alcohol, tobacco, and other drug addiction through the creation of collaborative and coordinated efforts among multiple key organizations and groups serving more than 250 individual local communities across the nation (Kaftarian and Hansen, 1994). Participant agencies include health, social service, criminal justice, and education agencies as well as voluntary and community organizations, private businesses, elected officials, the religious community, and grass roots groups.

The evaluation strategies and research experiences tied to these interventions may be able to guide improved evaluations of community-change interventions in the field of family violence. At this time, however, little is known about unique community factors or organizational arrangements that may facilitate or discourage the adaptation of this approach to family violence (Kaftarian and Hansen, 1994; Lorion et al., 1994; Hunt, 1994). Those who have studied service integration, comprehensive services, and community-change programs have emphasized the need for attention on the implementation process and the innovative efforts and resources needed to design and sustain these types of interventions. They also voice caution about integrating lessons drawn from diverse local community and program settings into a core program philosophy and guiding principles to reshape local projects. These studies demonstrate the difficulty of establishing long-term research programs within a culture of interventions that are focused strongly on empowering communities, short-term action, integrated and comprehensive services, and sustaining financial resources and organizational viability.

## IMPROVING EVALUATION

Chapter 3 contains the committee's major discussion of evaluation of community-based initiatives. Despite the paucity of evidence of the effectiveness of community interventions focused on family violence, evaluation studies in other fields are generating analytical frameworks, measurement tools, and data collection efforts that offer valuable insights. Community-based research is being pursued on children and families (Connell et al., 1995; Connell and Kubisch, 1996; Kahn and Kamerman, 1996), substance abuse prevention (Kaftarian and Hansen, 1994), and child maltreatment (Garbarino and Kostelny, 1994).

In the field of public health, several well-designed large-scale trials have been conducted in the last 15 years to test the impact of particular public health community intervention programs.[1] Yet few of these interventions have had significant impact in terms of widespread behavioral change; rigorous evaluations of most have shown meager effect sizes in relation to the effort expended (Susser, 1995). Four decades of experience with public health interventions in smoking prevention indicates that social movements directed toward behavioral change require extensive time to be effective. The experience with community

---

[1]The most notable of these interventions are the Multiple Risk Factor Intervention Trial, the Stanford Five-City Project, the Minnesota Heart Health Program, the 26-work-site Take Heart trial, and the 22-city COMMIT trials.

trials in changing smoking behavior also suggests that it is very difficult to detect change produced by interventions when large-scale programs are implemented after a social movement is under way. Small effect sizes for the interventions may simply show that the degree of change attainable by the program has already been reached by the progress of the social movement (Susser, 1995).

The experience with community trials also suggests that additional knowledge is required to improve their effectiveness with special target populations, such as youth or individuals who may be chemically addicted or chronically exposed to certain types of behavior and are thus more resistant to change than the general population.

A number of key questions must be explored in the evaluation of community change interventions:

1. Does the presence or absence of community interventions alter the motivation and behavior of at-risk individuals, particularly in terms of their willingness to participate or become involved in formal and informal groups or to use these groups to gain access to services in traditional agency settings?

2. Do changes in patterns of group participation or the creation of social and political networks in the community result in greater availability or use of agency services and support systems?

3. Does the presence or use of community services and support systems change child, family, or community outcomes? In what dimensions?

4. What levels of intensity and what time periods are needed in deprived communities to achieve significant changes in regional rates of family violence, especially among groups that experience multiple problems?

5. What are the most critical areas and what is the rate of change in child, family, and community outcomes that are associated with service integration, comprehensive service, and community-change interventions? Do these areas or rates accelerate or decline in the presence or absence of specific agencies or political leaders? How are they affected by the creation of new organizational structures, the extent of local community participation, or changing social norms?

## CONCLUSIONS

Although comprehensive community interventions are an area of growing interest and activity in the field of family violence, they represent one of the most difficult areas for evaluation research, and their impact remains unexamined in the research literature. Unique methodological challenges confront the development of studies of these interventions, and creative strategies are required to foster partnerships among researchers, service providers, and community residents to assess the strengths and limitations of these efforts to address family violence.

No single model of service integration, comprehensive services, or community change can be endorsed at this time; however, a range of interesting designs has emerged that have widespread popularity and support in local communities. Because their primary focus is often on prevention rather than treatment, comprehensive community interventions have the potential to reduce the scope and severity of family violence as well as contribute to remedies to other important social problems.

Despite their methodological challenges, these initiatives merit systematic evaluation that could focus on several key factors:

• What resource requirements and processes are necessary to implement comprehensive community interventions focused on family violence treatment and prevention?  What critical components contribute to their effectiveness in different social, political, and economic climates?

• Do comprehensive community interventions have greater impact on reducing risk factors, enhancing protective factors, or both?  Do adequate measures exist to examine the critical domains in which changes are expected to occur (such as the quality of social support for children, adults, and families or the timing of services) as a result of a community intervention?

• Is the impact of comprehensive community interventions stronger or weaker when their focus is restricted to a particular population, problem, or behavior?  Are the strategies that are developed in one area (such as domestic violence) useful in addressing other forms of family violence or the relationships between family and community violence?

• How can the evaluations of comprehensive community interventions for family violence draw lessons from evaluation experiences in other areas of prevention research, especially with regard to study design, sample recruitment and retention, and measurement?

# 8

# Cross-Cutting Issues

A vast share of the research literature on family violence interventions is organized in the context of the dominant institutional settings that characterize the field: social services, health care, criminal justice, and community-based programs. This organization facilitates a review of the ways in which service settings influence the development of interventions for the different types of family violence, but it discourages an analysis of the ways in which policies and practices in one institutional setting can affect interventions in the other institutional settings.

As communities move toward the integration and coordination of existing services and the development of community-wide interventions, stronger interest has emerged in the research, service, and policy sectors about the interactions *between* family violence interventions in different service settings. This discussion of cross-cutting concerns is intended to highlight these kinds of interactions. Focusing on these interactions may enable us to identify trends that are often overlooked in research syntheses that concentrate on a single service system or setting.

For example, the emerging integration of health and social service interventions for child maltreatment raises important questions about the threshold of risk or endangerment that should prompt treatment and prevention interventions. These service integration efforts also call attention to the interaction of concerns about privacy and confidentiality with the disclosure and documentation of child maltreatment. The role of the law enforcement and social service systems in identifying and meeting the needs of child witnesses to domestic violence is another example of service interactions that may shape the ways in which child protection, victim safety, mental health services, and family support interventions are developed in a particular community.

As agencies and communities develop comprehensive and collaborative interventions, fundamental tensions can arise from the goals, traditions, and cultures of the different institutional settings. These tensions may require particular attention to the effects of different service strategies (such as deterrence or treatment) in formulating a comprehensive approach to the problem of family violence.

This chapter supplements the committee's research reviews with an analysis of five key issues that arise repeatedly in the different service settings and in efforts to evaluate interventions based in these settings:

- The ecological context of family violence,
- Approaches to punishment and rehabilitation,
- The roles of autonomy and competence,
- Cultural factors and community representation, and
- Assessment of dangerousness and risk.

Some of these issues are unique to the field of family violence; others are more generally associated with violence research, criminal justice research, and community-based programs. Although the committee did not attempt to pursue these issues in great depth, the following discussion clarifies these issues, describes the relevant research, and examines their implications for the design of interventions and evaluations.

## THE ECOLOGICAL CONTEXT OF FAMILY VIOLENCE

Many theoretical frameworks seek to explain the causes of child maltreatment, domestic violence, and elder abuse. Evolving in different historical periods, these frameworks assign different levels of responsibility to individuals (including the parent, spouse, and child), the family, the community, and society in general (see Figure 8-1). Although no single theoretical framework dominates the field, both researchers and service providers are increasingly focused on the interactions that occur across multiple levels.

In the area of child maltreatment, early interventions focused on the individual characteristics of offenders and sought to explain maltreatment in terms of individual pathology (National Research Council, 1993a). However, only a very small percentage of child abuse and neglect cases involve parental psychosis (Pelton, 1989); the extent of less severe mental disorders is unknown.

More recent studies have yielded important distinctions between abusive and nonabusive parents in terms of expectations for their children, the extent to which parents view their children's behavior as stressful, and their view of themselves as inadequate or incompetent parents (Wolfe, 1991; National Research Council,

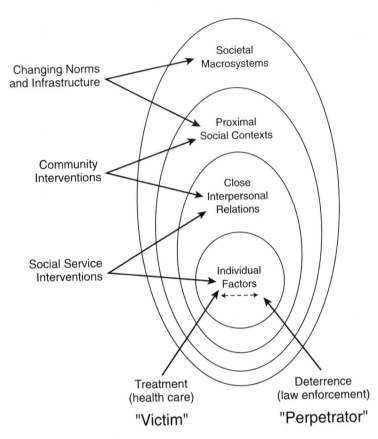

FIGURE 8-1 Systems that influence family violence and interventions to address them. SOURCE: Committee on the Assessment of Family Violence Interventions, National Research Council and Institute of Medicine, 1998.

1993a). What is not certain is how perceptions about adequate or competent parenting interact with the social ecology of the family, especially under conditions of poverty and economic distress. Many cases of child abuse and neglect involve disruptions of childrearing that coexist with other serious problems, such as poverty, substance abuse, transiency, and antisocial behavior (National Research Council, 1993a). Researchers and service providers have focused attention on the interactions between parenting behaviors and broader family or community factors that may contribute to the abuse or neglect.

The social ecology approach in child maltreatment interventions has stimulated interest in the need for concrete and supportive interventions for families (as opposed to educative and counseling interventions) to provide child care, housing assistance, job training, and employment referrals in addition to parenting education. These services are designed to improve the safety and protection of children, to enhance family interactions, and to strengthen community supports for families; they are increasingly offered in neighborhood-based settings as well as at traditional agency sites.

In a similar manner, studies of domestic violence and violence against women have shifted away from single-risk-factor approaches in favor of models that examine the interactions of factors across individual, social, and cultural domains (National Research Council, 1996). Domestic violence interventions in the criminal justice system initially encouraged a search for batterer profiles, based on psychopathology or individual personality traits, similar to that sought for child maltreatment in the 1970s. In more recent years, greater reliance has been placed on a series of multifactor models, testing new hypotheses regarding the relationship between domestic violence and other forms of violent behavior among adults (National Research Council, 1996). Some of these models conceptualize all forms of violence against women together (rape, incest, wife battering), rather than emphasizing the nature of family or intimate relationships as the pathway to violence (Counts et al., 1992; Levinson, 1989; Dobash and Dobash, 1979). Accordingly, domestic violence prevention advocates have emphasized the need to reform cultural attitudes toward gender in general and male attitudes toward women in particular as part of the social intervention process. Domestic violence interventions have also begun to stress the importance of addressing the material and financial needs of victims to help them to lead violence-free lives.

Although social ecology models have been used extensively in the development of interventions in the health care and social services domains, until recently they have had limited utility in law enforcement. Legal interventions such as investigative, arrest, and prosecution policies and practices have traditionally focused on individual motivation, standards of evidence, and the determination of criminal intent and behavior. With the development of drug courts, victim advocacy, and community policing programs, however, law enforcement agencies now pay more attention to the social context and settings in which violence occurs, prompting attention to family and community factors that accompany incidents and patterns of violence. This broader framework has encouraged the development of legal interventions that seek to enhance victim safety by improving the capacity of communities to care for their vulnerable members during times of distress and emergency need. In the area of domestic violence, the criminal justice system has been used extensively as an instrument of social change, designed not only to hold batterers accountable for their actions but also to serve as a referral source to enhance victim safety.

In the area of elder abuse, limited attention has been given to the ecological context of family violence. Rather, this field remains dominated by risk assessment models that focus on single risk and protective factors in the design of interventions.

The ecological framework, although still in an early stage of development, suggests that some forms of family violence may share risk factors and common origins and thus warrant common approaches—for example, training child welfare and law enforcement officials to recognize the relationships between domestic violence and child maltreatment. Other forms of family violence result from interactions among particular risk factors—for example, mental disorders and substance abuse—that can aggravate aggressive and injurious behavior. The presence of multiple risk factors in a household may require targeted interventions and risk assessment approaches to identify warning signals and dangerous settings from which the child or offending adult should be quickly removed in the interest of safety.

Achieving the right balance between comprehensive and targeted approaches requires knowledge of the strength of interactive relationships among the antecedents of family violence, particularly those that present extreme risks to the victim. Such knowledge can contribute to the development of community-based interventions as a form of primary prevention, an approach that can strengthen protective factors and reduce risk factors before cases or patterns of behavior require more intensive treatment. The interactive ecological models of family violence may have great potential for the development of theory to guide intervention efforts, but to date the research base has not developed the capacity to explain the multiple pathways involved.

This process of locating the level at which an intervention is focused has acquired new importance with the use of performance standards and outcome assessments in the management of human services agencies. Standards focused on reducing child deaths and injuries from abuse and neglect, for example, need to move beyond case report measures to take account of interim indicators, such as the availability and use of services and other interactions that may accompany or precede changes in child death and intentional injury trends. This approach emphasizes the importance of the availability and use of parent support services, the density and quality of community services and resources for low-income families, and the consistency of messages and norms in a social setting or community that encourage child safety and well-being and discourage the use of violence to resolve conflicts between spouses or in parent-child interactions. Evaluations of the impact of family support interventions, for example, could consider whether the presence and use of support services are associated with the patterns and level of violence in a community beyond their impact on specific clients or families.

## APPROACHES TO PUNISHMENT AND REHABILITATION

The development of family violence interventions has evolved in a social context that stresses the importance of both punishment and rehabilitation. Punishment is generally associated with law enforcement interventions, and it may include actions that are designed to deter as well as incapacitate offenders in the expectation that such efforts will foster individual and community safety. Punishment may also include acts of retribution that reflect society's belief that offenders must pay for serious acts of violence that violate basic principles of social conduct. Components of incapacitation, retribution, and deterrence theories are reflected in various proposals to address family violence, including mandatory sentencing procedures, increased prosecution and arrest practices, and attaching special conditions to protective orders (such as restrictions on access to firearms or a driver's license).

The criminalization of child maltreatment, domestic violence, and elder abuse classifies as criminal certain acts of family violence in the federal and state criminal and civil codes, fosters the creation of distinct categories of victims and perpetrators in the justice system, requires evidence of wrongdoing, and establishes a process to remove an offender or victim from the home environment without unreasonable delay. The criminal justice system has traditionally been reluctant to impose fines, sentences, and other punitive sanctions on individuals charged with child maltreatment, domestic violence, or elder abuse. Such cases are generally regarded as difficult to substantiate and to prosecute. Supporting evidence is often difficult to obtain, sometimes because witnesses are not willing to present evidence against those with whom they share a family or intimate relationship.

In contrast, the rehabilitation, or therapeutic, perspective is built around different assumptions that have guided the development of service interventions in social and health settings. This perspective often focuses on the multiple social problems that characterize the relationships and settings in which family violence occurs, such as substance abuse, unemployment, homelessness, and community crime. The rehabilitation approach further assumes that reducing the sources of stress or conflict in a family or intimate relationship will lead to more enduring reductions in violent behavior, although such efforts may involve extensive time and may require a temporary removal of the offender or victim. Rehabilitation interventions generally focus on changing perceptions and beliefs, such as inappropriate expectations about children's behavior or socialized belief systems that reflect male use of power and control over women. These multiple dysfunctions are seen as stressors that threaten healthy family functioning, disturb the development of parent-child and intimate partner relationships, and contribute to the use of violence in response to stressful situations.

The rehabilitation approach recognizes that, even when acts of violence occur in a family or intimate relationship, the ongoing nature of the relationships may provide many benefits as well as potential risks. The affected parties may want the violence to cease, but may also want the relationships to continue. These dual interests can foster ambivalence and uncertainty that may discourage some victims from seeking assistance from police or the courts because of their association with punitive interventions.

These two perspectives, which emphasize different ways of addressing the problem of family violence, can lead to very different types of interventions. Punitive interventions in law enforcement settings have generally been reserved for more severe cases of family violence. The rehabilitation and support services associated with social and health care settings are associated with the larger number of cases that involve child neglect or occasional or even chronic, but minor, incidents of violence. The shift in attention to the social settings and interactive nature of family violence, however, has stimulated a broad rethinking of the roles of law enforcement, social services, and health care, resulting in innovative approaches that seek to blend the deterrent capabilities of the law with the treatment and support resources of health and social service providers. This approach includes consideration of contextual and community factors, as well as client history, in the disposition of individual cases.

For example, punitive interventions, such as arrests and protective orders for domestic violence, can be important gateways to therapeutic treatment services for both offenders and victims, either as a complement or as an alternative to fines or incarceration. In this way, punitive interventions can take on aspects of respite services, providing opportunities for education, counseling, and concrete support services during the temporary removal of the offender.

The use of mandatory reporting and investigative systems that are designed to integrate social services and law enforcement interventions are regarded as another effort to blend punitive and support services, enabling appropriate authority to take action against the offender if necessary and to provide appropriate services for the victim. However, the threshold for intervention by the legal system is often higher than that for social and health interventions, requiring evidence of, rather than risk for, harm.

Service providers in various institutional settings must often determine which types of family violence cases and circumstances are appropriate for punishment (which includes deterrence, incapacitation, and compulsory treatment) or for therapeutic services (which include voluntary treatment and support programs). In making these distinctions, a host of ethical, legal, and economic issues arise that reflect competing goals and values. These issues often emerge acutely in risk assessment decisions and safety planning strategies, especially when the violence is severe, when the likelihood that it will recur is uncertain, and when the victim is particularly vulnerable or believed not to be competent to make decisions about his or her own well-being.

One area in which law and social service interventions seek to balance concerns about punishment and rehabilitation is court oversight of batterer treatment programs. Some research indicates that it does increase rates of completion (Dutton, 1995a), and completion has been linked to reductions in violent behavior, but the extent to which court oversight increases an individual offender's readiness to change remains elusive. Increasing the penalties for failure to comply with a treatment protocol is thought to ensure greater compliance and cooperation with the services system, although deterrence theory recognizes that there are limits to the influence over individual and group behavior of sanctions and controls—at some point, the perceived costs of compliance with a coercive treatment program may outweigh the benefits to be gained. Deterrence theory also suggests that law enforcement systems can be powerful instruments of social change if they hold batterers accountable for their behavior, protect victims, and foster deterrence throughout society. However, if law enforcement officials are not prepared to respond swiftly, or if resources are not available to support appropriate treatment services for less severe cases, the deterrent effects of the criminal justice response to family violence can be weakened.

Many uncertainties remain regarding the effectiveness of voluntary and coercive treatment programs in addressing different forms of family violence. These uncertainties are likely to continue until new knowledge or compelling theories can explain the probable outcomes associated with different types of treatment protocols. Experimental studies are needed that can compare the participation and completion rates, behavioral changes, and long-term effects of voluntary and coercive programs. The quality of the knowledge base will also be improved by studies that examine whether the use of sanctions enhances participation in batterers treatment programs, and whether treatment programs influence victim safety through the surveillance and monitoring of offenders. In the interim, the lack of clear research guidance in this area will foster an environment characterized by competing interests involving family integrity, community and victim safety, individual privacy, accountability, and the protection of vulnerable individuals.

## THE ROLES OF AUTONOMY AND COMPETENCE

Issues of autonomy and competence in family violence interventions arise in many settings and involve individuals who are engaged in family violence interventions, who are at risk of family violence, and who are involved in research evaluation studies. These issues involve the abilities of individuals across the life span to determine what is in their own interest or to determine the best interests of children or elders whose caregivers cannot fulfill their obligations. The compromised autonomy of elders and the functional incompetence of children are often cited as specific examples of these issues, although questions of autonomy and competence arise for mature adults as well. The experience of the law enforcement system with battered women who decline to press charges or who will not testify against their batterers, for example, has stimulated interventions designed to allow police and prosecutors to proceed with legal action even if the assault victim or witness does not cooperate. Women who have experienced continued violence in their family and intimate relationships may be extremely fearful for their safety or that of their children. They may not perceive themselves as victims and may be unwilling to request or support interventions from outside agencies. Shifting societal norms regarding the nature of violence between intimate partners have raised many questions regarding the extent to which law enforcement systems can or should intervene in cases in which victims refuse to hold their partners accountable for violent actions.

In evaluations of family violence interventions, two important issues have emerged: the problems of coercion and of the loss of privacy, both intentional and unintentional. Government regulations and professional standards that guide research on human subjects emphasize the principle of informed consent, based on the premise that subjects should be informed about the purpose and nature of research in which they will be asked to participate and that they should have an opportunity to consent to—or to refuse—such participation. Informed consent includes the principle that research subjects (or, in research involving children and minors, their parents or other custodial adults) should authorize the release of personal data and records regarding their own behavior or health status.

Many individuals who are the subjects of family violence interventions are either victims or perpetrators of child maltreatment, domestic violence, or elder abuse. These individuals may volunteer for treatment or support services, but in many cases they are referred for services without their consent. Individuals may also be arrested, removed from their home, or lose their rights as custodial parents as a result of court interventions. Research on family violence interventions therefore involves interactions with people who are in a highly vulnerable status, who may not be able to clearly discern distinctions between research and services, and who may not understand or wish to cooperate with the objectives of a research project. Individuals who are incarcerated, under court supervision, or dependent on public services may have a limited understanding of the ways in which they can exercise rights over the use of their personal records, or of the ways in which information disclosed in research interviews may be shared with others. This observation is particularly true when the research or evaluation studies are being conducted by public agencies or organizations that are involved in the delivery of the services.

The report from a series of meetings on ethical issues in violence research conducted by the National Institute of Mental Health from 1991 to 1993 observed that researchers who conduct violence studies must guard against unintentionally pressuring people to participate (National Institute of Mental Health, 1993). Participants who are clients in treatment programs, therapeutic day care centers, probation and corrections offices, and the courts may believe that negative consequences will result if they choose not to participate in or withdraw from a study on family violence. For example, participants recruited from a no-cost treatment program may believe they will be dropped from the program or asked to pay for services if they do not agree to participate in a research study.

Although the issue of confidentiality of research and the use of personal and public records has been examined in previous studies (National Research Council, 1985, 1993c), unique sensitivities arise in the context of family violence. Concerns involving stigma, bias, and labeling require special consideration in structuring group interviews, providing guidance and referrals for victims who have not been reported prior to their participation in a study, and assessing medical, child welfare, employment and police records. Furthermore, the safety of research subjects should be of paramount concern to the investigator. Individuals who are asked to participate in research studies should not be placed at greater risk as a result of their agreement—or refusal—to serve as a research subject.

## CULTURAL FACTORS AND COMMUNITY REPRESENTATION

Cultural factors and community representation are important issues in discussions of individual interventions and evaluations. Research in this area is based primarily on descriptive studies, and findings are preliminary in the absence of sound empirical data. The ways in which cultural practices, social class, and economic opportunities interact with intimate, parenting, and caregiving practices are only beginning to emerge in the research literature and scant attention has been given to them in the dynamics of family violence.

One study of ethnographies from 90 non-Western societies found wife-beating to be the most common form of family violence (found in 84 percent of the societies); physical punishment of children was found in 74 percent (Levinson, 1989). Although wife-beating is often associated with male control of wealth and decision making in the household, no single theory has emerged with sufficient power to explain the prevalence of this phenomenon in the modern world (Counts et al., 1992).

The social isolation of families, sometimes compounded through differences in race, legal status, and language, can interact with cultural and ethnic practices to generate conflict over male-female and parent-child role expectations—conflicts that in turn can stimulate the use of violence to resolve stressful situations. Studies of the role of cultural and ethnic practices as risk factors for family violence therefore need to consider the ways in which such practices interact with a broader set of variables involving child and family management practices and intimate behaviors. Efforts to focus on single ethnic practices or the authoritarian styles of parenting associated with some cultures can divert attention from the harder-to-understand ways in which culture interacts with social environments in a variety of settings to influence individual and family behaviors, especially during periods of danger, economic difficulty, and social change. The absence or presence of social networks that are bound by common ethnic heritage, language, or cultural practices is another important factor that may influence community responses to reports of family violence.

The Multi-Cultural Advisory Committee of the Washington State Risk Assessment Project has developed multicultural guidelines for assessing family strengths and risk factors in child protective services (English and Pecora, 1994). The guidelines help service providers differentiate child, parent, or family dysfunction that may be caused by poverty or the environment from that due to family circumstances or behaviors. However, the advisory committee cautions that there are limitations in current risk assessment research, and some items on their instrument and the scale structure have not been tested for predictive validity for all populations.

Another concern in this area involves issues of equity and fairness in gaining access to services in the conduct of research. In some disadvantaged communities, the introduction of a family violence research study may provide direct services to children and families that are not usually available in the community—such as pediatric and prenatal health care services, mental health and counseling services, and parent support programs. Many local health and social service agencies do not have the resources to continue such services when the evaluation study is completed. Community residents can become discouraged and develop negative perceptions of research if they believe their experiences or neighborhoods provide research materials without any clear benefit to those who reside in the community and who must remain when the researchers depart. Along these lines, at the February 1995 workshop for service providers organized by the committee as part of this study, one speaker emphasized that, in considering the merits of community-based approaches, researchers should be attentive to the absence of skilled resources in many deprived neighborhoods and consider in advance how to prepare communities to assume the responsibility and acquire the resources for family support efforts, especially during periods of extreme duress or chronic difficulty (Thomas, 1995).

Various mechanisms may facilitate the process of community representation in family violence research studies, including the creation of community advisory boards for research projects, the appointment of community leaders in institutional review board membership when family violence study designs are under review, basing the project staff in the community under study, purchasing research supplies and equipment from community-based vendors, and involving local students in the research activity. Such efforts would help ensure that evaluation studies are sensitive to the special needs and resources of local communities, especially those in which ethnic minorities are overrepresented as victims of violence.

Concerns about cultural factors and community representation have emerged in other forms of violence research as well. A study panel organized by the National Institutes of Health (NIH) has highlighted the need for improved coordination and community representation mechanisms in federal violence research programs, especially in the formulation of research questions, study design, data analysis and interpretation, peer review, and training (Stone, 1993). The NIH panel highlighted a critical need to increase the participation of minority institutions, researchers, and organizations in studies of violence, in order to involve representatives from communities who are often the subjects of violence-related research in the processes of study design and implementation. Such involvement would help ensure that the research community focuses on key questions that the communities affected by violence want to address. Greater community involvement may also strengthen attention to important issues relevant to ethnic and cultural competence in the selection of research instrumentation, the recruitment and retention of sample populations, and interpretation of survey responses.

## ASSESSMENT OF DANGEROUSNESS AND RISK

The assessment of dangerousness and severity in reported cases of family violence has become a major issue in selecting appropriate service interventions and assessing their effectiveness (Limandri and Sheridan, 1995). Child and adult protective service providers must decide whether it is safe to leave a client in a setting in which abuse is likely to recur or whether to recommend alternative placement. Law enforcement officers and judges seek a basis for judgments regarding the treatment or punishment of offenders, the placement of children and elders, and decisions regarding custody, visitation, and probation. Clinicians, counselors, and therapists have a "duty to warn" if, in their judgment, a patient or client is likely to inflict harm on another.

The development of service interventions for family violence has brought with it a gradual shift away from clinical assessments of danger and harm, which can be arbitrary and unreliable (Gottfredson and Gottfredson, 1988; Monahan, 1981), toward risk assessment instruments that are based on statistical measures and research on the causes of family violence. The assessment of dangerousness has become a major focal point in mental health law, public health, social work, and police and law enforcement studies, as illustrated by the work of the Network on Law and Mental Health of the John D. and Catherine T. MacArthur Foundation in Chicago. Monahan and Steadman (1994) have suggested seven characteristics to guide the next generation of research in this field:

1. The concept of dangerousness includes several components, including risk factors that can predict future violence, the severity and type of violence being predicted (harm), and the likelihood that harm will occur (risk).

2. An array of risk factors in multiple domains should be chosen that are theory-generated.

3. Harm should be scaled in terms of seriousness and assessed with multiple measures.

4. Risk should be treated as a probability estimate that changes over time and context.

5. Priority should be given to actuarial research (based on statistical models) that establishes a relationship between risk factors and harm.

6. Large representative samples of subjects at multiple, coordinated sites should participate in the research.

7. Managing risk as well as assessing risk should be a goal of the research.

These characteristics have significant implications for the development of risk assessment instruments and decision-making processes in both social services and law enforcement systems. Statistical prediction depends on the construction of risk assessment instruments that can be tested for reliability and validity in various social settings. The development of risk assessment measures for family violence is still in its infancy, and the ability of such instruments to predict who is likely to harm or harm again has not been established. Most "danger assessment" measures have not been validated with different populations (Campbell, 1995). Such instruments establish base rates for a specific behavior, identify specific domains of risk factors that are thought to be predictive for family violence, calculate the likelihood of true and false positives, and test the instrument on varied populations over time to confirm its ability to discriminate between known abusers and a control population.

In child maltreatment investigations and research studies, multiple risk assessment instruments are being used and they are often administered as part of a comprehensive needs assessment process (Campbell, 1995; Cicchinelli, 1991). The state of Washington, for example, has developed a research-based risk assessment instrument for child maltreatment that can assess 32 separate items related to individual characteristics (both parent and child), family functioning factors, and environmental characteristics. Caseworkers rate the importance and identify the "highest" risk factor in an individual case. Research is being conducted on caseworker assessments to examine which risk factors were associated with high overall risk ratings and more serious outcomes such as placement.

A risk prediction instrument for cases involving sexual offenses against children has recently been constructed using a sample of rapists and child molesters released from a maximum security psychiatric facility (Quinsey et al., 1995). The researchers found that recidivism for sexual abuse was well predicted by previous criminal history, psychopathy ratings, and phallometric assessment data. They recommend the use of the instrument to guide clinical judgment.

In the area of domestic violence, Saunders (1995) has summarized research findings on risk factors that distinguish cases involving severe assault from other forms of intimate partner violence. Homicide predictions involving battered women have used several different lists of predictive factors, including Campbell's danger assessment instrument, based on retrospective studies of risk factors in cases in which battered women killed or were seriously injured or killed by their abusers (Campbell, 1995). The instrument has been tested among ethnically diverse groups and has achieved sufficient statistical support for use in clinical settings.

In 1991, the Navy Family Advocacy program adopted a risk assessment model for use in investigating reports of child abuse and domestic violence. It includes 23 variables grouped into 7 risk domains, which include incident characteristics, victim characteristics, alleged offender characteristics, victim-perpetrator interaction, environmental characteristics, nonoffending caretaker characteristics, and nonoffending caretaker-victim interaction (English, 1995). A review of the literature to determine research support for the risk domains included in the Navy model concluded that no single factor can predict the risk of future harm, that risk is produced by an interaction among factors, and that the weight given to an individual risk factor or risk domain may vary depending on the interaction among factors (English, 1995).

In the area of elder abuse, the Illinois Department on Aging has developed a risk assessment process to determine the extent to which a client is in danger of harm, injury, or loss; 23 factors are included (Neale et al., 1996). It also can be used after a designated time period (i.e., 90 days) and at the close of case management to assess change in level of risk over the period of agency involvement.

The growing reliance on risk assessment instruments is an indication of the gradual integration of family violence research findings into service guidelines and practices. These instruments can provide important tools to guide health and social service and law enforcement decisions for individual clients, and they can make an important contribution to more effective evaluations of interventions.

Risk assessment instruments have not been sufficiently validated, however, either for general or specific populations (such as age or ethnic groups). Instruments that do not recognize cultural variation or consider language or distrust of institutional resources as potential environmental barriers to cooperation with recommended services run the risk of falsely labeling certain protective behaviors or attitudes as abusive when they may not be.

The use of risk assessment instruments that have established interrater validity in both research and service provider decisions can provide a consistent baseline for measuring areas of change among both victims and offenders. These measurements can enhance understanding of the pathways and sequences in which behavioral changes occur, contribute to theory-building and data collection, and assist with the screening of clients in evaluation studies to determine who should receive usual-care services (assumed to be safest), so that high-risk individuals are not assigned to innovative but unevaluated interventions.

## CONCLUSIONS

The recognition that no single risk factor can explain or predict the majority of cases of family violence, and no single service program or system can be responsible for treatment and prevention, has stimulated numerous efforts to integrate services and research studies, but the complexity of this task in addressing family violence is daunting. The need for efforts that can offer individual and group support, as well as assess for dangerousness and risk in the development of service systems, requires consideration of a broad range of social science, health, and law enforcement research, including clinical research findings based on case reports as well as community-based studies that can identify broad trends in groups and neighborhoods.

New emphasis is being given to the role of cultural norms, social networks, and community change in shaping individual behavior, family and other relationship practices, and service system designs. These new areas of research, in turn, are stimulating the involvement of local community representatives in evaluation studies and experimentation with innovative study designs, data collection efforts, and the testing of instrumentation.

The next generation of interventions and evaluations in the field of family violence, especially in the area of comprehensive community services, is likely to focus attention on the ways in which different service systems provide consistent or contradictory messages in their interactions with clients and communities. Fundamental differences in attitudes and beliefs about the causes and consequences of family violence, and the purpose and roles of different service sectors, can be expected to provoke discussions about the relative importance—and timing—of punishment, oversight, rehabilitation, retribution, deterrence, treatment, and the use of mandatory and voluntary services in addressing child maltreatment, domestic violence, and elder abuse.

These discussions will benefit from research studies and exchanges among researchers and service providers to clarify areas in which the knowledge base is strong enough to guide agency practices and, when appropriate, establish performance standards to assess their effectiveness. The shift from practices based on ideology and habit to ones that are shaped by empirical research will not be easy; many conflicts can be expected to emerge when research findings diverge from conventional wisdom in areas such as child protection, batterer treatment, victim safety, and community well-being, or when research instruments are not strong enough to capture hard-to-measure factors that influence interactions among individuals, families, and communities. Concerns for privacy, autonomy, justice, and care for vulnerable individuals and groups will require particular consideration in the development of measures of risk assessment and dangerousness that are compatible with community norms and general principles of social governance.

The absence of minority researchers involved in evaluation studies in this field is problematic. Improving the situation will require special attention to training programs, research opportunities, minority research supplement efforts, and career development strategies to diversify the ethnic and cultural representation of the research expertise focused on family violence.

Finally, it is important to clarify the ethical principles that can provide design strategies for research investigators as they probe more deeply into the parenting practices, intimate relationships, service use patterns, and social networks of those who are affected by violence in families.

# 9

# Conclusions and Recommendations

The problems of child maltreatment, domestic violence, and elder abuse have generated hundreds of separate interventions in social service, health, and law enforcement settings. This array of interventions has been driven by the urgency of the different types of family violence, client needs, and the responses of service providers, advocates, and communities. The interventions now constitute a broad range of institutional services that focus on the identification, treatment, prevention, and deterrence of family violence.

The array of interventions that is currently in place and the dozens of different types of programs and services associated with each intervention represent a valuable body of expertise and experience that is in need of systematic scientific study to inform and guide service design, treatment, prevention, and deterrence. The challenge for the research community, service providers, program sponsors, and policy makers is to develop frameworks to enhance critical analyses of current strategies, interventions, and programs and identify next steps in addressing emerging questions and cross-cutting issues. Many complexities now characterize family violence interventions and challenge the development of rigorous scientific evaluations. These complexities require careful consideration in the development of future research, service improvements, and collaborative efforts between researchers and service providers. Examples of these complexities are illustrative:

• The interventions now in place in communities across the nation focus services on discrete and isolated aspects of family violence. They address different aspects of child maltreatment, domestic violence, and elder abuse. Some interventions have an extensive history of experience, and others are at a very early stage of development.

• Many interventions have not been fully implemented because of limited funding or organizational barriers. Thus in many cases it is too early to expect that research can determine whether a particular intervention or strategy (such as deterrence or prevention) is effective because the intervention may not yet have sufficient strength to achieve its intended impact.

• The social and institutional settings of many interventions present important challenges to the design of systematic scientific evaluations. The actual strength or dosage of a particular program can be directly influenced by local or national events that stimulate changes in resources, budgets, and personnel factors that influence its operation in different service settings. Variations in service scope or intensity caused by local service practices and social settings are important sources of "noise" in cross-site research studies; they can directly affect evaluation studies in such key areas as definitions, eligibility criteria, and outcome measures.

• Emerging research on the experiences of family violence victims and offenders suggests that this is a complex population composed of different types of individuals and patterns of behavior. Evaluation studies thus need to consider the types of clients served by particular services, the characteristics of those who benefited from them, and the attributes of those who were resistant to change.

In this chapter the committee summarizes its overall conclusions and proposes policy and research recommendations. A key question for the committee was whether and when the research evidence is sufficient to guide a critical examination of particular interventions. In some areas, the body of research is sufficient to inform policy choices, program development, evaluation research, data collection, and theory-building; the committee makes recommendations for current policies and practices in these areas below. In other areas, although the research base is not yet mature enough to guide policy and program development, some interventions are ready for rigorous evaluation studies. For this second tier of interventions, the committee makes recommendations for the next generation of evaluation studies. The committee then identifies a set of four topics for basic research that reflect current insights into the nature of family violence and trends in family violence interventions. A final section makes some suggestions to increase the effectiveness of collaborations between researchers and service providers.

## CONCLUSIONS

The committee's conclusions are derived from our analysis of the research literature and discussions with service providers in the workshops and site visits, rather than from specific research studies. This analysis takes a client-oriented approach to family violence interventions, which means that we focus on how existing services in health, social services, and law enforcement settings affect the individuals who come in contact with them.

1. The urgency of the need to respond to the problem of family violence and the paucity of research to guide service interventions have created an environment in which insights from small-scale studies are often adopted into policy and professional practice without sufficient independent replication or reflection on their possible shortcomings. Rigorous evaluations of family violence interventions are confined, for the most part, to small or innovative programs that provide an opportunity to develop a comparison or control study, rather than focusing on the major existing family violence interventions.

This situation has fostered a series of trial-and-error experiences in which a promising intervention is later found to be problematic when employed with a broader and more varied population. Major treatment and prevention interventions, such as child maltreatment reporting systems, casework, protective orders, and health care for victims of domestic violence, battered women's shelters, and elder abuse interventions of all types, have not been the subjects of rigorous evaluation studies. The programmatic and policy emphasis on single interventions as panaceas to the complex problems of family violence, and the lack of sufficient opportunity for learning more about the service interactions, client characteristics, and contextual factors that could affect the impact of different approaches, constitute formidable challenges to the improvement of the knowledge base and prevention and treatment interventions in this field.

2. In all areas of family violence, after-the-fact services predominate over preventive interventions. For child maltreatment and elder abuse, case identification and investigative services are the primary form of intervention; services designed to prevent, treat, or deter family violence are relatively rare in social service, health, and criminal justice settings (with the notable exceptions of foster care and family preservation services). For domestic violence, interventions designed to treat victims and offenders and deter future incidents of violence are more common, but preventive services remain relatively underdeveloped.

The current array of family violence interventions (especially in the areas of child maltreatment and elder abuse) is a loosely coupled network of individual programs and services that are highly reactive in nature, focused primarily on the detection of specific cases. It is a system largely driven by events, rather than one that is built on theory, research, and data collection. Interventions are oriented toward the identification of victims and the substantiation and documentation of their experiences, rather than the delivery of recommended services to reduce the incidence and consequences of family violence in the community overall. As a result, enormous resources are invested to develop evidence that certain victims or offenders need treatment, legal action, or other interventions, and comparatively limited funds are available for the treatment and support services themselves—a situation that results in lengthy waiting lists, discretionary decision-making processes in determining which cases are referred for further action, and extensive variation in a service system's ability to match clients with appropriate interventions.

3. The duration and intensity of the mental health and social support services needed to influence behaviors that result from or contribute to family violence may be greater than initially estimated. Family violence treatment and preventive interventions that focus on single incidents and short periods of support services, especially in such areas as parenting skills, mental health, and batterer treatment, may be inadequate to deal with problems that are pervasive, multiple, and chronic. Many programs for victims involve short-term treatment services— less than 6 weeks. Services for offenders are also typically of short duration. Yet research suggests that short-term programs designed to alter violent behavior are often the least likely to succeed, because of the difficulties of changing behavior that has persisted for a period of years and has become part of an established pattern in relationships. Efforts to address fundamental sources of conflict, stress, and violence that occur repeatedly over time within the family environment may require extensive periods of support services to sustain the positive effects achieved in short-term interventions.

4. The interactive nature of family violence interventions constitutes a major challenge to the evaluation of interventions because the presence or absence of policies and programs in one domain may directly affect the implementation and outcomes of interventions in another. Research suggests that the risk and protective factors for child maltreatment, domestic violence, and elder abuse interact across multiple levels. The uncoordinated but interactive system of services requires further attention and consideration in future evaluation studies. Such evaluations need to document the presence and absence of services that affect members of the same family unit but offer treatment for specific problems in separate institutions characterized by different service philosophies and resources.

For example, factors such as court oversight or mandatory referrals may influence individual participation in treatment services and the outcomes associated with such participation. The culture and resources of one agency can influence the quality and timing of services offered by another. Yet little information is available regarding the extent or quality of interventions in a community. Clients who receive multiple interventions (especially children) are often not followed through different service settings. Limited information is available to distinguish key features of innovative interventions from those usually offered in a community; to describe the stages of implementation of specific family violence programs, interventions, or strategies; to explain rates of attrition in the client base; or to capture case characteristics that influence the ways in which clients are selected for specific treatment programs.

5. The emergence of secondary prevention interventions specifically targeted to serve children, adults, and communities with characteristics that are

thought to place them at greater risk of family violence than the general population, along with the increasing emphasis on the need for integration and coordination of services, has the potential to achieve significant benefits. However, the potential of these newer interventions to reduce the need for treatment or other support services over the lifetime of the client has not yet been proven for large populations.

Secondary preventive interventions, such as those serving children exposed to domestic violence, have the potential to reduce future incidents of family violence and to reduce the existing need for services in such areas as recovery from trauma, substance abuse, juvenile crime, mental health and health care. However, evaluation studies are not yet available to determine the value of preventive interventions for large populations in terms of reduction of the need for treatment or other support services over a client's lifetime.

The shortage of service resources and the emphasis on reactive, short-term treatment have directed comparatively little attention to interventions for people who have experienced or perpetrated violent behavior but who have not yet been reported or identified as offenders or victims. Efforts to achieve broader systemic collaboration, comprehensive service integration, and proactive interventions require attention to the appropriate balance among enforcement, treatment, and prevention interventions in addressing family violence at both state and national levels. Such efforts also need to be responsive to the particular requirements of diverse ethnic communities with special needs or unique resources that can be mobilized in the development of preventive interventions. Because they extend to a larger population than those currently served by treatment centers, secondary prevention efforts can be expensive; their benefits may not become apparent until many years after the intervention occurs.

6. Policy leadership is needed to help integrate family violence treatment, enforcement and support actions, and preventive interventions and also to foster the development of evaluations of comprehensive and cross-problem interventions that have the capacity to consider outcomes beyond reports of future violent behavior.

7. Creative research methodologies are also needed to examine the separate and combined effects of cross-problem service strategies (such as the treatment of substance abuse and family violence), follow individuals and families through multiple service interventions and agency settings, and examine factors that may play important mediating roles in determining whether violence will occur or continue (such as the use of social networks and support services and the threat of legal sanctions).

Most evaluations seek to document whether violent behavior decreased as a result of the intervention, an approach that often inhibits attention to other factors that may play important mediating roles in determining whether violence will occur. The individual victim or offender is the focus of most interventions and the unit of analysis in evaluation studies, rather than the family or the community in which the violence occurred.

Integrated approaches have the potential to illuminate the sequences and ways in which different experiences with violence in the family do and do not overlap with each other and with other kinds of violence. This research approach requires time to mature; at present, it is not strong enough to determine the strengths or limitations of strategies that integrate different forms of family violence compared with approaches that focus on specific forms of family violence. Service integration efforts focused on single forms of family violence may have the potential to achieve greater impact than services that disregard the interactive nature of this complex behavior, but this hypothesis also remains unproven.

## RECOMMENDATIONS FOR CURRENT POLICIES AND PRACTICES

It is premature to offer policy recommendations for most family violence interventions in the absence of a research base that consists of well-designed evaluations. However, the committee has identified two areas (home visitation and family preservation services) in which a rigorous set of studies offers important guidance to policy makers and service providers. In four other areas (reporting practices, batterer treatment programs, record keeping, and collaborative law enforcement approaches) the committee has drawn on its judgment and deliberations to encourage policy makers and service providers to take actions that are consistent with the state of the current research base.

These six interventions were selected for particular attention because (1) they are the focus of current policy attention, service evaluation, and program design; (2) a sufficient length of time has elapsed since the introduction of the intervention to allow for appropriate experience with key program components and measurement of outcomes; (3) the intervention has been widely adopted or is under consideration by a large number of communities to warrant its careful analysis; and (4) the intervention has been described and characterized in the research literature (through program summaries or case studies).

### Reporting Practices

All 50 states have adopted laws requiring health professionals and other service providers to report suspected child abuse and neglect. Although state laws vary in terms of the types of endangerment and evidentiary standards that warrant a report to child protection authorities, each state has adopted a procedure that requires designated professionals—or, in some states, all adults—to file a report if they believe that a child is a victim of abuse or neglect. Mandatory reporting is thought to enhance early case detection and to increase the likelihood that services will be provided to children in need.

For domestic violence, mandatory reporting requirements for professional groups like health care providers have been adopted by the state of California and are under consideration in several other states. Mandatory reports are seen as a method by which offenders who abuse multiple partners can be identified through the health care community for law enforcement purposes. Early detection is assumed to lead to remedies and interventions that will prevent further abuse by holding the abuser accountable and helping to mitigate the consequences of family violence.

Critics have argued that mandatory reporting requirements may damage the confidentiality of the therapeutic relationship between health professionals and their clients, disregard the knowledge and preferences of the victim regarding appropriate action, potentially increase the danger to victims when sufficient protection and support are not available, and ultimately discourage individuals who wish to seek physical or psychological treatment from contacting and disclosing abuse to health professionals. In many regions, victim support services are not available or the case requires extensive legal documentation to justify treatment for victims, offenders, and families.

For elder abuse, 42 states have mandatory reporting systems. Several states have opted for voluntary systems after conducting studies that considered the advantages and disadvantages of voluntary and mandatory reporting systems, on the grounds that mandatory reports do not achieve significant increases in the detection of elder abuse cases.

In reviewing the research base associated with the relationship between reporting systems and the treatment and prevention of family violence, the committee has observed that no existing evaluation studies can demonstrate the value of mandatory reporting systems compared with voluntary reporting procedures in addressing child maltreatment or domestic violence. For elder abuse, studies suggest that a high level of public and professional awareness and the availability of comprehensive services to identify, treat, and prevent violence is preferable to reporting requirements in improving rates of case detection.

The absence of a research base to support mandatory reporting systems raises questions as to whether they should be recommended for all areas of family violence. The impact of mandatory reporting systems in the area of child maltreatment and elder abuse remains unexamined. The committee therefore suggests that it is important for the states to proceed cautiously at this time and to delay adopting a mandatory reporting system in the area of domestic violence, until the positive and negative impacts of such a system have been rigorously examined in states in which domestic violence reports are now required by law.

**Recommendation 1: The committee recommends that states initiate evaluations of their current reporting laws addressing family violence to examine whether and how early case detection leads to improved outcomes for the victims or families and promote changes based on sound research. In**

**particular, the committee recommends that states refrain from enacting mandatory reporting laws for domestic violence until such systems have been tested and evaluated by research.**

In dealing with family violence that involves adults, federal and state government agencies should reconsider the nature and role of compulsory reporting policies. In the committee's view, mandatory reporting systems have some disadvantages in cases involving domestic violence, especially if the victim objects to such reports, if comprehensive community protections and services are not available, and if the victim is able to gain access to therapeutic treatment or support services in the absence of a reporting system.

The dependent status of young children and some elders provides a stronger argument in favor of retaining mandatory reporting requirements where they do exist. However, the effectiveness of reporting requirements depends on the availability of resources and service personnel who can investigate reports and refer cases for appropriate treatment, as well as clear guidelines for processing reports and determining which cases qualify for services. Greater discretion may be advised when the child and family are able to receive therapeutic treatment from health care or other service providers and when community resources are not available to respond appropriately to their cases. The treatment of adolescents especially requires major consideration of the pros and cons of mandatory reporting requirements. Adolescent victims are still in a vulnerable stage of development: they may or may not have the capacity to make informed decisions regarding the extent to which they wish to invoke legal protections in dealing with incidents of family violence in their homes.

## Batterer Treatment Programs

Four key questions characterize current policy and research discussions about the efficacy of batterer treatment, one of the most challenging problems in the design of family violence interventions: Is treatment preferable to incarceration, supervised probation, or other forms of court oversight for batterers? Does participation in treatment change offenders' attitudes and behavior and reduce recidivism? Does the effectiveness of treatment depend on its intensity, duration, or the voluntary or compulsory nature of the program? Is treatment what creates change, or is change in behavior reduced by multiple interventions, such as arrest, court monitoring of client participation in treatment services, and victim support services?

Descriptive research studies suggest that there are multiple profiles of batterers, and therefore one generic approach is not appropriate for all offenders. Treatment programs may be helpful in changing abusive behavior when they are part of an overall strategy designed to recognize and reduce violence in a relationship, when the batterer is prepared to learn how to control aggressive impulses, and when the treatment plan emphasizes victim safety and provides for frequent interactions with treatment staff.

Research on the effectiveness of treatment programs suggests that the majority of subjects who complete court-ordered treatment programs do learn basic cognitive and behavioral principles taught in their course. However, such learning requires appropriate program content and client participation in the program for a sufficient time to complete the necessary training. Very few studies have examined matched groups of violent offenders who are assigned to treatment and control groups or comparison groups (such as incarceration or work-release). As a result, the comparative efficacy of treatment is unknown in reducing future violence. Differing client populations and differing forms of court oversight are particularly problematic factors that inhibit the design of rigorous evaluation studies in this field.

The absence of strong theory and common measures to guide the development of family violence treatment regimens, the heterogeneity of offenders (including patterns of offending and readiness to change) who are the subjects of protective orders or treatment, and low rates of attendance, completion, and enforcement are persistent problems that affect both the evaluation of the interventions and efforts to reduce the violence. A few studies suggest that court oversight does appear to increase completion rates, which have been linked to enhanced victim safety in the area of domestic violence, but increased completion rates have not yet led to a discernible effect on recidivism rates in general.

Further evaluations are needed to examine the outcomes associated with different approaches and programmatic themes (such as cognitive-behavioral principles: issues of power, control, and gender; personal accountability). Completion rates have been used as an interim outcome to measure the success of batterer treatment programs; further studies are needed to determine if completers can be identified readily, if program completion by itself is a critical factor in reducing recidivism, and if participation in a treatment program changes the nature, timing, and severity of future violent behavior.

The current research base is inadequate to identify the conditions under which mandated referrals to batterer treatment programs offer a clear advantage over incarceration or untreated probation supervision in reducing recidivism for the general population of male offenders. Court officials should monitor closely the attendance, participation, and completion rates of offenders who are referred to batterer treatment programs in lieu of more punitive sentences. Treatment staff should inform law enforcement officials of any significant behavior by the offender that might represent a threat to the victim. Mandated treatment referrals may be effective for certain types of batterers, especially if they increase completion rates. The research is inconclusive, however, as to which types of individuals should be referred for treatment rather than more punitive sanctions. In selecting individuals for treatment, attention should be given to client history (first-time offenders are more likely to benefit), motivation for treatment, and likelihood of completion.

Mandated treatment referrals for batterers do appear to provide benefits to victims, such as intensive surveillance of offenders, an interlude to allow planning for safety and victim support, and greater community awareness of the batterer's behavior. These outcomes may interact to deter and reduce domestic violence in the community, even if a treatment program does not alter the behavior of a particular batterer. Treatment programs that include frequent interactions between staff and victims also provide a means by which staff can help educate victims about danger signals and support them in efforts to obtain greater protection and legal safeguards, if necessary.

**Recommendation 2: In the absence of research that demonstrates that a specific model of treatment can reduce violent behavior for many domestic violence offenders, courts need to put in place early warning systems to detect failure to comply with or complete treatment and signs of new abuse or retaliation against victims, as well as to address unintended or inadvertent results that may arise from the referral to or experience with treatment.**

Further research evaluation studies are needed to review the outcomes for both offenders and victims associated with program content and levels of intensity in different treatment models. This research will help indicate whether treatment really helps and what mix of services are more helpful than others. Improved research may also help distinguish those victims and offenders for whom particular treatments are most beneficial.

### Record Keeping

Since experience with family violence appears to be associated with a wide range of health problems and social service needs, service providers are recognizing the importance of documenting abuse histories in their client case records. The documentation in health and social service records of abuse histories that are self-reported by victims and offenders can help service providers and researchers to determine if appropriate referrals and services have been made and the outcomes associated with their use. The exchange of case records among service providers is essential to the development of comprehensive treatment programs, continuity of care, and appropriate follow-up for individuals and families who appear in a variety of service settings. Such exchanges can help establish greater accountability by service systems for responding to the needs of identifiable victims and offenders; health and social service records can also provide appropriate evidence for legal actions, in both civil and criminal courts and child custody cases.

Research evaluations of service interventions often require the use of anonymous case records. The documentation of family violence in such records will enhance efforts to improve the quality of evaluations and to understand more about patterns of behavior associated with violent behaviors and victimization experiences. Although documentation of abuse histories can improve evaluations and lead to integrated service responses, such procedures require safeguards so that individuals are not stigmatized or denied therapeutic services on the basis of their case histories. Insurance discrimination, in particular, which may preclude health care coverage if abuse is judged to be a preexisting condition, requires attention to ensure that professional services are not diminished as a result of voluntary disclosures. Creative strategies are needed to support integrated service system reviews of medical, legal, and social service case records in order to enhance the quality and accountability of service responses. Such reviews will need to meet the expectations of privacy and confidentiality of both individual victims and the community, especially in cases in which maltreatment reports are subsequently regarded as unfounded.

Documentation of abuse histories that are voluntarily disclosed by victims or offenders to health care professionals and social service providers must be distinguished from screening efforts designed to trigger such disclosures. The committee recommends screening as a strong candidate for future evaluation studies (see discussion in the next section).

**Recommendation 3: The committee recommends that health and social service providers develop safeguards to strengthen their documentation of abuse and histories of family violence in both individual and group records, regardless of whether the abuse is reported to authorities.**

The documentation of histories of family violence in health records should be designed to record voluntary disclosures by both victims and offenders and to enhance early and coordinated interventions that can provide a therapeutic response to experiences with abuse or neglect. Safeguards are required, however, to ensure that such documentation does not lead to stigmatization, encourage discriminatory practices, or violate assurances of privacy and confidentiality, especially when individual histories become part of patient group records for health care providers and employers.

## Collaborative Law Enforcement Strategies

In the committee's view, collaborative law enforcement strategies that create a web of social control for offenders are an idea worth testing to determine if such efforts can achieve a significant deterrent effect in addressing domestic violence. Collaborative strategies include such efforts as victim support and offender tracking systems designed to increase the likelihood that domestic violence cases will be prosecuted when an arrest has been made, that sanctions and treatment services will be imposed when evidence exists to confirm the charges brought against the offender, and that penalties will be invoked for failure to comply with treatment conditions. The attraction of collaborative strategies is based on their potential ability to establish multiple interactions with offenders across a large domain of interactions that reinforce social standards in the community and establish penalties for violations of those standards. Creating the deterrent effect, however, requires extensive coordination and reciprocity between victim support and offender monitoring efforts involving diverse sectors of the law enforcement community. These efforts may be difficult to implement and evaluate. Further studies are needed to determine the extent to which improved collaboration among police officers, prosecutors, and judges will lead to improved coordination and stronger sanctions for offenders and a reduction in domestic violence.

The absence of empirical research findings of the results of a collaborative law enforcement approach in addressing domestic violence makes it difficult to compare the costs and benefits of increased agency coordination with those achieved by a single law enforcement strategy (such as arrest) in dealing with different populations of offenders and victims. Even though relatively few cases of arrest are made for any form of family violence, arrest is the most common and most studied form of law enforcement intervention in this area. Research studies conducted in the 1980s on arrest policies in domestic violence cases are the strongest experimental evaluations to date of the role of deterrence in family violence interventions. These experiments indicate that arrest may be effective for some, but not most, batterers in reducing subsequent violence by the offender. Some research studies suggest that arrest may be a deterrent for employed and married individuals (those who have a stake in social conformity) and may lead to an escalation of violence among those who do not, but this observation has not been tested in studies that could specifically examine the impact of arrest in groups that differ in social and economic status. The differing effects (in terms of a reduction of future violence) of arrest for employed/unemployed and married/unmarried individuals raise difficult questions about the reliance of law enforcement officers on arrest as the sole or central component of their response to domestic violence incidents in communities where domestic violence cases are not routinely prosecuted, where sanctions are not imposed by the courts, or where victim support programs are not readily available.

The implementation of proarrest policies and practices that would discriminate according to the risk status of specific groups is challenged by requirements for equal protection under the law. Law enforcement officials cannot tailor arrest policies to the marital or employment status of the suspect or other characteristics that may interact with deterrence efforts. Specialized training efforts may help alleviate the tendency of police officers to arrest both suspect and victim, however, and may alert law enforcement personnel to the need to review both criminal and civil records in determining whether an arrest is advisable in response to a domestic violence case.

Two additional observations merit consideration in examining the deterrent effects of arrest. First, in the research studies conducted thus far, the implementation of legal sanctions was minimal. Most offenders in the replication studies were not prosecuted once arrested, and limited legal sanctions were imposed on those cases that did receive a hearing. Some researchers concluded that stronger evidence of effectiveness might be obtained from proarrest policies if they are implemented as part of a law enforcement strategy that expands the use of punitive sanctions for offenders—including conviction, sentencing, and intensive supervised probation.

Second is the issue of reciprocity between formal sanctions against the offender and informal support actions for the victims of domestic violence. The effects of proarrest policies may depend on the extent to which victims have access to shelter services and other forms of support, demonstrating the interactive dimensions of community interventions. A mandatory arrest policy, by itself, may be an insufficient deterrent strategy for domestic violence, but its effectiveness may be enhanced by other interventions that represent coordinated law enforcement efforts to deter domestic violence—including the use of protective orders, victim advocates, and special prosecution units. Coordinated efforts may help reduce or prevent domestic violence if they represent a collaborative strategy among police, prosecutors, and judges that improves the certainty of the use of sanctions against batterers.

**Recommendation 4: Collaborative strategies among caseworkers, police, prosecutors, and judges are recommended as law enforcement interventions that have the potential to improve the batterer's compliance with treatment as well as the certainty of the use of sanctions in addressing domestic violence.**

The impact of single interventions (such as mandatory arrest policies) is difficult to discern in the research literature. Such practices by themselves can neither be recommended nor rejected as effective measures in addressing domestic violence on the basis of existing research studies.

## Home Visitation and Family Support Services

Home visitation and family support programs constitute one of the most promising areas of child maltreatment prevention. Studies in this area have experimented with different levels of treatment intensity, duration, and staff expertise. For home visitation, the findings generally support the principle that early intervention with mothers who are at risk of child maltreatment makes a difference in child outcomes. Such interventions may be difficult to implement and maintain over time, however, and their effectiveness depends on the willingness of the parents to participate. Selection criteria for home visitation should be based on a combination of social setting and individual risk factors.

In their current form, home visitation programs have multiple goals, only one of which is the prevention of child abuse and neglect. Home visitation and family support programs have traditionally been designed to improve parent-child relations with regard to family functioning, child health and safety, nutrition and hygiene, and parenting practices. American home visiting programs are derived from the British system, which relies on public health nurses and is offered on a universal basis to all parents with young children. Resource constraints, however, have produced a broad array of variations in this model; most programs in the United States are now directed toward at-risk families who have been reported to social services or health agencies because of prenatal health risks or risks for child maltreatment. Comprehensive programs provide a variety of services, including in-home parent education and prenatal and early infant health care, screening, referral to and, in some cases, transportation to social and health services. Positive effects include improved childrearing practices, increased social supports, utilization of community services, higher birthweights, and longer gestation periods.

Researchers have identified improvements in cognitive and parenting skills and knowledge as evidence of reduced risk for child maltreatment; they have also documented lower rates of reported child maltreatment and number of visits to emergency services for home-visited families. The benefits of home visitation appear most promising for young, first-time mothers who delay additional pregnancies and thus reduce the social and financial stresses that burden households with large numbers of young children. Other benefits include improved child care for infants and toddlers and an increase in knowledge about the availability of community services for older children. The intervention has not been demonstrated to have benefits for children whose parents abuse drugs or alcohol or those who are not prepared to engage in help-seeking behaviors. The extent to which home visitation benefits families with older children, or families who are already involved in abusive or neglectful behaviors, remains uncertain.

**Recommendation 5: As part of a comprehensive prevention strategy for child maltreatment, the committee recommends that home visitation programs should be particularly encouraged for first-time parents living in social settings with high rates of child maltreatment reports.**

The positive impact of well-designed home visitation interventions has been demonstrated in several evaluation studies that focus on the role of mothers in child health, development, and discipline. The committee recommends their use in a strategy designed to prevent child maltreatment. Home visitation programs do require additional evaluation research, however, to determine the factors that may influence their effectiveness. Such factors include (1) the conditions under which home visitation should be provided as part of a continuum of family support programs, (2) the types of parenting behaviors that are most and least amenable to change as a result of home visitation, (3) the duration and intensity of services (including amounts and types of training for home visitors) that are necessary to achieve positive outcomes for high-risk families, (4) the experience of fathers in general and of families in diverse ethnic communities in particular with home visitation interventions, and (5) the need for follow-up services once the period of home visitation has ended.

## Intensive Family Preservation Services

Intensive family preservation services represent crisis-oriented, short-term, intensive case management and family support programs that have been introduced in various communities to improve family functioning and to prevent the removal of children from the home. The overall goal of the intervention is to provide flexible forms of family support to assist with the resolution of circumstances that stimulated the child placement proposal, thus keeping the family intact and reducing foster care placements.

Eight of ten evaluation studies of selected intensive family preservation service programs (including five randomized trials and five quasi-experimental studies) suggest that, although these services may delay child placement for families in the short term, they do not show an ability to resolve the underlying family dysfunction that precipitated the crisis or to improve child well-being or family functioning in most families. However, the evaluations have shortcomings, such as poorly defined assessment of child placement risk, inadequate descriptions of the interventions provided, and nonblinded determination of the assignment of clients to treatment and control groups.

Intensive family preservation services may provide important benefits to the child, family, and community in the form of emergency assistance, improved family functioning, better housing and environmental conditions, and increased collaboration among discrete service systems. Intensive family preservation services may also result in child endangerment, however, when a child remains in a family environment that threatens the health or physical safety of the child or other family members.

**Recommendation 6: Intensive family preservation services represent an important part of the continuum of family support services, but they should not be required in every situation in which a child is recommended for out-of-home placement.**

Measures of health, safety, and well-being should be included in evaluations of intensive family preservation services to determine their impact on children's outcomes as well as placement rates and levels of family functioning, including evidence of recurrence of abuse of the child or other family members. There is a need for enhanced screening instruments that can identify the families who are most likely to benefit from intensive short-term services focused on the resolution of crises that affect family stability and functioning.

The value of appropriate post-reunification (or placement) services to the child and family to enhance coping and the ability to make a successful transition toward long-term adjustment also remains uncertain. The impact of post-reunification or post-placement services needs to be considered in terms of their relative effects on child and family functioning compared with the use of intensive family preservation services prior to child removal. In some situations, one or the other type of services might be recommended; in other cases, they might be used in some combination to achieve positive outcomes.

## RECOMMENDATIONS FOR THE NEXT GENERATION OF EVALUATIONS

Determining which interventions should be selected for rigorous and in-depth evaluations in the future will acquire increased importance as the array of family violence interventions expands in social services, law, and health care settings. For this reason, clear criteria and guiding principles are necessary to guide sponsoring agencies in their efforts to determine which types of interventions are suitable for evaluation research. Recognizing that all promising interventions cannot be evaluated, public and private agencies need to consider how to invest research resources in areas that show programmatic potential as well as an adequate research foundation. Future allocations of research investments may require agencies to reorganize or to develop new programmatic and research units that can inform the process of selecting interventions for future evaluation efforts, determine the scope of adequate funding levels, and identify areas in which program integration or diversity may contribute to a knowledge base that can inform policy, practice, and research. Such agencies may also consider how to sustain an ongoing dialogue among research sponsors, research scientists, and service providers to inform these selection efforts and to disseminate evaluation results once they are available.

In the interim, the committee offers several guiding principles to help inform the evaluation selection process.

*(1) An intervention should be mature enough to warrant evaluation.* Evidence is needed, based on descriptive studies, that an existing intervention has been or has the capacity to be fully implemented and that it can attract and retain clients over an extended period. Prior to the conduct of a rigorous evaluation, preliminary research studies are necessary to provide an understanding of the flow and selection effects of participants and to identify variations that may exist in the intervention process as a result of time, client or contextual characteristics, or other factors.

Program maturity does not imply that evaluations of effectiveness should be restricted to areas with a clear track record in the research literature; such a conservative tactic would unnecessarily slow the pace of service innovation and evaluation research. What is more important is that the intervention is able to meet the preconditions for experimentation that are described in the other principles outlined below.

(2) *An intervention should be different enough from existing services that its critical components can be evaluated.* Prior to the evaluation study, key aspects of usual care must be described so that the effects of the intervention can be measured. An appropriate comparison or control group should be similar in character to those who will receive the intervention but it should receive services that are measurably different.

(3) *Service providers should be willing to collaborate with the researchers and appropriate data should be accessible in the service records.* Sufficient support for a sound evaluation effort from relevant service providers is essential to the execution of a rigorous evaluation. If service providers are unwilling to cooperate, or do not understand or support the importance of maintaining an independent study, they can seriously compromise the subject selection and assignment process and create sources of bias within the study. If appropriate data are not accessible in the service records, service providers who wish to cooperate may not be able to provide the basic information necessary for the conduct of the study.

(4) *Satisfactory measurement processes should exist to assess client outcomes.* The rationale for change embedded in the intervention should be clearly understood so that researchers can identify and observe the relevant domains in which results are likely to occur. Research measures that can assess these changes over time also need to be in place prior to the initiation of an evaluation, so that appropriate data can be collected and critical pathways can be explored in areas in which long-term results may not be easily obtained.

(5) *Adequate time and resources should be available to conduct a quality assessment.* A funding source should be in place, prior to the initiation of an in-depth evaluation, that can provide stability and consistency for the study over the period of data collection and analysis. The analysis of long-term outcomes, in particular, requires extensive time, resources, and creative research management to examine whether the intervention has achieved enduring effects for a significant proportion of the client population.

With these principles in mind, the committee has identified a set of interventions that are the focus of current policy attention and service innovation efforts but have not received significant attention from research. In the committee's judgment, each of these nine interventions has reached a level of maturation and preliminary description in the research literature to justify their selection as strong candidates for future evaluation studies.

## Training for Service Providers and Law Enforcement Officials

Training in basic educational programs and continuing education on all aspects of family violence has expanded for professionals in the health care, legal, and social service systems.  Such efforts can be expected to enhance skills in identifying individual experiences with family violence, but improvements in training may improve other outcomes as well, including the patterns and timing of service interventions, the nature of interactions with victims of family violence, linkage of service referrals, the quality of investigation and documentation for reported cases, and, ultimately, improved health and safety outcomes for victims and communities.

Training programs alone may be insufficient to change professional behavior and service interventions unless they are accompanied by financial and human resources that emphasize the role of psychosocial issues and support the delivery of appropriate treatment, prevention, and referral services in different institutional and community settings.  Evaluations of their effectiveness therefore need to consider the institutional culture and resource base that influence the implementation of the training program and the abilities of service providers to apply their knowledge and skills in meeting the needs of their clients.

Evaluation research is needed to assess the impact of training programs on counseling and referral practices and service delivery in health care, social service, and law enforcement settings.  This research should include examination of the effects of training on the health and mental health status of those who receive services, including short- and long-term outcomes such as empowerment, freedom from violence, recovery from trauma, and rebuilding of life.  Evaluations should also examine the role of training programs as catalysts for innovative and collaborative services.  They should consider the extent to which training programs influence the behavior of agency personnel, including the interaction of service providers with professionals from other institutional settings, their participation in comprehensive community service programs, and the exposure of personal experiences in institutions charged with providing interventions for abuse.

## Universal Screening in Health Care Settings

The significant role of health care and social service professionals in screening for victimization by all forms of family violence deserves critical analysis and rigorous evaluation. Early detection of child maltreatment, spousal violence, and elder abuse is believed to lead to an infusion of treatment and preventive services that can reduce exposure to harm, mitigate the negative consequences of abuse and neglect, improve health outcomes, and reduce the need for future health services.  Screening programs can also enhance primary prevention efforts by providing information, education, and awareness of resources in the community. The benefits associated with early detection need to be balanced against risks presented by false positives and false negatives associated with large-scale screening efforts and programs characterized by inadequate staff training and responses.

Such efforts also need to consider whether appropriate treatment, protection, and support services are available for victims or offenders once they have been detected.

The use of enhanced screening instruments also requires attention to the need for services that can respond effectively to the large caseloads generated by expanded detection activities. The child protective services literature suggests that increased reporting can diminish the capacity of agencies to respond effectively if additional resources are not available to support enhanced services as well as screening.

The use of screening instruments in health care and social service settings for batterer identification and treatment is more problematic, given the lack of knowledge about factors that enhance or discourage their violent behavior. Screening only victims may be insufficient to provide a full picture of family violence; however, screening batterers may increase the danger for their victims, especially if batterer treatment interventions are not available or are not reliable in providing effective treatment and if support services are not available for victims once a perpetrator is identified. Screening adults for histories of childhood abuse, which may help prevent future victimization of the patient or others, may also be problematic without adequate training or mental health services to deal with the possible resurgence of trauma.

Evaluation studies of family violence screening efforts could build on the lessons derived from screening research in other health care areas (such as HIV detection, lead exposure, sickle cell, and others). This research could provide data that would support or contradict the theory that early identification is a useful secondary prevention intervention, especially in areas in which appropriate services may not be available or reliable. The cost issues associated with universal screening need to be considered in terms of their implications for savings in possible cost reductions from consequent conditions (such as the health consequences of HIV infection, sexually transmitted diseases, unplanned pregnancy, substance abuse, post-traumatic stress disorder, depression, and the exacerbation of other medical conditions) that may occur in other health care areas. Finally, the risks associated with screening (such as the establishment of a preexisting condition that may influence insurance eligibility) require consideration; such issues are already being addressed by some advocacy groups, insurance corporations, and regulatory bodies in the health care area.

## Mental Health and Counseling Services

Little is known at present regarding the comparative effectiveness of different forms of therapeutic services for victims of family violence. Findings from recent studies of child physical and sexual abuse suggest that certain approaches (specifically cognitive-behavioral programs) are associated with more positive outcomes for parents, such as reducing aggressive/coercive behavior, compared with family therapy and routine community mental health services. No treatment outcome studies have been conducted in the area of child neglect. Interventions in this field generally draw on approaches for dealing with other childhood and adolescent problems with similar symptom profiles.

For domestic violence, research evaluations are in the early stages of design and empirical data are not yet available to guide analyses of the effectiveness of different approaches. Major challenges include the absence of agreement regarding key psychosocial outcomes of interest in assessing the effectiveness of interventions, variations in the use of treatment protocols designed for post-traumatic stress for individuals who may still be experiencing traumatic situations, tensions between protocol-driven models of treatment (which are easier to evaluate) and those that are driven by the needs of the client or the context in which the violence occurred, the co-occurrence of trauma and other problems (such as prior victimization, depression, substance abuse, and anxiety disorders) that may have preceded the violence but require mental health services, and the difficulty of involving victims in follow-up studies after the completion of treatment. Variations in the context in which mental health services are provided for victims of domestic violence (such as isolated services, managed care programs, and services that are incorporated into an array of social support programs, including housing and job counseling) also require attention. Topics of special interest include contextual issues, such as the general lack of access to quality mental health services for women without sufficient independent income, and the danger of psychiatric diagnoses being used against battered women in child custody cases.

Collaborative efforts are needed to provide opportunities for the exchange of methodology, research measures, and designs to foster the development of controlled studies that can compare the results of innovative treatment approaches with routine counseling programs in community services.

### Comprehensive Community Initiatives

Evaluations of batterer treatment programs, protective orders, and arrest policies suggest that the role of these individual interventions may be enhanced if they are part of a broad-based strategy to address family violence. The development of comprehensive, community-based interventions has become extremely widespread in the 1990s; examples include domestic violence coordinating councils, child advocacy centers, and elder abuse task forces. A few communities (most notably Duluth, Minnesota, and Quincy, Massachusetts) have developed systemwide strategies to coordinate their law enforcement and other service responses to domestic violence.

Comprehensive community-based interventions must confront difficult challenges, both in the design and implementation of such services, and in the selection of appropriate measures to assess their effectiveness. Many evaluations of comprehensive community-based interventions have focused primarily on the design and implementation process, to determine whether an individual program had incorporated sufficient range and diversity among formal and informal networks so that it can achieve a significant impact in the community. This type of process evaluation does not necessarily require new methods of assessment or analysis, although it can benefit from recent developments in the evaluation literature, such as the empowerment evaluations discussed in Chapter 3.

In contrast, the evaluation challenges that emerge from large-scale community-based efforts are formidable. First, it may be difficult to determine when an intervention has reached an appropriate stage of implementation to warrant a rigorous assessment of its effects. Second, the implementation of a community-wide intervention may be accompanied by a widespread social movement against family violence, so that it becomes difficult to distinguish the effects of the intervention itself from the impact of changing cultural and social norms that influence behavior. In some cases, the effects attributed to the intervention may appear weak, because they are overwhelmed by the impact of the social movement itself. Third, the selection of an appropriate comparison or control group for community-wide interventions presents formidable problems in terms of matching social and structural characteristics and compensating for community-to-community variation in record keeping.

These challenges require close attention to the emerging knowledge associated with the evaluation of comprehensive community-wide interventions in areas unrelated to family violence, so that important design, theory, and measurement insights can be applied to the special needs of programs focused on child maltreatment, domestic violence, and elder abuse. Although no single model of service integration, comprehensive services, or community change can be endorsed at this time, a range of interesting community service designs has emerged that have achieved widespread popularity and support at the local level. Because their primary focus is often on prevention, rather than treatment, comprehensive community interventions have the potential to achieve change across multiple levels of interactions affecting individuals, families, communities, and social norms and thus reduce the scope and severity of family violence as well as contribute to remedies to other important social problems.

A growing research literature has appeared in other fields, particularly in the area of substance abuse and community development, that identifies the conceptual frameworks, data collection, and methodological issues that need to be considered in designing evaluation studies for community-based and systemwide interventions. As an example, the Center for Substance Abuse Prevention in the federal Substance Abuse and Mental Health Services Administration has funded a series of studies designed to improve methodologies for the evaluation of community-based substance abuse prevention programs that offer important building blocks for the field of family violence interventions.

Developing effective evaluation strategies for comprehensive and systemwide programs is one of the most challenging issues for the research community in this field. No evaluations have been conducted to date to examine the relative advantages of comprehensive and systemwide community initiatives compared with traditional services. Evaluations need to consider the mix of components in comprehensive interventions that determine their effectiveness and successful implementation; the comparative strengths and limitations of inter- and intra-agency interventions; community factors, such as political leadership, historical tensions, diversity of ethnic/cultural composition, and resource allocation strategies; and the impact of comprehensive interventions on the capacity of service agencies to provide traditional care and effective responses to reports of family violence.

### Shelter Programs and Other Domestic Violence Services

Over time, most battered women's shelters have expanded their services to encompass far more than the provision of refuge. Today, many shelters have support groups for women residents, support groups for child residents, emergency and transitional housing, and legal and welfare advocacy. Nonresidential services also have expanded, so that any battered woman in the community is able to attend a support group or request advocacy services. Many agencies now offer educational groups for men who batter, as well as programs dealing with dating violence. Some communities have never opened a shelter yet are able to offer support groups, advocacy, crisis intervention, and safe homes (neighbors sheltering a neighbor, for example) to help battered women and their families in times of crisis. In addition to providing services for victims, the battered women service organizations also define their goal as transforming the conditions and norms that support violence against women. Thus these organizations work as agents of social change in their communities to improve the community-wide response to battered women and their children.

Shelter services and battered women's support organizations are ready for evaluations that can identify program outcomes and compare the effectiveness of different service interventions. Research studies are also needed that can describe the multiple goals and theories that shape the program objectives of these interventions, provide detailed histories of the ways in which different service systems have been implemented, and examine the characteristics of the women who do or do not use or benefit from them.

### Protective Orders

Protective orders can be an important part of the prevention strategy for domestic violence and help document the record of assaults and threatening actions. The low priority traditionally assigned to the handling of protective orders, which are usually treated as civil matters in police agencies, requires attention, as do the procedural requirements of the legal system. Courts have accepted alternative forms of due process, including public notice, notice by mail, and other forms of notification that do not require personal contact. Efforts are needed now to compare the effectiveness of short-term (30-day) restraining orders with a longer (1-year) protective order in reducing violent behavior by offenders and securing access to legal and support services for the complainants.

In-depth case studies and interviews with victims who have had police and court contacts because of domestic violence are needed to highlight individual, social, and institutional factors that facilitate or inhibit victim use of and perpetrator compliance with protective orders in different community settings. Such studies could (1) reveal patterns of help-seeking contacts and services that affect the use of protective orders and compliance with their requirements, (2) highlight the forms of sanctions that are appropriate to ensure compliance and to deter future violent behavior, (3) explore the extent to which the effects of protective orders are enhanced in reducing violence if victim advocates, shelter services, or other social support resources are available and are used by the victim in redefining the terms of her relationship with her partner, and (4) examine the extent to which protective orders can mitigate the consequences of violence for children who may have been assaulted or who may have witnessed an assault against their mother.

## Child Fatality Review Panels

The emergence of child fatality review teams in 21 states since 1978 represents an innovative effort in many communities to address systemwide implications of severe violence against children and infants. Child fatality review teams involve a multiagency effort to compile and integrate information about child deaths and to review and evaluate the record of caseworkers and agencies in providing services to these children when a report of abuse or neglect had been made prior to a child's death. These review teams can provide an opportunity to examine the quality of a community's total approach to child abuse and neglect prevention and treatment.

The experience of child fatality review teams in identifying systemic features that enhance or weaken agency efforts to protect children needs to be evaluated and made accessible to individual service providers in health, legal, and social service agencies. Key research issues include: the effect of review team actions on the protection of family members of children who have died as a result of child maltreatment; the impact of child fatality review reports on the prosecution of offenders; the influence of review team efforts on the routine investigation, treatment, and prevention activities of participating agencies; the impact of review teams on other community child protection and domestic violence prevention efforts; and the identification of early warning signals that emerge in child homicide investigations that represent opportunities for preventive interventions.

## Child Witness to Violence Programs

Child witness programs represent an important development in the evolution of comprehensive approaches to family violence, but they have not yet been evaluated. Evaluation studies of these programs should examine the experience with symptomatology among children who witness family violence, to determine whether and for whom early intervention influences the course of development of social and mental health consequences, such as depression, anxiety, emotional detachment, aggression and violence, and post-traumatic stress symptoms. Such studies could also compare variations in the developmental histories of children who witness violence with those of children who are injured or otherwise are directly victimized by their parents or who witness violence in their communities. Evaluation studies should consider the recommended forms of treatment for these children, the standards of eligibility that determine their placement in treatment programs, and the impact of institutional setting (hospital, shelter, or social service agency) and reimbursement plans on the quality of the treatment.

## Elder Abuse Services

Only seven program evaluation studies have been published on elder abuse interventions, none of which includes random groups and most of which involve small sample sizes. Three major issues challenge effective interventions in this area: the degree of dependence between perpetrators and victims, restricted social services budgets, general public distrust of social welfare programs, and the relationship between judgments about competence and the application of the principles of self-determination and privacy to the problem of elder abuse.

Evaluation studies should consider the different types and multiple dimensions of elder abuse in the development of effective interventions. The benefits of specific programs need to be compared with integrated service systems that are designed to foster the well-being of the elderly population without regard to special circumstances. Evaluation research should be integrated into community service programs and agency efforts on behalf of elderly persons to foster studies that involve the use of comparison and control groups, common measures, and the assessment of outcomes associated with different forms of service interventions.

## TOPICS FOR BASIC RESEARCH

The committee identified four basic research topics that require further development to inform policy and practice. These topics raise fundamental questions about the approaches that should be used in designing treatment, prevention, and enforcement strategies. As such, they highlight important dimensions of family violence that should be addressed in a research agenda for the field.

*1. Cross-problem research.* Richer knowledge of the complex origins and ramifications of family violence has called attention to the need for research that can examine ways in which family violence contributes to, and is influenced by, health and other social problems. Substance abuse and alcoholism are prime candidates for initiating cross-issue research in family violence studies. The co-occurrence of family violence and substance abuse or alcoholism has been documented in public health and social work research, and some communities have taken steps to integrate components of substance abuse treatment and domestic violence prevention programs.

Other candidates are the links between family violence and community violence, which warrant study given growing interest in community-based approaches to injury control and prevention, and pressing questions regarding the interactive effects on children and adults of exposure to violence both inside and outside the home. Research on mental disorders is another opportunity for cross-problem studies that could integrate research on family violence with studies of depression, stress disorders, suicide, antisocial conduct, and related problems.

This research needs to explore critical issues such as the forms and sequence of overlap between family violence and associated problems and disorders; the existence of common pathways that lead to the occurrence of multiple problems and the implications of this research for prevention and treatment; the processes by which the existence of co-occurring problems influence the outcomes and consequences of family violence; and the impact of cultural and social settings that mediate the experience and impact of abuse, service utilization, and outcomes of interventions.

*2. Studies of family dynamics and processes.* Children who are victimized by witnessing family violence have only recently been the subject of research. Although this literature has identified a range of consequences, it has also revealed that many children exposed to violence do not develop marked problems. This relatively young area of research has the potential to take the family as the unit of analysis and integrate the largely separate strands of research on child maltreatment, domestic violence, and elder abuse. For this reason, the committee strongly urges that this line of research be continued in a fashion that cuts across these areas of study.

One productive next step would be to broaden theoretical frameworks for studying how children are brought into violent adult interactions in families and how they cope with and interpret violence in their homes. From the adult perspective, for example, how often are children the "reason why" parents fight and in what ways does this situation exacerbate the effects on children who are exposed to violence? How often do children perceive themselves to be the cause of marital conflict and violence?

Another useful approach would be an examination of the links between family formation and development and the onset and intensification of family violence, looking specifically at stressful stages of family life, such as pregnancy, birth, infancy, and adolescence. Other issues linked to family formation include the use of corporal punishment in child discipline, gender roles, privacy, and strategies for resolving conflict among adults or siblings.

A third approach would be studies to discern the protective factors inside and outside families that enable some children who are exposed to violence to not only survive but also to develop coping mechanisms that serve them well later in life. This analysis would have widespread implications for assessing the impact of biological and experiential factors in specific domains, such as fear, anxiety, self-blame, identity formation, helplessness, and help-seeking behaviors. Such research could also identify abuse-related coping strategies (such as excessive distrust of or overdependence on others) that may contribute to other problems that emerge in the course of adolescent and adult development.

*3. Cost analysis and service system studies.* The economic and social costs of family violence remain virtually undocumented. Cost analysis studies are needed that can distinguish between direct and indirect service costs; the impact of family violence on its victims and offenders; cost implications for health, social service, and law enforcement agencies and community programs; the costs and benefits associated with integrated service records and more comprehensive record management, especially in managed care settings; the extent to which episodes and histories of violence can be tracked within families or across generations; and the relationships between the need or demand for services and the available supply in specific communities. These economic and social indicators will become increasingly important with the enhanced use of performance measures by health care, public health, and social service agencies.

Programmatic research is needed that can identify whether certain characteristics of selected family violence treatment and prevention interventions (such as the mixture, scope, and intensity of services; the philosophy and training of service providers; and levels of institutional support) are related to improved outcomes for particular groups of clients. The effectiveness of family support services (including intensive family preservation and home visitation services) for reducing child and elder maltreatment needs to be studied through the development and critical assessment of models (1) to determine program goals that can be converted to interim and long-term operational measures (especially in the domains of family cooperation and receptivity to services), (2) to examine multiple program outcomes, such as attitudinal changes, improvements in family functioning, environmental issues related to housing and safety, child well-being, and consumer satisfaction, rather than focusing solely on program-specific goals, such as rates of placement or maltreatment, and (3) to clarify program components that appear to contribute directly to positive outcomes and require attention in future certification standards. The advantages and limitations of targeted interventions need to be compared with integrated service systems, especially in dealing with specific age groups and populations (such as the elderly, adolescents, first-time parents, victims and offenders who have substance abuse histories, etc.)

*4. Social setting issues.* In numerous family violence interventions, key social setting issues arise that warrant study because of their implications for the design of treatment, support, prevention, and law enforcement strategies. These issues include ways in which the mandatory or voluntary character of reporting and treatment systems influences service provider behavior and institutional practices; conditions and factors in the criminal justice system that foster deterrence, especially among individuals who have a history of violent behavior and who have little stake in social conformity; psychological, social, and institutional factors that facilitate or inhibit victim use of and perpetrator compliance with protective orders, treatment programs, mental health services, and other interventions in different community settings; classification of groups of offenders that can distinguish offenders who use violence only against certain family members from those who pose a general threat to others inside and outside their family; and behavioral or cognitive processes associated with "natural improvements" or "spontaneous change" (without intervention) in comparison populations of offenders and victims in the different areas of family violence.

## FORGING PARTNERSHIPS BETWEEN
## RESEARCH AND PRACTICE

Although it is premature to expect research to offer definitive answers about the relative effectiveness of the array of current service and enforcement strategies, the committee sees valuable opportunities that now exist to accelerate the rate by which service providers can identify the types of individuals, families, and communities that may benefit from certain types or combinations of service and enforcement interventions. Major challenges must be addressed, however, to improve the overall quality of the evaluations of family violence interventions and to provide a research base that can inform policy and practice. These challenges include issues of study design and methodology as well as logistical concerns that must be resolved in order to conduct research in open service systems where the research investigator is not able to control factors that may weaken the study design and influence its outcome. The resolution of these challenges will require collaborative partnerships between researchers, service providers, and policy makers to generate common approaches and data sources.

The integration of research and practice in the field of family violence, as in many other areas of human services, has occurred on a haphazard basis. As a result, program sponsors, service providers, clients, victims, researchers, and community representatives have not been able to learn in a systematic manner from the diverse experiences of both large and small programs. Mayors, judges, police officers, caseworkers, child and victim advocates, health professionals, and others must make life-or-death decisions each day in the face of tremendous uncertainty, often relying on conflicting reports, anecdotal data, and inconsistent information in judging the effectiveness of specific interventions.

The development of creative partnerships between the research and practice communities would greatly improve the targeting of limited resources to specific clients who can benefit most from a particular type of intervention. Yet significant barriers inhibit the development of such partnerships, including disagreements about the nature and origins of family violence, broad variations in the conceptual frameworks that guide service delivery, differences over the relative merits of service and research, a lack of faith in the ability of research to inform and improve services, a lack of trust in the ability of service providers to inform the design of research experiments and the formation of theoretical frameworks, and concerns about fairness and safety in including victims and offenders in experimental treatment groups. These fundamental differences obscure identification of outcomes of interest in the development of evaluation studies, which are further complicated by limitations in study design and access to appropriate subjects that are necessary for the conduct of research.

Even if greater levels of trust fostered more interaction between the research community and service providers, collaborative efforts would be challenged by factors such as the lack of funding for empirical studies, the availability of limited resources to support studies over appropriate time frames, and the social and economic characteristics of some of the populations served by family violence interventions that make them difficult to follow over extended periods of time (chaotic households, high mobility of the client population, concerns for safety, lack of telephones and permanent residences, etc.).

Service providers and program sponsors have often been skeptical of efforts to evaluate the impact of a selected intervention, knowing that critical or premature assessments could jeopardize the program's future and restrict future opportunities for service delivery. Service providers have also been less than enthusiastic in seeking program evaluations, knowing that the programs to be evaluated have been underfunded and are understaffed and present a less than ideal situation; in their view, the assessment may diminish future resources and affect the development of a particular strategy or programmatic approach. The tremendous demand for services and the limited availability of staff resources create a pressured environment in which the staff time involved in filling out forms for research purposes is seen as being sacrificed from time that might be used to serve people in need. In some cases, research funds support demonstration programs that are highly valued by a community, yet few resources are available to support them once the research phase has been completed.

Researchers and service providers need to resolve the programmatic tensions that have sometimes surfaced in contentious debates over the type of services that should be put into place in addressing problems of family violence. The mistrust and skepticism present major challenges that need to resolved before the technical challenges to effective evaluations can be addressed. A reformulation of the research process is needed so that, while building a long-term capacity to focus on complex issues and conduct rigorous studies, researchers can also provide useful information to service providers.

The committee has identified three major principles to help integrate research and practice in the field of family violence interventions:

- **Evaluation should be an integral part of any major intervention, particularly those that are designed to be replicated in multiple communities.** Interventions have often been put into place without a research base to support them or rigorous evaluation efforts to guide their development. Evaluation research based on theoretical models is needed to link program goals and operational objectives with multiple program components and outcomes. Intensive marketing and praise for a particular intervention or program should no longer be a substitute for empirical data in determining the effectiveness of programs that are intended to be replicated in multiple sites.

- **Coordinating policy, program, and research agendas will improve family violence interventions.** Evaluation research will help program sponsors and managers clarify program goals and experience and identify areas in need of attention because of the difficulties of implementation, the use of resources, and changes in the client base. Research and data-based analysis can guide ongoing program and policy efforts if evaluation studies are integrated into the design and development of interventions. The knowledge base can be improved by (1) framing key hypotheses that can be tested by existing or new services, (2) building statistical models to explore the system-wide effects of selected interventions and compare these effects with the consequences of collaborative and comprehensive approaches, (3) using common definitions and measures to facilitate comparisons across individual studies, (4) using appropriate comparison and control groups in evaluation studies, including random assignment, when possible, (5) developing culturally sensitive research designs and measures, (6) identifying relevant outcomes in the assessment of selected interventions, and (7) developing alternative designs when traditional design methodology cannot be used for legal, ethical, or practical reasons.

- **Surmounting existing barriers to collaboration between research and practice communities requires policy incentives and leadership to foster partnership efforts.** Many interventions are not evaluated because of limited funds, because the individuals involved in service delivery consider research to be peripheral to the needs of their clients, because the researchers are disinterested in studying the complexity of service delivery systems and the impact of violence in clients' lives, or because research methods are not yet available to assess outcomes that result from the complex interaction of multiple systems. This situation will continue until program sponsors and policy officials exercise leadership to build partnerships between the research and practice communities and to provide funds for rigorous evaluations in the development of service and law enforcement interventions. Additional steps are required to foster a more constructive dialogue and partnership between the research and practice communities.

Partnership efforts are also needed to focus research attention on the particular implementation of an individual program rather than the strategy behind the program design. Promising intervention strategies may be discarded prematurely because of special circumstances that obstructed full implementation of the program. Conversely, programs that offer only limited effectiveness may appear to be successful on the basis of evaluation studies that did not consider the significant points of vulnerability and limitations in the service design or offer a comparative analysis with the benefits to be derived from routine services.

**The establishment and documentation of a series of consensus conferences on relevant outcomes, and appropriate measurement tools, will strengthen and enhance evaluations of family violence interventions and lead to improvements in the design of programs, interventions, and strategies.** Many opportunities currently exist for research to inform the design and assessment of treatment and prevention interventions. In addition, service providers can help guide researchers in the identification of appropriate domains in which program effects may occur but are currently not being examined. Ongoing dialogues can guide the identification and development of instruments and methods that can capture the density and distribution of relevant effects that are not well understood. The organization of a series of consensus conferences by sponsors in public and private agencies that are concerned with the future quality of family violence interventions would be an important contribution to the development of this field.

# References

Abbott J., R. Johnson, J. Koziol-McLain, and S.R. Lowenstein
  1995   Domestic violence against women: Incidence and prevalence in an emergency department population. *Journal of the American Medical Association* 273(22):1763-1767.
Adams, S.L.
  1994   Restraining order trend analysis and defendant profile. *Executive Exchange* 2-3.
Agency for Health Care Policy and Research
  1996   Domestic Violence Identification: Outcomes/Effectiveness. Grant number HSO7568. Prepared by Robert S. Thompson and Frederick Rivara. Washington, D.C.: U.S. Department of Health and Human Services.
Alexander, P.C., R.A. Neimeyer, V.M. Follette, M.K. Moore, and S. Harter
  1989   A comparison of group treatments of women sexually abused as children. *Journal of Consulting and Clinical Psychology* 57(4):479-483.
Alexander, P.C., R.A. Neimeyer, and V.M. Follette
  1991   Group therapy for women sexually abused as children: A controlled study and investigation of individual differences. *Journal of Interpersonal Violence* 6(2):218-231.
Alexander, R.C.
  1990   Education of the physician in child abuse. *The Pediatric Clinics of North America* 37(4): 971-981.
Alliance Elder Abuse Project
  1981   An Analysis of States' Mandatory Reporting Laws on Elder Abuse. Unpublished document, Alliance Elder Abuse Project, Syracuse, N.Y.
Amaro, H., L.E. Fried, H. Cabral, and B. Zuckerman
  1990   Violence during pregnancy and substance use. *American Journal of Public Health* 80(5): 575-579.
American Academy of Pediatrics, Committee on Child Abuse and Neglect
  1991   Guidelines for the evaluation of sexual abuse of children. *Pediatrics* 87(2):254-259.
American Humane Association
  1979   *National Analyses of Official Child Neglect and Abuse.* Denver, Colo.: American Humane Association.

American Medical Association
1992a *Diagnostic and Treatment Guidelines on Child Physical Abuse and Neglect.* Chicago, Ill.: American Medical Association.
1992b *Diagnostic and Treatment Guidelines on Child Sexual Abuse.* Chicago, Ill.: American Medical Association.
1992c Violence against women: Relevance for medical practitioners. *Journal of the American Medical Association* 267(23):3184-3189.
1992d *Diagnostic and Treatment Guidelines on Elder Abuse and Neglect.* Chicago: American Medical Association.
1995 *Diagnostic and Treatment Guidelines on Mental Health Effects of Family Violence.* Chicago, Ill.: American Medical Association.
American Psychiatric Association
1994 *Diagnostic and Statistical Manual of Mental Disorders, Fourth Edition.* Washington, D.C.: American Psychiatric Association.
Ammerman, R.T.
1989 Child abuse and neglect. Pp. 353-394 in M. Hersen, ed., *Innovations in Child Behavior Therapy.* New York: Springer.
Andrews, D.A., I. Zinger, R.D. Hoge, J. Bonta, P. Gendreau, and F.T. Cullen
1990 Does correctional treatment work? A clinically relevant and psychologically informed meta-analysis. *Criminology* 28:369-397.
Anetzberger, G.J.
1995 Adult protective services: Intervening on behalf of dependent elder abuse victims. In *Service Provider Perspectives on Family Violence Interventions: Proceedings of a Workshop.* Committee on the Assessment of Family Violence Interventions. Washington, D.C.: National Academy Press.
Ansello, E.F., N.R. King, and G. Taler
1986 The Environmental Press Model: A theoretical model for intervention in elder abuse. Pp. 314-330 in K.A. Pillemer and R.S. Wolf, eds., *Elder Abuse: Conflict in the Family.* Dover, Mass.: Auburn House.
AuClaire, P., and I.M. Schwartz
1986 An Evaluation of the Effectiveness of Intensive Home-Based Services as an Alternative to Placement for Adolescents and Their Families. Unpublished document, Hennepin County Community Services Department, Minneapolis, Minnesota.
Azar, S.T.
1988 Methodological considerations in treatment outcome research in child maltreatment. Pp. 288-298 in J.T. Hotaling, D. Finkelhor, J.T. Kirkpatrick, and M.A. Straus, eds., *Coping with Family Violence: Research and Policy Perspectives.* Beverly Hills, Calif.: Sage.
Bachman, R., and L.E. Saltzman
1995 *Violence Against Women: Estimates from the Redesigned Survey.* NCJ-154348. Washington, D.C.: Bureau of Justice Statistics.
Ball, M.
1977 Issues of violence in family casework. *Social Casework* 58(1):3-12.
Bard, M., and J. Zacker
1971 The prevention of family violence: Dilemmas of community interaction. *Journal of Marriage and the Family* 33:677-682.
Barnett, O.W., C.L. Miller-Perrin, and R.D. Perrin
1997 *Family Violence Across the Lifespan.* Thousand Oaks, Calif: Sage.
Barth, R.P.
1990 *Preventing Adolescent Abuse: Effective Intervention Strategies and Techniques.* Lexington, Mass.: Lexington Books.

1991    An experimental evaluation of in-home child abuse prevention services. *Child Abuse and Neglect* 15:363-375.

Barth, R.P., and D. Derezotes

1990    *Preventing Adolescent Abuse: Effective Interventions, Strategies and Techniques.* Lexington, Mass.: Lexington Books.

Barth, R.P., S. Hacking, and J.R. Ash

1988    Preventing child abuse: An experimental evaluation of the Child Parent Enrichment Project. *Journal of Primary Prevention* 8(4):201-217.

Barth, R.P., M. Courtney, J.D. Berrick, and V. Albert

1994    *From Child Abuse to Permanency Planning: Child Welfare Services Pathways and Placements.* New York: Aldine de Gruyter.

Barton, K.

1994    Healing at home can be cost effective. *California Agriculture* 48(7):36-38.

Bates, B.C., D.J. English, and S. Kouidou-Giles

1995    Residential treatment and its alternatives: A review of the literature. *Child and Youth Care Forum* 26:7-51.

Bath, H.I., and D.A. Haapala

1993    Intensive family preservation services with abused and neglected children: An examination of group differences. *Child Abuse and Neglect* 17:213-225.

Becker, J.V., and J.A. Hunter

1992    Evaluation of treatment outcome for adult perpetrators of child sexual abuse. *Criminal Justice and Behavior* 19(1):74-92.

Bell, C.C., and E.J. Jenkins

1991    Traumatic stress and children. *Journal of Health Care for the Poor and Underserved* 2(1):175-185.

Belle, D., ed.

1989    *Children's Social Networks and Social Supports.* New York: Wiley.

Belsky, J.

1980    Child maltreatment: An ecological integration. *American Psychologist* 35:320-335.

1993    Etiology of child maltreatment: A developmental-ecological analysis. *Psychological Bulletin* 114(3):413-434.

Belsky, J., and J. Vondra

1989    Lessons from child abuse: The determinants of parenting. Pp. 153-202 in D. Cicchetti and V. Carlson, eds., *Current Research and Theoretical Advances in Child Maltreatment.* Cambridge, England: Cambridge University Press.

Bennett, G.

1987    Group therapy for men who batter women: Some promising developments. *Holistic Nursing Practice* 1(2):33-42.

Bennett, L., and M. Lawson

1994    Barriers to cooperation between domestic-violence and substance-abuse programs. *Journal of Contemporary Human Services* May:277-286.

Bergman, B., and B. Brismar

1991    A 5-year follow-up study of 117 battered women. *American Journal of Public Health* 81(11):1486-1489.

Bergquist, C., D. Szwejda, and G. Pope

1993    Evaluation of Michigan's Families First Program: Summary Report. Unpublished document, Michigan Department of Social Services, Lansing, Michigan.

Berk, R.A., P.J. Newton, and S.F. Berk

1986    What a difference a day makes: An empirical study of the impact of shelters for battered women. *Journal of Marriage and the Family* 48(3):431-490.

Berk, R.A., A. Campbell, R. Klap, and B. Western
  1992a  A Bayesian analysis of the Colorado Springs spouse abuse experiment. *Journal of Crimi-
         nal Law and Criminology* 83(1):170-200.
  1992b  The deterrent effect of arrest in incidents of domestic violence: A Bayesian analysis of
         four field experiments. *American Sociological Review* 57:698-708.
Berliner, L., and B. Saunders
  1996   Treating fear and anxiety in sexually abused children: Results of a controlled 2-year
         follow-up study. *Child Maltreatment* 1(4):294-309.
Besharov, D.
  1994   Responding to child sexual abuse: The need for a balanced approach. *Future of Children*
         4(2):135-155.
Beutler, L.E., R.E. Williams, and H.A. Zetzer
  1994   Efficacy of treatment for victims of child sexual abuse. *The Future of Children* 4(2):156-
         175.
Binder, A., and J.W. Meeker
  1992   Implications of the failure to replicate the Minneapolis experimental findings. *American
         Sociological Review* 58:886-888.
Blakely, B.E., and R. Dolon
  1991   Area agencies on aging and the prevention of elder abuse: The results of a national study.
         *Journal of Elder Abuse and Neglect* 3(2):21-40.
Bland, R., and H. Orn
  1986   Family violence and psychiatric disorder. *Canadian Journal of Psychiatry* 31(2):129-
         137.
Blythe, B.J.
  1983   A critique of outcome evaluation in child abuse treatment. *Child Welfare* 62(4):325-335.
Bond, L.M.
  1995   Healthy Families America. In *Service Provider Perspectives on Family Violence Inter-
         ventions.* Proceedings of a Workshop, Committee on the Assessment of Family Violence
         Interventions. Washington, D.C.: National Academy Press.
Borland, E., and E. Brady
  1985   *The Prosecution of Felony Arrests, 1980.* Washington, D.C.: U.S. Department of Justice.
Boruch, R.F.
  1994   The future of controlled randomized experiments: A briefing. *Evaluation Practice* 15(3):
         265-274.
Brayden, R.M., W.A. Altemeier, M.S. Dietrich, D.D. Tucker, M.J. Christensen, F.J. McLaughlin,
and K.B. Sherrod
  1993   A prospective study of secondary prevention of child maltreatment. *Pediatrics* 122(4):
         511-516.
Briere, J.N.
  1996   Treatment outcome research with abused children: Methodological considerations in three
         studies. *Child Maltreatment* 14:348-352.
Bronfenbrenner, U.
  1979   *The Ecology of Human Development.* Cambridge, Mass.: Harvard University Press.
Brooks-Gunn, J.
  1990   Promoting healthy development in young children: What educational interventions work?
         Pp. 125-145 in D.E. Rodgers and E. Ginzberg, eds., *Improving the Life Chances of Chil-
         dren at Risk.* Boulder, Colo.: Westview Press.
Brosig, C.L., and S.C. Kalichman
  1992   Child abuse reporting decisions: Effects of statutory wording of reporting requirements.
         *Professional Psychology, Research and Practice* 23(6):486-492.

Bross, D.C.
1995    Terminating the parent-child legal relationship as a response to child sexual abuse. *Loyola University of Chicago Law Journal* 26(2):287-319.

Brown, J.
1997    Working toward freedom from violence: The process of change in battered women. *Violence Against Women* 3:5-26.

Browne, A., and K.R. Williams
1993    Gender, intimacy, and lethal violence: Trends from 1976 through 1987. *Gender and Society* 7(1):78-98.

Brunk, M., S. Henggeler, and J.P. Whelan
1987    Comparison of multisystemic therapy and parent training in the brief treatment of child abuse and neglect. *Journal of Consulting and Clinical Psychology* 55(2):171-178.

Bulkley, J.
1988    Recommendations for improving legal intervention in intrafamily child sexual abuse cases. Pp. 397-403 in E.B. Nicholson and J. Bulkley, eds., *Sexual Abuse Allegations in Custody and Visitation Cases*. Washington, D.C.: American Bar Association.

Bulkley, J., J.N. Feller, P. Stern, and R. Roe
1996    Child abuse and neglect law and legal proceedings. Pp. 271-296 in J. Briere, J. Bulkley, C. Jenny, and T. Reid, eds., *The APSAC Handbook on Child Maltreatment*. Thousand Oaks, Calif: Sage.

Bullock, L., J. McFarlane, L.H. Bateman, and V. Miller
1989    The prevalence and characteristics of battered women in a primary care setting. *Nurse Practitioner* 14(6):47-54.

Burch, G., and V. Mohr
1980    Evaluating a child abuse intervention program. *Social Casework* February:90-99.

Burchard, J.D., and R.T. Clarke
1989    Individualized approaches to treatment: Project Wraparound. Pp. 51-57 in A. Adgarin, R. Friedman, A. Duchnowski, K. Kutash, S. Silver, and M. Johnson, eds., *Second Annual Conference Proceedings from the Children's Mental Health Services and Policy Conference: Building a Research Base*. Tampa: Research and Training Center for Children's Mental Health, University of South Florida.

Burchard, J.D., S.N. Burchard, R. Sewell, and J. Van den Berg
1993    *One Kid at a Time: Evaluative Case Studies and Description of the Alaska Youth Initiative Demonstration Project*. Washington D.C.: CASSP Technical Assistance Center, Georgetown University Press.

Bureau of Justice Statistics
1994    *Selected Findings: Violence Between Intimates*. NCJ-149259. Prepared by M.W. Zawitz. Washington, D.C.: U.S. Department of Justice.

Byers, B., J.E. Hendricks, and D. Wiese
1993    An overview of adult protective services. Pp. 3-31 in B. Byers and J.E. Hendricks, eds., *Adult Protective Services: Research and Practice*. Springfield, Ill.: Charles C Thomas.

Calhoun, K.S., and B.M. Atkenson
1991    *Treatment of Rape Victims: Facilitating Psychosocial Adjustment*. New York: Pergamon Press.

Cameron, G.
1990    Child maltreatment: Challenges in expanding our concept of helping. Pp. 277-285 in M. Rothery and G. Cameron, eds., *Maltreatment: Expanding Our Concept of Helping*. Hillsdale, N.J.: Lawrence Erlbaum Associates.

Campbell, D.T., and J.C. Stanley
1966    *Experimental and Quasi-Experimental Designs for Research*, 2nd ed. Chicago, Ill.: Rand McNally.

Campbell, J.C., ed.
1995    *Assessing Dangerousness: Violence by Sexual Offenders, Batterers, and Child Abusers.*
        Thousand Oaks, Calif.: Sage.
Campbell, J.C., and B. Parker
· 1992   Battered women and their children. Pp. 77-95 in *Annual Review of Nursing Research.*
        New York: Springer.
Campbell, J.C., J. Kub, R.A. Belknap, and T. Templin
1997    Predictors of depression in battered women. *Violence Against Women* 3(3):271-293.
Campbell, R., C.M. Sullivan, and W.S. Davidson
1995    Women who use domestic violence shelters: Changes in depression over time. *Psychology of Women Quarterly* 19(2):237-255.
Campbell, R.V., S. O'Brien, A.D. Bickett, and J.R. Lutzker
1983    In home parent training, treatment of migraine headaches, and marital counseling as an
        ecobehavioral approach to prevent child abuse. *Journal of Behavioral Therapy and Experimental Psychiatry* 14(2):147-154.
Carr, K., G. Dix, and T. Fulmer
1986    An elder abuse assessment team in an acute hospital setting. *The Gerontologist* 25:115-118.
Carroll, L.A., R.G. Miltenberger, and H.K. O'Neill
1992    A review and critique of research evaluating child sexual abuse prevention programs.
        *Education and Treatment of Children* 15(4):335-354.
Cascardi M., and K.D. O'Leary
1992    Depressive symptomatology, self-esteem, and self-blame in battered women. *Journal of Family Violence* 7:249-259.
Ceci, S.J., D. Ross, and M. Toglia
1987    Age differences in suggestibility: Narrowing the uncertainties. Pp. 79-91 in S.J. Ceci,
        M.P. Toglia, and D.F. Ross, eds., *Children's Eyewitness Memory.* New York: Springer-Verlag.
Chadwick, D.L.
1994    Falls and childhood deaths: Sorting real falls from inflicted injuries. *APSAC Advisor* 7(4).
Chamberlain, P., S. Moreland, and K. Reid
1992    Enhanced services and stipends for foster parents: Effects on retention rates and outcomes
        for children. *Child Welfare* 71(5):387-401.
Chapman, J.R., and B.E. Smith
1987    *Child Sexual Abuse: An Analysis of Case Processing.* Washington, D.C.: American Bar
        Association.
Chen, H.T., and P.H. Rossi
1983    Evaluating with sense: The theory-driven approach. *Evaluation Review* 7:283-302.
Chen, H.T., C. Bersani, S.C. Myers, and R. Denton
1989    Evaluating the effectiveness of a court sponsored abuser treatment program. *Journal of Family Violence* 4(4):309-322.
Christoffel, K.
1990    Violent death and injury in U.S. children and adolescents. *American Journal of Diseases of Children* 144:697-706.
Cicchetti, D.
1989    How research on child maltreatment has informed the study of child development: Perspectives from developmental psychopathology. Pp. 377-431 in D. Cicchetti and V. Carlson, eds., *Child Maltreatment: Theory and Research on the Causes and Consequences of Child Abuse and Neglect.* New York: Cambridge University Press.

Cicchetti, D., and V. Carlson, eds.

1989    *Current Research and Theoretical Advances in Child Maltreatment.* Cambridge, England: Cambridge University Press.

Cicchinelli, L.

1991    Risk assessment: Expectations, benefits, and realities. Pp. 7-18 in *Fourth National Roundtable on CPS Risk Assessment.* Washington, D.C.: American Public Welfare Association.

Clark, H.B., M.E. Prange, B. Lee, A. Boyd, B.A. McDonald, and E.S. Stewart

1994    Improving adjustment outcomes for foster children with emotional and behavioral disorders: Early findings from a controlled study on individualized services. *Journal of Emotional and Behavioral Disorders* 2(4):207-218.

Cochran, D.

1994    Domestic violence: The invisible problem. *Executive Exchange* 1-2.

Cohen, J.A., and A.P. Mannarino

1996    A treatment outcome study for sexually abused preschool children: Initial findings. *Journal of the American Academy of Child and Adolescent Psychiatry* 35(1):42-50.

Cohen, S.

1988    *Statistical Power Analysis for the Behavioral Sciences,* 2nd ed. Hillsdale, N.J.: Lawrence Erlbaum Associates.

Cohen, S., E. Gray, and M. Wald

1984    Preventing Child Maltreatment: A Review of What We Know. Working Paper No. 024. National Committee to Prevent Child Abuse, Chicago, Ill.

Cohn, A.H., and D. Daro

1987    Is treatment too late: What ten years of evaluative research tell us. *Child Abuse and Neglect* 11:433-442.

Colditz, G.A., E. Burdick, and F. Mosteller

1995    Heterogeneity in meta-analysis of data from epidemiologic studies: A commentary. *Epidemiology* 142(4):371-382.

Coleman, D.H., and M.A. Straus

1986    Marital power, conflict, and violence in a nationally representative sample of American couples. *Violence and Victims* 1:141-157.

Collins, A.H., and D.L. Pancoast

1976    *Natural Helping Networks: A Strategy for Prevention.* Washington, D.C.: National Association of Social Workers.

The Commonwealth Fund

1996    *Prevention and Women's Health: A Shared Responsibility.* Policy report of the Commonwealth Fund Commission on Women's Health. New York: The Commonwealth Fund.

Connell, J.P., and A.C. Kubisch

1996    Applying Theories of Change Approach to the Evaluation of Comprehensive Community Initiatives: Progress, Prospects and Problems. Unpublished document, The Aspen Institute, New York.

Connell, J.P., A.C. Kubisch, L.B. Schorr, and C.H. Weiss, eds.

1995    *New Approaches to Evaluating Community Initiatives: Concepts, Methods, and Contexts.* New York: The Aspen Institute.

Connelly, C.D., and M.A. Straus

1992    Mother's age and risk for physical abuse. *Child Abuse and Neglect* 16(5):709-718.

Conte, J.R., C. Rosen, L. Saperstein, and R. Shermack

1985    An evaluation of a program to prevent the sexual victimization of young children. *Child Abuse and Neglect* 9:319-328.

Cook R., J. Roehl, C. Oros, and J. Trudeau
    1994    Conceptual and methodological issues in the evaluation of community-based substance
            abuse prevention coalitions: Lessons learned from the national evaluation of the commu-
            nity partnership program. *Journal of Community Psychology Monograph Series*. Bran-
            don, Vt.: Clinical Psychology Publishing Company, Inc.
Cook, T.D., and D.T. Campbell
    1979    *Quasi-Experimentation: Design and Analysis Issues for Field Settings*. Boston, Mass.:
            Houghton-Mifflin.
Cook, T.D., and W.R. Shadish
    1994    Social experiments: Some developments over the past fifteen years. *Annual Review of
            Psychology* 45:545-580.
Cordray, D.S.
    1986    Quasi-experimental analysis: A mixture of methods and judgment. *New Directions for
            Program Evaluation* 31:9-27.
    1993    Synthesizing evidence and practice. *Evaluation Practice* 14(1):1-8.
Cordray, D.S., and G.M. Pion
    1993    Psycho-social rehabilitation assessment: A broader perspective. Pp. 215-240 in R.
            Glueckauf, G. Bond, L. Sechrest, and E.C. McDonel, eds., *Improving Assessment in
            Rehabilitation and Health*. Newbury Park, Calif.: Sage.
Counts, D., J. Brown, and J. Campbell
    1992    *Sanctions and Sanctuary: Cultural Perspectives on the Beating of Wives*. Boulder, Colo.:
            Westview Press.
Cox, J.W., and C.D. Stoltenberg
    1991    Evaluation of a treatment program for battered wives. *Journal of Family Violence*
            6(4):395-413.
Cronbach, L.J., and R.E. Snow
    1981    *Aptitudes and Instructional Methods: A Handbook for Research on Interactions*. New
            York: Irvington Publishers.
Culp, R.E., V. Little, D. Letts, and H. Lawrence
    1991    Maltreated children's self-concept: Effects of a comprehensive treatment program. *Ameri-
            can Journal of Orthopsychiatry* 61(1):14-21.
Daro, D.
    1988    *Enhancing Child Abuse Prevention Effects: Research Priorities for the 1990's*. Chicago,
            Ill.: National Committee to Prevent Child Abuse.
Daro, D., and K. McCurdy
    1994    Preventing child abuse and neglect: Programmatic interventions.    *Child Welfare*
            73(5):405-430.
Davis, R.C., and B. Smith
    1995    Domestic violence reforms: Empty promises or fulfilled expectations? *Crime and Delin-
            quency* 41(4):541-552.
Davis, R.C., and B. Taylor
    1995    A Joint Social Service and Police Response to Domestic Violence: The Results of a
            Randomized Experiment. Unpublished document, Victim Services Agency, New York.
Dayaratna, S.
    1992    Social Problems and Rising Health Care Costs in Pennsylvania. Unpublished document,
            Pennsylvania Blue Shield Institute.
Deblinger, E., J. Lippman, and R. Steer
    1996    Sexually abused children suffering posttraumatic stress symptoms: Initial treatment out-
            come findings. *Child Maltreatment* 1(4):310-321.
Dennis-Small, L., and K. Washburn
    1986    Family-Centered, Home-Based Intervention Project for Protective Services Clients. Un-
            published document, Texas Department of Human Services, Austin.

DePanfilis, D.
  1996    Social isolation of neglectful families: A review of social support assessment and inter-
          vention models. *Child Maltreatment* 1(1):37-52.
Dobash, R.E., and R.P. Dobash
  1979    *Violence Against Wives: A Case Against the Patriarchy.* New York: The Free Press.
Dobash, R.E., R.P. Dobash, M. Wilson, and M. Daly
  1992    The myth of sexual symmetry in marital violence. *Social Problems* 39(1):71-91.
Dollard, N., M.E. Evans, J. Lubrecht, and D. Schaeffer
  1994    The use of flexible service dollars in rural community-based programs for children with
          serious emotional disturbance and their families. *Journal of Emotional and Behavioral
          Disorders* 2(2):117-112.
Downing, J., S.J. Jenkins, and G.L. Fisher
  1988    A comparison of psychodynamic and reinforcement treatment with sexually abused chil-
          dren. *Elementary School Guidance and Counseling* 22:291-299.
Downing, J.D., S.J. Wells, and J. Fluke
  1990    Gatekeeping in child protective services: A survey of screening policies. *Child Welfare*
          69(4):357-369.
Dubowitz, H.
  1990    Costs and effectiveness of interventions in child maltreatment. *Child Abuse and Neglect*
          14:177-186.
Dubowitz, H., M. Black, R.H. Starr, Jr., and S. Zuravin
  1993    A conceptual definition of child neglect. *Criminal Justice and Behavior* 20(1):8-26.
Duchnowski, A.J., M.K. Johnson, K.S. Hall, K. Kutash, and R.M. Friedman
  1993    The alternatives to residential treatment study: Initial findings. *Journal of Emotional and
          Behavioral Disorders* (1):17-26.
Dunford, F.W., D. Huizinga, and D.S. Elliott
  1990    The role of arrest in domestic assault: The Omaha experiment. *Criminology* 28:183-206.
Durfee, M.
  1994    Fatal child abuse: Intervention and prevention. In *Child Fatality Review Teams: A Multi-
          Agency National Training Conference,* February 16-17. Washington, D.C.: Office of Jus-
          tice Programs, U.S. Department of Justice.
Durfee, M.J., G.A. Gellert, and D. Tilton-Durfee
  1992    Origins and clinical relevance of child death review teams. *Journal of the American
          Medical Association* 267(23):3172-3175.
Dutton, D.G.
  1986    The outcome of court-mandated treatment for wife assault: A quasi-experimental evalua-
          tion. *Violence and Victims* 1(3):163-175.
  1988    Profiling of wife assaulters: Preliminary evidence for a trimodal analysis. *Violence and
          Victims* 3(1):5-29.
  1994    The origin and structure of the abusive personality. *Journal of Personality Disorders*
          8(3):181-191.
  1995a   *The Domestic Assault of Women,* 2nd ed. Boston, Mass.: Allyn-Bacon.
  1995b   Trauma symptoms and PTSD-like profiles in perpetrators of intimate abuse. *Journal of
          Traumatic Stress* 8(2):299-316.
Dutton, D.G., and A.J. Starzomski
  1993    Borderline personality in perpetrators of psychological and physical abuse. *Violence and
          Victims* 8(4):327-337.
Dutton, D.G., K. Saunders, A. Starzomski, and K. Bartholomew
  1994    Intimacy-anger and insecure attachments as precursors of abuse in intimate relationships.
          *Journal of Applied Social Psychology* 24:1367-1386.

Dutton, M.A.

1992   *Empowering and Healing the Battered Woman: A Model for Assessment and Intervention.* New York: Springer.

Edleson, J.L., and R.J. Grusznski

1989   Treating men who batter: Four years of outcome data from the Domestic Abuse Project. *Journal of Social Service Research* 12:3-22.

Edleson, J.L., and M. Syers

1990   The relative effectiveness of group treatments for men who batter. *Social Work Research and Abstracts* 26(2):10-17.

Edleson, J.L., and R.M. Tolman

1992   *Interventions for Men Who Batter: An Ecological Approach.* Newbury Park, Calif.: Sage.

Edna McConnell Clark Foundation

1985   *Keeping Families Together: The Case for Family Preservation.* New York: Edna McConnell Clark Foundation.

Egan, K.J.

1983   Stress management and child management with abusive parents. *Journal of Clinical Child Psychology* 12(3):292-299.

Egeland, B., and B. Vaughan

1981   Failure of "bond formation" as a cause of abuse, neglect, and maltreatment. *American Journal of Orthopsychiatry* 51(1):78-84.

Egeland, B., D. Jacobvitz, and K. Papatola

1987   Intergenerational continuity of abuse. Pp. 255-276 in R.J. Gelles and J.B. Lancaster, eds., *Child Abuse and Neglect: Biosocial Dimensions.* Hawthorne, N.Y.: Aldine de Gruyter.

Ehrlich, P., and G. Anetzberger

1991   Survey of state public health departments on procedures for reporting elder abuse. *Public Health Reports* 106(2):151-154.

Eisenberg, H.B.

1991   Combatting elder abuse through the legal process. *Journal of Elder Abuse and Neglect* 3(1):65-96.

Eisikovits, Z.C., and J.L. Edleson

1989   Intervening with men who batter: A critical review of the literature. *Social Service Review* Sept.: 384-414.

Elmer, E.

1986   Outcome of residential treatment for abused and high-risk infants. *Child Abuse and Neglect* 10:351-360.

Elmer, E., and G.S. Gregg

1967   Developmental characteristics of abused children. *Pediatrics* 40(4):596-602.

Emerson, R.E.

1983   Holistic effects in social control decision making. *Law & Society Review* 17:425-455.

Emery, R.E.

1989   Family violence. *American Psychologist* 44(2):321-328.

English, D.J.

1994   Grant Application: Longitudinal Use of Services by At-Risk Children. Department of Social and Health Services, Children's Administration, State of Washington, Olympia, Wash.

1995   *A Review of the Research Literature: The Navy Risk Assessment Model on Child Maltreatment and Domestic Violence, Module 1.* Washington, D.C.: U.S. Navy Family Advocacy Program.

English, D.J., and S. Aubin

1991    *Impact of Investigations:  Outcomes for Child Protective Services Cases Receiving Differential Levels of Service.* National Center on Child Abuse and Neglect. Washington, D.C.: U.S. Department of Health and Human Services.

English, D.J., and P.J. Pecora

1994    Risk assessment as a practice method in child protective services. *Child Welfare* 73(5):451-473.

Ensign, K.

1991    *Prevention Services in Child Welfare: An Exploratory Paper on the Evaluation of Family Preservation and Family Support Programs.* Washington, D.C.: U.S. Department of Health and Human Services.

Eth, S., and R.S. Pynoos

1985    Psychiatric intervention with children traumatized by violence. Pp. 285-309 in D.H. Schetky and E.P. Benedek, eds., *Issues in Child Psychiatry and the Law.* New York: Brunner/Mazel, Inc.

Fagan, J.

1989    Cessation from family violence: Deterrence and dissuasion. Pp. 357-426 in L. Ohlin and M. Tonry, eds., *Family Violence, Volume 11 of Crime and Justice: An Annual Review of Research.* Chicago, Ill.: University of Chicago Press.

1990    Contributions of research to criminal justice policy on wife assault. Pp. 53-81 in D.J. Besharov, ed., *Family Violence: Research and Public Policy Issues.* Washington, D.C.: American Enterprise Institute Press.

Fagan, J., and A. Browne

1994    Violence between spouses and intimates: Physical aggression between women and men in intimate relationships. Pp. 115-292 in National Research Council, *Understanding and Preventing Violence,* Vol. 3. Washington, D.C.: National Academy Press.

Fagan, J., E. Friedman, S. Wexler, and V.O. Lewis

1984    *Final Report:  National Family Violence Evaluation.* Grant 80-JN-AX-0004, Office of Juvenile Justice and Delinquency Prevention. Washington, D.C.: U.S. Department of Justice.

Fanshel, D.

1992    Foster care as a two-tiered system. *Children and Youth Services Review* 14(1/2):49-60.

Fanshel, D., and E. Shinn

1978    *Children in Foster Care: A Longitudinal Investigation.* New York: Columbia University Press.

Fanshel, D., S.J. Finch, and J.F. Grundy

1992    Serving the urban poor: A study of child welfare preventive services. *Child Welfare* 71:197-211.

Fantuzzo, J., and C.T. Twentyman

1986    Child abuse and psychotherapy research: Merging social concerns with empirical investigation. *Child Abuse and Neglect* 17(5):375-380.

Fantuzzo, J.W., A. Stovall, D. Schachtel, C. Goins, and R. Hall

1987    The effects of peer social initiations on social behavior of withdrawn maltreated preschool children. *Journal of Behavioral Therapy and Experiential Psychiatry* 18:357-363.

Fantuzzo, J.W., L. Jurecic, A. Stovall, A.D. Hightower, and C. Goins

1988    Effects of adult and peer social initiations on the social behavior of withdrawn, maltreated preschool children. *Journal of Consulting and Clinical Psychology* 56:34-39.

Fantuzzo, J., L. DePaola, L. Lambert, and T. Martino

1991    Effect of interpersonal violence on the psychological adjustment and competencies of young children. *Journal of Consulting and Clinical Psychology* 59:258-265.

Fantuzzo, J.W., R. Boruch, A. Beriama, M. Atkins, and S. Marcus
    1997    Domestic violence and children: Prevalence and risk in five major U.S. cities. *Journal of the American Academy of Child and Adolescent Psychiatry* 36(1):116-122.

Feazell, C.S., R.S. Mayers, and J. Deschner
    1984    Services for men who batter: Implications for programs and policies. *Family Relations* 33:217-223.

Federal Bureau of Investigation
    1993    *Uniform Crime Reports.* Washington, D.C.: U.S. Department of Justice.

Feldman, L.H.
    1991    Assessing the Effectiveness of Family Preservation Services in New Jersey Within an Ecological Context. Unpublished document, Department of Human Services, New Jersey Division of Youth and Family Services, Trenton.

Felitti, V.J.
    1991    Long-term medical consequences of incest, rape, and molestation. *Southern Medical Journal* 84:328-331.

Fergusson, D.M., J. Fleming, and D.P. O'Neill
    1972    *Child Abuse in New Zealand.* Wellington, New Zealand: Department of Social Welfare.

Festinger, T.
    1983    *No One Ever Asked Us....A Postscript to Foster Care.* New York: Columbia University Press.

Fetterman, D., S.J. Kaftarian, and A. Wandersman, eds.
    1996    *Empowerment Evaluation.* Thousand Oaks, Calif.: Sage.

Filinson, R.
    1993    An evaluation of a program of volunteer advocates for elder abuse victims. *Journal of Elder Abuse and Neglect* 5(1):77-93.

Fink, A., and L. McCloskey
    1990    Moving child abuse and prevention programs forward: Improving program evaluations. *Child Abuse and Neglect* 14:187-206.

Finkelhor, D.
    1983    Removing the child—prosecuting the offender in cases of sexual abuse: Evidence from the national reporting system for child abuse and neglect. *Child Abuse and Neglect* 7:195-205.
    1984    Child sexual abuse in a sample of Boston families. In D. Finkelhor, ed., *Child Sexual Abuse: New Theory and Research.* New York: The Free Press.

Finkelhor, D., and L. Berliner
    1995    Research on the treatment of sexually abused children: A review and recommendations. *Journal of the American Academy of Child and Adolescent Psychiatry* 34(11):1408-1423.

Finkelhor, D., and G.L. Zellman
    1991    Commentary: Flexible reporting options for skilled child abuse professionals. *Child Abuse and Neglect* 15(4):335-341.

Finkelhor, D., G. Hotaling, I.A. Lewis, and C. Smith
    1990    Sexual abuse in a national survey of adult men and women: Prevalence, characteristics, and risk factors. *Child Abuse and Neglect* 14:19-28.

Flitcraft, A.
    1993    Physicians and domestic violence: Challenges for prevention. *Health Affairs* 12(4):154-161.

Foege, W.
    1986    Violence and public health. Chap. 4 in *Surgeon General's Workshop on Violence and Public Health Report*, Leesburg, Va., October 27-29, 1985. Washington, D.C.: Office of Juvenile Justice and Delinquency Prevention and Office of the Surgeon General and Public Health Service.

Ford, D.A.
  1991    Prosecution as a victim power source: A note on empowering women in violent conjugal relationships. *Law & Society Review* 25(2):313-334.
Ford, D.A., and M.J. Regoli
  1993    The Indianapolis Domestic Violence Prosecution Experiment. Final Report, Grant 86-IJ-CX-0012 to the National Institute of Justice. Indianapolis, Ind.: Indiana University.
Forst, B.E., and J.C. Hernon
  1985    The criminal justice response to victim harm. In *National Institute of Justice Research in Brief*. Washington, D.C.: U.S. Department of Justice.
Frankel, H.
  1988    Family-centered, home-based services in child protection: A review of the research. *Social Service Review* March:137-157.
Fraser, M., P. Pecora, and D. Haapala
  1991    *Families in Crisis: The Impact of Intensive Family Preservation Services.* Hawthorne, N.Y.: Aldine de Gruyter.
Fredriksen, K.I.
  1989    Adult protective services: Changes with the introduction of mandatory reporting. *Journal of Elder Abuse and Neglect* 1(2):59-70.
Freeman-Longo, R.E., and F.H. Knopp
  1992    State-of-the-art sex offender treatment: Outcome and issues. *Annals of Sex Research* 5(3):141-160.
Friedman, L.S., J.H. Samet, M.S. Roberts, M. Hudlin, and P. Hans
  1992    Inquiry about victimization experiences. A survey of patient preferences and physician practices. *Archives of International Medicine* 1:39-47.
Friedrich, W.N., and J.A. Boriskin
  1976    Ill-health and child abuse. *Lancet* 1(7960):649-650.
Fryer, G.E., S.K. Kraizer, and T. Miyoshi
  1987    Measuring actual reduction of risk to child abuse: A new approach. *Child Abuse and Neglect* 11:173-179.
Fulmer, T., D.J. McMahon, M. Baer-Hines, and B. Forget
  1992    Abuse, neglect, abandonment, violence, and exploitation: An analysis of all elderly patients seen in one emergency department during a six-month period. *Journal of Emergency Nursing* 18(6):505-510.
Fulmer, T.T., and T.A. O'Malley
  1987    *Inadequate Care of the Elderly: A Health Care Perspective on Abuse and Neglect.* New York: Springer.
Furby, L., M.R. Weinrott, and L. Blackshaw
  1989    Sex offender recidivism: A review. *Psychological Bulletin* 105(1):3-30.
Gabinet, L.
  1983    Shared parenting: A new paradigm for the treatment of child abuse. *Child Abuse and Neglect* 7(4):403-411.
Gamache, D.J., J.L. Edleson, and M.D. Schock
  1988    Coordinated police, judicial, and social service response to woman battering: A multiple baseline evaluation across three communities. Pp. 193-209 in G.T. Hotaling, D. Finkelhor, J.T. Kirkpatrick, and M.A. Straus, eds., *Coping with Family Violence: Research and Policy Perspectives.* Newbury Park, Calif.: Sage.
Garbarino, J.
  1977    The human ecology of child maltreatment: A conceptual model for research. *Journal of Marriage and the Family* 39:721-735.
  1986    Can we measure success in preventing child abuse? Issues in policy, programming, and research. *Child Abuse and Neglect* 10:143-156.

1987    Family support and the prevention of child maltreatment. In S. Kagan, R. Powell, B. Weissbourd, and E. Zigler, eds., *America's Family Support Programs.* New Haven, Conn.: Yale University Press.

Garbarino, J., and K. Kostelny

1994    Neighborhood-based programs. Pp. 304-352 in G. Melton and F. Barry, eds., *Protecting Children from Abuse and Neglect.* New York: Guilford Press.

Garmezy, N.

1985    Stress-resistant children: The search for protective factors. In J.E. Stevenson, ed., *Recent Research in Developmental Psychopathology.* Oxford, England: Pergamon Press.

1993    Children in poverty: Resilience despite risk. *Psychiatry* 56:127-136.

Garner, J., J. Fagan, and C. Maxwell

1995    Published findings from the Spouse Assault Replication Program: A critical review. *Journal of Quantitative Criminology* 11(1):3-28.

Gaudin, J.M.

1979    Mothers' Perceived Strength of Primary Group Networks and Maternal Child Abuse. Unpublished doctoral dissertation, Florida State University, Tallahassee.

Gaudin, J.M., J.S. Wodarski, M.K. Arkinson, and L.S. Avery

1991    Remedying child neglect: Effectiveness of social network interventions. *Journal of Applied Social Sciences* 15(1):97-123.

Gaudin, J.M., N.A. Polansky, A.C. Kilpatrick, and P. Shilton

1993    Loneliness, depression, stress, and social supports in neglectful families. *American Journal of Orthopsychiatry* 63:597-605.

Gazmararian, J.A., S. Lazorick, A.M. Spitz, T.J. Ballard, L.E. Saltzman, and J.S. Marks

1996    Prevalence of violence during pregnancy: A review of the literature. *Journal of the American Medical Association* 275(24):1915-1920.

Gebotys, R.J., D. O'Connor, and K.J. Mair

1992    Public perceptions of elder physical mistreatment. *Journal of Elder Abuse and Neglect* 4(1/2):151.

Gelles, R.J.

1975    The social construction of child abuse. *American Journal of Orthopsychiatry* 45(3):363-371.

1980    A profile of violence toward children in the United States. Pp. 82-105 in G. Gerbner et al., eds., *Child Abuse: An Agenda for Action.* New York: Oxford University Press.

1987    *The Violent Home.* Newbury Park, Calif.: Sage.

Gelles, R.J., and W.A. Hargreaves

1981    Maternal employment and violence towards children. *Journal of Family Issues* 2:509-530.

Gelles, R.J., and M.A. Straus

1974    Toward an integrated theory of intrafamily violence. Kingston: Department of Sociology and Anthropology, Rhode Island University

1979    Determinants of violence in the family: Toward a theoretical integration. Pp. 549-581 in W. Burr et al., eds., *Contemporary Theories About the Family.* New York: The Free Press.

1988    Compassion or control: Legal, social, and medical services. Pp. 160-182 in *Intimate Violence: The Definitive Study of the Causes and Consequences of Abuse in the American Family.* New York: Simon and Schuster.

Gielen, A.C., P.J. O'Campo, and X. Xue

1994    Interpersonal conflict and physical violence during the childbearing years. *Social Science and Medicine* 39(6):781-787.

Gil, D.G.

1971    Violence against children. *Journal of Marriage and the Family* 33(4):637-638.

Giles-Sims, J.
    1983    *Wife Battering. A Systems Theory Approach.*  New York: Guilford Press.

Gin, N.E., L. Ruker, S. Frayne, R. Cygan, and F.A. Hubbell
    1991    Prevalence of domestic violence among patients in three ambulatory care internal medicine clinics. *Journal of General Internal Medicine* 6:317-322.

Giovannoni, J.M., and A. Billingsley
    1970    Child neglect among the poor: A study of parental adequacy in families of three ethnic groups. *Child Welfare* 49(April):196-204.

Gleason, W.J.
    1993    Mental disorders in battered women: An empirical study. *Violence and Victims* 8(1):53-68.

Goerge, R.M., K.M. Casey, and S.H. Grant
    1992    *Substitute Care in Illinois: 1976-1991.*  Chicago, Ill.: Children's Policy Project, Chapin Hall Center for Children.

Goerge, R., F. Wulczyn, and D. Fanshel
    1994a    A foster care research agenda for the '90s. *Child Welfare* 73(5):525-549.

Goerge, R.M., J. Van Voorhis, and B.J. Lee
    1994b    Illinois' longitudinal and relational child and family research database. *Social Science Computer Review* 12(3).

Goldkamp, J.
    1996    *The Role of Drug and Alcohol Abuse in Domestic Violence and Its Treatment: Dade County's Domestic Violence Court Experiment.*  Philadelphia: Crime and Justice Research Institute.

Goldson, E.
    1987    Child development and the response to maltreatment. Pp. 3-20 in D.C. Bross and L.F. Michaels, eds., *Foundations of Child Advocacy.* Longmont, Colo.: Bookmakers Guild, Inc.

Gomes-Schwartz, B., J.M. Horowitz, and A.P. Cardarelli
    1990    *Child Sexual Abuse: The Initial Effects.* Newbury Park, Calif.: Sage.

Gondolf, E.W.
    1988    Who are those guys? Toward a behavioral typology of batterers. *Violence and Victims* 3:187-203.
    1991    A victim-based assessment of court-mandated counseling for batterers. *Criminal Justice Review* 16(2):214-228.
    1995    Batterers programs: What we know and what we need to know. Presented at the Violence Against Women Strategic Planning Meeting, National Institute of Justice, U.S. Department of Justice, Washington, D.C. March 31.

Gondolf, E.W., and E.R. Fisher
    1988    *Battered Women as Survivors: An Alternate to Treating Learned Helplessness.* Lexington, Mass.: Lexington Books.

Goodman, G.S.
    1984    The child witness: Conclusions and future directions for research and legal practice. *Journal of Social Issues* 40:157-175.

Goodman, G.S., and R.S. Reed
    1986    Age difference in eyewitness testimony. *Law and Human Behavior* 10(4):317-332.

Goodman, G.S., C. Aman, and J. Hirschman
    1987    Child sexual and physical abuse: Children's testimony. Pp. 3-23 in S.J. Ceci, M.P. Toglia, and D.F. Ross, eds., *Children's Eyewitness Memory.* New York: Springer-Verlag.

Gottfredson, S.D., and D.M. Gottfredson
    1988    Violence prediction methods: Statistical and clinical strategies. *Violence and Victims* 3(4):303-324.

Gottlieb, B.H.
 1980    The role of individual and social support in preventing child maltreatment. Pp. 37-60 in
         J. Garbarino and S.H. Stocking, eds., *Protecting Children from Abuse and Neglect.* San
         Francisco, Calif.: Jossey-Bass.
Granik, L.A., M. Durfee, and S.J. Wells
 1992    *Child Death Review Teams: A Manual for Design and Implementation.* Washington,
         D.C.: American Bar Association and the American Academy of Pediatrics.
Green, S.B., and D.P. Byar
 1984    Using observational data from registries to compare treatments: The fallacy of
         omnimetrics. *Statistics in Medicine* 3:361-370.
Groves, B., and B. Zuckerman
 1997    Interventions with parents and community care givers. In J.D. Osofsky, ed., *Children in
         a Violent Society.* New York: Guilford Press.
Groves, B., B. Zuckerman, S. Marans, and D. Cohen
 1993    Silent victims: Children who witness violence. *Journal of the American Medical Asso-
         ciation* 269:262-264.
Halper, G., and M.A. Jones
 1981    *Serving Families at Risk of Dissolution: Public Preventive Services in New York City.*
         New York: Human Resources Administration, Special Services for Children.
Halpern, R.
 1990    Community-based early intervention. Pp. 469-498 in S. Meisels and J. Shonkoff, eds.,
         *Handbook of Early Childhood Intervention.* New York: Cambridge University Press.
 1994    Neighborhood-based strategies to address poverty-related social problems: An historical
         perspective. Chap. 2 in A. Kahn and S.B. Kamerman, eds., *Children and Their Families
         in Big Cities.* New York: School of Social Work, Columbia University.
Hamberger, L.K., and J.E. Hastings
 1986    Personality correlates of men who batter and non-violent men: A cross validational
         study. *Journal of Family Violence* 1:323-346.
 1988    Skills training for treatment of spouse abusers: An outcome study. *Journal of Family
         Violence* 3(2):121-130.
 1989    Counseling male spouse abusers: Characteristics of treatment completers and dropouts.
         *Violence and Victims* 4(4):275-286.
 1991    Personality correlates of men who batter and non-violent men: Some continuities and
         discontinuities. *Journal of Family Violence* 6:131-147.
Hamberger, L.K., and D.G. Saunders
 1991    Battered Women in Non-Emergency Medical Settings: Incidence, Prevalence, Physician
         Interventions. Paper presented at the American Psychological Association Meeting, San
         Francisco, Calif., August 18.
Hamilton, C.J., and J.J. Collins
 1985    The role of alcohol in wife beating and child abuse: A review of the literature. Pp. 253-
         287 in J.J. Collins, ed., *Drinking and Crime: Perspectives on the Relationship Between
         Alcohol Consumption and Criminal Behavior.* New York: Guilford.
Hampton, R.L., and E.H. Newberger
 1985    Child abuse incidence and reporting by hospitals: Significance of severity, class, and race.
         *American Journal of Public Health* 75(1):56-60.
Harari, T.
 1980    Teenagers Exiting Family Foster Care: A Retrospective Look. Unpublished doctoral
         dissertation, University of California, Berkeley.
Harford, T.C., and D.A. Parker
 1994    Antisocial behavior, family history, and alcohol dependence symptoms. *Alcoholism Clini-
         cal and Experimental Research* 18(2):265-268.

Harrell, A.
1992    *The Impact of Court-Ordered Treatment for Domestic Violence Offenders.*  Washington, D.C.: The Urban Institute.
Harrell, A., B. Smith, and L. Newmark
1993    *Court Processing and the Effects of Restraining Orders for Domestic Violence Victims.* Washington, D.C.: The Urban Institute.
Harris, J., S. Savage, T. Jones, and W. Brooke
1988    A comparison of treatments for abusive men and their partners within a family-service agency. *Canadian Journal of Community Mental Health* 7:147-155.
Hart, B.J.
1995    Coordinated Community Approaches to Domestic Violence. Paper presented at the Strategic Planning Workshop on Violence Against Women, National Institute of Justice, Washington, D.C., March 31. Battered Women's Justice Project, Pennsylvania Coalition Against Domestic Violence, Reading.
Hart, S.D., D.G. Dutton, and T. Newlove
1993    The prevalence of personality disorder among wife assaulters. *Journal of Personality Disorders* 7(4):328-340.
Hartman, A.
1978    Diagrammatic assessments of family relationships. *Social Casework* 59:465-476.
Harvey, P., R. Forehand, C. Brown, and T. Holmes
1988    The prevention of sexual abuse: Examination of the effectiveness of a program with kindergarten-age children. *Behavior Therapy* 19:429-435.
Hawkins, R.P., P. Meadowcroft, B.A. Trout, and W.C. Luster
1985    Foster family-based treatment. *Journal of Clinical Child Psychology* 3:220-228.
Hawkins, R., C. Almeida, and M. Samet
1989    Comparative evaluation of foster-family-based treatment and five other placement choices: A preliminary report. Pp. 98-119 in A. Algarin, R. Friedman, A. Duchnowski, K. Kutash, S. Silver, and M. Johnson, eds., *Second Annual Conference Proceedings from the Children's Mental Health Services and Policy Conference: Building a Research Base.* Tampa: Research and Training Center for Children's Mental Health, University of South Florida.
Hazzard, A., C. Webb, C. Kleemeier, L. Angert, and J. Pohl
1991    Child sexual abuse prevention: Evaluation and one-year follow-up. *Child Abuse and Neglect* 15:123-138.
Hegar, R.L., and J.J. Youngman
1989    Toward a causal typology of child neglect. *Children and Youth Services Review* 11(3):203-220.
Heneghan, A.M., S.M. Horwitz, and J.M. Leventhal
1996    Evaluating intensive family preservation programs: A methodological review. *Pediatrics* 97(4):535-542.
Henton, J., et al.
1983    Romance and violence in dating relationships. *Journal of Family Issues* 4(3):467-482.
Hilberman, E.
1980    Overview: The "wife beater's wife" reconsidered. *American Journal of Psychiatry* 137: 1336-1347.
Hilberman, E., and K. Munson
1977    Sixty battered women. *Victimology* 2(3-4):460-470.
Hirschel, J.D., and I.W. Hutchison III
1992    Female spouse abuse and the police response: The Charlotte, North Carolina experiment. *Journal of Criminal Law and Criminology* 83(1):73-119.

Hollister, R.G., and J. Hill
    1995    Problems in the evaluation of community-wide initiatives. Pp. 127-172 in J.P. Connell, A.C. Kubisch, L.B. Schorr, and C.H. Weiss, eds., *New Approaches to Evaluating Community Initiatives.* New York: The Aspen Institute.

Hornick, J.P., and M.E. Clarke
    1986    A cost-effectiveness evaluation of lay therapy treatment for child abusing and high risk parents. *Child Abuse and Neglect* 10:309-318.

Hotaling, G.T., and D.B. Sugarman
    1986    An analysis of risk markers in husband to wife violence: The current state of knowledge. *Violence and Victims* 1:101-124.
    1990    A risk marker analysis of assaulted wives. *Journal of Family Violence* 5(1):1-13.

Hotaling, G.T., J.H. Ascheim, and D. Sugarman
    no      The Children's Community Bridge Project: Outcome Evaluation Results. Unpublished
    date    manuscript, Division of Public Health Services, Office of Family and Community Health, Concord, N.H.

Hudson, M.F.
    1994    Elder abuse: Its meaning to middle-aged and older adults. Part II: Pilot results. *Journal of Elder Abuse and Neglect* 6(1):55.

Hunt, G.P.
    1994    Ethnography and the pursuit of culture: The use of ethnography in evaluating the community partnership program. In *Journal of Community Psychology Monograph Series.* Brandon, Vt.: Clinical Psychology Publishing Company, Inc.

Hurd, G., E.M. Pattison, and J.E. Smith
    1981    Test, re-test reliability of social network self reports: The Pattison Psychosocial Inventory (PPI). Paper presented at the Sun Belt Social Networks Conference, Tampa, Florida.

Hurley, D.J., and P. Jaffe
    1990    Children's observations of violence. II. Clinical implications for children's mental health professionals. *Canadian Journal of Psychiatry* 35(6):471-476.

Hyman, A., D. Schillinger, and B. Lo
    1995    Laws mandating reporting of domestic violence: Do they promote patient well-being? *Journal of the American Medical Association* 273(22):1781-1787.

Illinois Department on Aging
    1990    *Elder Abuse Intervention: Guidelines for Practice.* Springfield, Ill.: Illinois Department on Aging.

Infante-Rivard, C., G. Filion, M. Baumgarten, M. Bourassa, J. Labelle, and M. Messier
    1989    A public health home intervention among families of low socioeconomic status. *Child Health Care* 18(2):102-107.

Institute of Medicine
    1988    *The Future of Public Health.* Washington, D.C.: National Academy Press.
    1994    *Reducing Risks for Mental Disorders: Frontiers for Intervention Research,* P.J. Mrazek and R.J. Haggerty, eds. Report of the Committee on the Prevention of Mental Disorders. Washington, D.C.: National Academy Press.
    1997    *Improving Health in the Community: A Role for Performance Monitoring,* J.S. Durch, L.A. Bailey, and M.A. Stoto, eds. Report of the Committee on Using Performance Monitoring to Improve Community Health. Washington, D.C.: National Academy Press.

Irazuzta, J.E., J.E. McJunkin, K. Danadian, F. Arnold, and J. Zhang
    1997    Outcome and cost of child abuse. *Child Abuse and Neglect* 21(8):751-757.

Irueste-Montes, A.M., and F. Montes
    1988    Court-ordered vs. voluntary treatment of abusive and neglectful parents. *Child Abuse and Neglect* 12:33-39.

Jacob, H.
1983 Courts as organizations. In L. Mather and K. Boyum, eds., *Empirical Theories About the Courts.* New York: Longman.
Jaffe, P., D.A.Wolfe, S. Wilson, and L. Zak
1986a Emotional and physical health problems of battered women. *Canadian Journal of Psychiatry* 31(7): 625-629.
1986b Family violence and child adjustment: A comparative analysis of girls' and boys' behavioral symptoms. *American Journal of Psychiatry* 143(1):74-77.
Jaffe, P.G., M. Sudermann, D. Reitzel, and S.M. Killip
1992 An evaluation of a secondary school primary prevention program on violence in intimate relationships. *Violence and Victims* 7(2):129-146.
James, B., and M. Masjleti
1983 *Treating Sexually Abused Children and Their Families.* Palo Alto, Calif.: Consulting Psychologists Press.
Jenson, J.M., J.D. Hawkins, and R.F. Catalano
1986 Social support in aftercare services for troubled youth. *Children and Youth Services Review* 8:323-347.
Johnson, C.L.
1974 *Child Abuse in the Southeast: Analysis of 1172 Reported Cases.* Athens: Georgia University and Regional Institute of Social Welfare Research.
Johnson, M.K., and M.A. Foley
1984 Differentiating fact from fantasy: The reliability of children's memory. *Journal of Social Issues* 40:33-50.
Jones, L.E.
1991 The Minnesota School Curriculum Project: A statewide domestic violence prevention project in secondary schools. Pp. 258-266 in B. Levy, ed., *Dating Violence: Young Women in Danger.* Seattle, Wash.: Seal Press.
Jones, M.A.
1985 *A Second Chance for Families. Five Years Later. Follow-up of a Program to Prevent Foster Care.* New York: Child Welfare League of America.
1991 Measuring outcomes. Pp. 33-46 in K. Wells and D. Biegel eds., *Family Preservation Services: Research Evaluation.* Newbury Park, Calif.: Sage.
Jones, M.A., and B. Moses
1984 *West Virginia's Former Foster Children: Their Experiences in Care and Their Lives as Young Adults.* New York: Child Welfare League of America.
*Journal of the American Medical Association*
1990 From the Centers for Disease Control and Prevention. Family and other intimate assaults—Atlanta, 1984. *Journal of the American Medical Association* 264(10): 1243-1244.
Kaftarian, S.J., and W.B. Hansen, eds.
1994 Community Partnership Program. In *Journal of Community Psychology Monograph Series* . Brandon, Vt.: Clinical Psychology Publishing, Inc.
Kahn, A., and S. Kamerman
1996 *Starting Right: How America Neglects Its Youngest Children and What We Can Do About It.* New York: School of Social Work, Columbia University.
Kalichman, S.C.
1993 *Mandated Reporting of Suspected Child Abuse.* Washington, D.C.: American Psychological Association.
Kantor, G.K.
1993 Refining the brush strokes in portraits on alcohol and wife assaults. Pp. 281-290 in *Alcohol and Interpersonal Violence: Fostering Multidisciplinary Perspectives.* NIAA Monograph 24. Rockville, Md.: National Institute on Alcohol Abuse and Alcoholism.

Kantor, G.K., and M.A. Straus
   1987   The "drunken bum" theory of wife beating. *Social Problems* 34(3):213-230.
Kashani, J., A.E. Daniel, A.C. Dandoy, and W.R. Holcomb
   1992   Family violence: Impact on children. *Journal of the American Academy of Child and Adolescent Psychiatry* 31:181-182.
Kaufman, J., and E. Zigler
   1987   Do abused children become abusive parents? *American Journal of Orthopsychiatry* 57(2): 186-192.
Keilitz, S.L., P.L. Hannaford, and H.S. Efkeman
   1996   Civil Protection Orders: The Benefits and Limitations for Victims of Domestic Violence. National Center for State Courts, Williamsburg, Virginia.
Keller, R.A., L.F. Ciccinelli, and D.M. Gardner
   1989   Characteristics of child sexual abuse treatment programs. *Child Abuse and Neglect* 13:361-368.
Kelly, R.J.
   1982   Behavioral reorientation of pedophiliacs: Can it be done? *Clinical Psychology Review* 2:387-408.
Kempe, C.H., F.N. Silverman, B. Steele, W. Droegemueller, and H.R. Silver
   1962   The battered child syndrome. *Journal of the American Medical Association* 181(1):17-24.
Kendall-Tackett, K.A., L.M. Williams, and D. Finkelhor
   1993   *The Impact of Sexual Abuse on Children: A Review and Synthesis of Recent Empirical Studies.* San Diego, Calif.: American Professional Society on the Abuse of Children.
Kennedy, E.
   1991   *Child Abuse, Domestic Violence, Adoption and Family Services Act of 1991.* Report No. 102-164. Washington, D.C.: U.S. Senate Committee on Labor and Human Resources.
Kinard, E.M., and L.V. Klerman
   1980   Teenage parenting and child abuse. Are they related? *American Journal of Orthopsychiatry* 50(3):481-488.
Kinderknecht, C.H.
   1986   In-home social work with abused or neglected elderly: An experiential guide to assessment and treatment. *Journal of Gerontological Social Work* 9(3):29-42.
King, C.A., L. Radpour, and E.N. Jouriles
   1995   Parent's marital functioning and adolescent psychopathology. *Journal of Consulting and Clinical Psychology* 63(5):749.
Kinney, J.J., B. Madsen, T. Flemming, and D. Haapala
   1977   Homebuilders: Keeping families together. *Journal of Consulting Clinical Psychology* 45:667-673.
Kinney, J., D. Haapala, and C. Booth
   1991   *Keeping Families Together: The Homebuilders Model.* Hawthorne, N.Y.: Aldine de Gruyter.
Kleemeier, C., C. Webb, A. Hazzard, and J. Pohl
   1988   Child sexual abuse prevention: Evaluation of a teacher training model. *Child Abuse and Neglect* 12(4):555-561.
Klein, A.R.
   undated   Re-abuse in a Population of Court-Restrained Male Batterers. Unpublished document, Quincy Court Domestic Violence Program, Quincy, Mass.
Klein, C.F., and L.E. Orloff
   1996   Civil protection orders. Pp. 4-1 to 4-9 in D.M. Goelman, F.L. Lehrman, and R.L. Valente, eds., *The Impact of Domestic Violence on Your Legal Practice: A Lawyer's Handbook.* Washington, D.C.: The American Bar Association.

Kolko, D.
  1987 Treatment of child sexual abuse: Programs, progress, and prospects. *Journal of Family Violence* 2:303-318.
  1988 Educational programs to promote awareness and prevention of child sexual victimization: A review and methodological critique. *Clinical Psychology Review* 8:195-209.
  1996a Individual Cognitive-Behavioral Treatment and Family Therapy for Physically Abused Children and Their Offending Parents: A Comparison of Clinical Outcomes. Unpublished manuscript, University of Pittsburgh.
  1996b Clinical monitoring of treatment course in child physical abuse: Psychometric characteristics and treatment comparisons. *Child Abuse and Neglect* 20(1):23-43.

Kolko, D.J., J.T. Moser, and J. Hughes
  1989 Classroom training in sexual victimization awareness and prevention skills: An extension of the Red Flag/Green Flag People Program. *Journal of Family Violence* 4(1):25-45.

Korbin, J.E., G.J. Anetzberger, R. Thomasson, and C. Austin
  1991 Abused elders who seek legal recourse against their adult offspring: Findings from an exploratory study. *Journal of Elder Abuse and Neglect* 3(3):1-18.

Koss, M.P., P.G. Koss, and W.J. Woodruff
  1991 Deleterious effects of criminal victimization on women's health and medical utilization. *Archives of Internal Medicine* 151:342-347.

Koss, M.P., L.A. Goodman, A. Browne, L.F. Fitzgerald, G.P. Keita, and N.F. Russo
  1994 *No Safe Haven: Male Violence Against Women at Home, at Work, and in the Community.* Washington, D.C.: American Psychological Association.

Krajewski, S.S., M.F. Rybarik, M.F. Dosch, and G.D. Gilmore
  1996 Results of a curriculum intervention with seventh graders regarding violence in relationships. *Journal of Family Violence* 11(2):93-112.

Krugman, R.D., M. Lenherr, L. Betz, and G.E. Fryer
  1986 The relationship between unemployment and physical abuse of children. *Child Abuse and Neglect* 10(3):415-418.

Kurz, D.
  1987 Emergency department responses to battered women: Resistance to medicalization. *Social Problems* 34(1):69-81.

Lachs, M.S., and K. Pillemer
  1995 Abuse and neglect of elderly persons. *New England Journal of Medicine* 332(7):437-443.

Laner, M.R.
  1989a Competition and combativeness in courtship: Reports from men. *Journal of Family Violence* 4(1):47-62.
  1989b Competition and combativeness in courtship: Reports from women. *Journal of Family Violence* 4(2):181-195.

Lang, R.A., G.M. Pugh, and R. Langevin
  1988 Treatment of incest and pedophilic offenders: A pilot study. *Behavioral Sciences and the Law* 6(2):239-255.

Lanyon, R.I.
  1986 Theory and treatment in child molestation. *Journal of Consulting and Clinical Psychology* 54:176.

Larson, C.P.
  1980 Efficacy of prenatal and postpartum home visits on child health and development. *Pediatrics* 66(2):191-197.

Lavoie, F., L. Vezina, C. Piche, and M. Boivin
  1995 Evaluation of a prevention program for violence in teen dating relationships. *Journal of Interpersonal Violence* 10(4):516-524.

Legal Counsel for the Elderly, Inc.
  1987    *Decision-Making, Incapacity, and the Elderly: A Protective Services Manual.* Washing-
          ton, D.C.: American Association of Retired Persons.
Leonard, K.E., and H.T. Blane
  1992    Alcohol and marital aggression in a national sample of young men. *Journal of Interper-
          sonal Violence* 7(1):19-30.
Leonard, K.E., and M. Senchak
  1993    Alcohol and premarital aggression among newlywed couples. *Journal of Studies of Alco-
          hol* 11:96-108.
Lerman L.G.
  1981    *Legal Help for Battered Women.* Washington, D.C.: Center for Women Policy Studies.
Leventhal, J.M.
  1981    Risk factors for child abuse: Methodologic standards in case-control studies. *Pediatrics*
          68(5):684-690.
Levine, M., J. Freeman, and C. Compaan
  1994    Maltreatment-related fatalities: Issues of policy and prevention. *Law & Policy* 16(4):449-
          471.
Levinson, D.
  1989    *Family Violence in Cross Cultural Perspective.* Newbury Park, Calif.: Sage.
Limandri, B.J., and D.J. Sheridan
  1995    Prediction of intentional interpersonal violence: An introduction. Pp. 1-19 in J.C.
          Campbell, ed., *Assessing Dangerousness: Violence by Sexual Offenders, Batterers, and
          Child Abusers.* Thousand Oaks, Calif.: Sage.
Lindsey, D.
  1994    Family preservation and child protection: Striking a balance. *Children and Youth Ser-
          vices Review* 16(5/6):279.
Lipsey, M.W.
  1990    *Design Sensitivity: Statistical Power for Experimental Research.* Newbury Park, Calif.:
          Sage.
Lipsey, M.W., and D. Wilson
  1993    The efficacy of psychological, educational and behavioral treatment: Confirmation from
          meta-analysis. *American Psychologist* 48(12):1181-1209.
Lipsey, M.W., D.S. Cordray, and D.E. Berger
  1981    Evaluation of a juvenile diversion program: Using multiple lines of evidence. *Evaluation
          Review* 5:283-306.
Lipsey, M.W., S. Crosse, J. Dunkle, J. Pollard, and G. Stobart
  1985    Evaluation: The state of the art and the sorry state of the science. In D.S. Cordray, ed.,
          *Utilizing Prior Research in Evaluation Planning.* San Francisco: Jossey-Bass.
Lorion, R.P., T.G. Myers, C. Bartels, and A. Dennis
  1994    Preventive intervention research: Pathways for extending knowledge of child/adolescent
          health and pathology. *Advances in Clinical Child Psychology* 16:109-139.
Lundstrom, M., and R. Sharpe
  1991    Getting away with murder. *Public Welfare* xx:18-29.
Lutzker, J.R., D. Wesch, and J.M. Rice
  1984    A review of Project 12 Ways: An ecobehavioral approach to the treatment and prevention
          of child abuse and neglect. *Advances in Behavioral Research and Therapy* 6:63-73.
Lynn, M., N. Jacob, and L. Pierce
  1988    Child sexual abuse: A follow-up study of reports to a protective services hotline. *Chil-
          dren and Youth Services Review* 10:151-165.
MacMurray, B.K.
  1989    Criminal determination for child sexual abuse. *Journal of Interpersonal Violence* 4:233-
          244.

Makepeace, J.M.
    1981    Courtship violence among college students. *Family Relations* 30(1):97-102.
    1983    Life events stress and courtship violence. *Family Relations* 32(1):101-109.

Malamuth, N.M., C.L. Heavey, and D. Linz
    1993    Predicting men's antisocial behavior against women: The interaction model of sexual aggression. Pp. 63-97 in G.N. Hall, R. Hirschman, J. Graham, and M. Zaragoza, eds., *Sexual Aggression: Issues in Etiology, Assessment, and Treatment.* Washington, D.C.: Hemisphere.

Malinosky-Rummell, R., and D.J. Hansen
    1993    Long-term consequences of childhood physical abuse. *Psychological Bulletin* 114(1):68-79.

Marcenko, M.O., and M. Spence
    1994    Home visitation services for at-risk pregnant and post-partum women. *American Journal of Orthopsychiatry* 64(3):468-478.

Marciniak, E.
    1994    Community Policing of Domestic Violence: Neighborhood Differences in the Effect of Arrest. Ph.D. dissertation, Institute of Criminal Justice and Criminology, University of Maryland, College Park.

Margolin, L.
    1990    Fatal child neglect. *Child Welfare* 69(4):309-319.

Marshall, W.L., and H.E. Barbaree
    1988    The long-term evaluation of a behavioral treatment program for child molesters. *Behavioral Research and Therapy* 26(6):499-511.

Marshall, W.L., R. Jones, T. Ward, P. Johnston, and H.E. Barbaree
    1991    Treatment outcome with sex offenders. *Clinical Psychology Review* 11:465-485.

Martens, H.L.
    1992    *Community Ministry with Ex-Offenders: An Eco-Systemic Approach to Family Violence and Related Recidivism.* Ontario, Canada: Ministry of the Solicitor General of Canada.

Martin, D.
    1976    *Battered Wives.* San Francisco: Glide Publications.

McCauley, J., D.E. Kern, K. Kolodner, L. Dill, A.F. Schroeder, H.K. DeChant, J. Ryden, E.B. Bass, and L.R. Deragotis
    1995    The "battering syndrome": Prevalence and clinical characteristics of domestic violence in primary care internal medicine practices. *Annals of Internal Medicine* 123(10):737-746.

McClain, P.W., J.J. Sacks, R.G. Froehlke, and B.G. Weigman
    1993    Estimates of fatal child abuse and neglect, United States, 1979 through 1988. *Pediatrics* 91(2):338-343.

McCord, J.
    1983    A forty year perspective on effects of child abuse and neglect. *Child Abuse and Neglect* 7:265-270.

McCroskey, J., and W. Meezan
    1993    Outcomes of home-based services: Effects on family functioning, child behavior, and child placement. *Social Work* November:32 pp.

McCurdy, K.
    1995    Summary of Research on Home Visiting. Unpublished manuscript, National Center on Child Abuse and Neglect, Washington, D.C.

McCurdy, K., and D. Daro
    1994    Child maltreatment: A national survey of reports of fatalities. *Journal of Interpersonal Violence* 9(1):75-94.

McDonald, T.P., R.I. Allen, A. Westerfelt, and I. Piliavin
  1993   *Assessing the Long-Term Effects of Foster Care: A Research Synthesis.* Institute of Research on Poverty Special Report Series #57. Madison: University of Wisconsin.
McDonald, W.R., C.E. Wheeler, D. Struckman-Johnson, and M. Rivest
  1990   *Evaluation of AB 1562 In-Home Care Demonstration Projects, Volume I: Final Report.* Sacramento, Calif.: Office of Child Abuse Prevention, Department of Social Services.
McFarlane, J., B. Parker, K. Soeken, and L. Bullock
  1992   Assessing for abuse during pregnancy: Severity and frequency of injuries and associated entry into prenatal care. *Journal of the American Medical Association* 267(23):3176-3178.
McGrath, P., M. Cappelli, D. Wiseman, N. Khalil, and B. Allan
  1987   Teacher awareness program on child abuse: A randomized controlled trial. *Child Abuse and Neglect* 11:125-132.
McLeer, S.V., and R. Anwar
  1989   A study of women presenting in an emergency department. *American Journal of Public Health* 79(1):65-66.
McLeer, S.V., R. Anwar, S. Herman, and K. Maquiling
  1989   Education is not enough: A systems failure protecting battered women. *Annals of Emergency Medicine* 18(6):651-653.
Meddin, B., and I. Hansen
  1985   The services provided during a child abuse and/or neglect case investigation and the barriers that exist to service provision. *Child Abuse and Neglect* 9:175-182.
Melnick, B., and J.R. Hurley
  1969   Distinctive personality of child-abusing mothers. *Journal of Consulting and Clinical Psychology* 33:746-749.
Melton, G.B.
  1985   Sexually abused children and the legal system: Some policy recommendations. *American Journal of Family Therapy* 13:61-67.
Melton, G.B., G.S. Goodman, S.C. Kalichman, M. Levine, K.J. Saywitz, and G.P. Koocher
  1995   Empirical research on child maltreatment and the law. Report of the American Psychological Association Working Group on Legal Issues related to Child Abuse and Neglect. *Journal of Clinical Child Psychology* 24(Suppl.): 47-77.
Mercy, J.A., M.L. Rosenberg, K.E. Powell, C.V. Broome, and W.L. Roper
  1993   Public health policy for preventing violence. *Health Affairs* 12(4):7-29.
Metcalf, C.E., and C. Thornton
  1992   Random assignment. *Children and Youth Services Review* 14:145-156.
Meyer, H.
  1992   The billion dollar epidemic. *American Medical News* 35(1):7.
Miller, B.A., W.R. Downs, and D.M. Gondoli
  1989   Spousal violence among alcoholic women as compared to a random household sample of women. *Journal of Studies on Alcohol* 50(6):533-540.
Miller, T.R, M.A. Cohen, and B. Wiersema
  1994   Crime in the United States: Victim Costs and Consequences. Unpublished manuscript, National Public Services Research Institute, Washington, D.C.
Miltenberger, R.G., and E. Thiesse-Duffy
  1988   Evaluation of home-based program for teaching personal safety skills to children. *Journal of Applied Behavioral Analysis* 21(1):81-87.
Missouri Department of Health, Bureau of Dental Health
  1995   *What Is the PANDA Coalition to Prevent Child Abuse/Neglect?* St. Louis National Center on Child Abuse and Neglect. St. Louis: Missouri Department of Health.

Monahan, J.
  1981    *Predicting Violent Behavior.* Beverly Hills, Calif.: Sage.
Monahan, J., and H.J. Steadman
  1994    *Violence and Mental Disorder: Developments in Risk Assessment.* Chicago, Ill: University of Chicago Press.
Morley, R.
  1994    Wife beating and modernization: The case of Papua New Guinea. *Journal of Comparative Family Studies* 25(1):25-52.
Murphy, M., M. Jellinek, D. Quinn, G. Smith, F.G. Poitrast, and M. Goshko
  1991    Substance abuse and serious child mistreatment: Prevalence, risk, and outcome in a court sample. *Child Abuse and Neglect* 15:197-211.
Myers, J.E.
  1994    Medicine, mental health, and the legal system: Critical partners in responding to family violence. *Work Group on Assessment, National Conference on Family Violence: Health and Justice, Washington, D.C.* Sacramento, Calif.: University of the Pacific.
National Center on Child Abuse and Neglect
  1983a   *Collaborative Research of Community and Minority Group Action to Prevent Child Abuse and Neglect. Volume I: Perinatal Interventions. Part II. Perinatal Positive Parenting.* Washington, D.C.: U.S. Department of Health and Human Services.
  1983b   *Collaborative Research of Community and Minority Group Action to Prevent Child Abuse and Neglect: Pride in Parenthood.* Washington, D.C.: U.S. Department of Health and Human Services.
  1988    *Study Findings: Study of National Incidence and Prevalence of Child Abuse and Neglect.* Washington, D.C.: U.S. Department of Health and Human Services.
  1996a   *The Third National Incidence Study of Child Abuse and Neglect.* Washington, D.C.: U.S. Department of Health and Human Services.
  1996b   *Child Maltreatment 1994: Reports from the States to the National Child Abuse and Neglect Data System.* Washington, D.C.: U.S. Department of Health and Human Services.
  1996c   *Child Abuse and Neglect Case-Level Data 1993: Working Paper 1.* Washington, D.C.: U.S. Department of Health and Human Services.
National Center on Elder Abuse and Neglect
  1995    *The National Elder Abuse Incidence Study.* Washington, D.C.: National Center on Elder Abuse and Neglect.
National Committee to Prevent Child Abuse
  1991    *Current Trends in Child Abuse Reporting and Fatalities: The Results of the 1990 Annual Fifty State Survey.* Chicago, Ill.: National Committee to Prevent Child Abuse.
  1996    Intensive Home Visitation: A Randomized Trial, Follow-Up, and Risk Assessment Study of Hawaii's Healthy Start Program. Chicago, Ill.: National Committee to Prevent Child Abuse.
National Institute of Mental Health
  1992    *Family Violence. National Workshop on Violence: Analyses and Recommendations.* Prepared by Daniel O'Leary and Angela Browne. Violence and Traumatic Stress Research Branch. Bethesda, Md.: National Institute of Mental Health.
  1993    Ethical Considerations in Violence-Related Research. Unpublished document, National Institute of Mental Health, Bethesda, Md.
National Research Council
  1985    *Sharing Research Data.* S.E. Fienberg, M.E. Martin, and M.L. Straf, eds. Committee on National Statistics. Washington, D.C.: National Academy Press.

1993a  *Understanding Child Abuse and Neglect.* Panel on Research on Child Abuse and Neglect. Washington, D.C.: National Academy Press.

1993b  *Understanding and Preventing Violence,* A.J. Reiss, Jr. and J.A. Roth, eds. Panel on the Understanding and Control of Violent Behavior. Washington D.C.: National Academy Press.

1993c  *Private Lives and Public Policies: Confidentiality and Accessibility of Government Statistics,* G.T. Duncan, T.B. Jabine, and V. de Wolf, eds. Panel on Confidentiality and Data Access. Washington, D.C.: National Academy Press.

1995  *Preventing HIV Transmission: The Role of Sterile Needles and Bleach,* J. Normand, D. Vlahov, and L.E. Moses, eds. Panel on Needle Exchange and Bleach Distribution Programs, National Research Council and Institute of Medicine. Washington, D.C.: National Academy Press.

1996  *Understanding Violence Against Women,* N.A. Crowell and A.W. Burgess, eds. Panel on Research on Violence Against Women. Washington, D.C.: National Academy Press.

National Resource Center on Family Based Services

1986  Evaluation of Fourteen Child Placement Prevention Projects in Wisconsin, 1983-1985. Unpublished document, School of Social Work, University of Iowa, Iowa City.

Neale, A.V., M.A. Hwalek, C.S. Goodrich, and K.M. Quinn

1996  The Illinois elder abuse system: Program description and administrative findings. *Gerontologist* 36(4):502-511.

Nelson, K.E.

1988  *Factors Contributing to Success and Failure in Family-Based Child Welfare Services: Executive Summary.* Unpublished document, School of Social Work, University of Iowa, Iowa City.

Newberger, E., R. Reed, J. Daniel, J. Hyde, and M. Kotelchuck

1977  Pediatric social illness: Toward an etiological classification. *Pediatrics* 60:178-185.

Oates, R.K., B.I. O'Toole, and G. Cooney

1994  Stability and change in outcomes for sexually abused children. *Journal of the American Academy of Child and Adolescent Health* 33(7):945-953.

O'Connor, A.

1995  Evaluating comprehensive community initiatives: A view from history. Pp. 23-63 in J.P. Connell, A.C. Kubisch, L.B. Schorr, and C.H.Weiss, eds., *New Approaches to Evaluating Community Initiatives: Concepts, Methods, and Contexts.* New York: The Aspen Institute.

O'Donohue, W.T., and A.N. Elliott

1992  Treatment of the sexually abused child: A review. *Journal of Clinical Child Psychology* 21(3):218-228.

Office of Juvenile Justice and Delinquency Prevention

1994  *OJJDP Model Programs 1990. Preserving Families to Prevent Delinquency.* Washington, D.C.: U.S. Department of Justice.

Ohlin, L., and M. Tonry

1989  Family violence in perspective. Pp. 1-18 in M.D. Pagelow, ed., *Family Violence.* Chicago, Ill.: University of Chicago Press.

Olds, D.L.

1992  Home visitation for pregnant women and parents of young children. *American Journal of Diseases of Children* 146(6):704-708.

Olds, D., and C.R. Henderson

1990  The prevention of maltreatment. Pp. 722-763 in D. Cicchetti and V. Carlson, eds., *Child Maltreatment.* New York: Cambridge University Press.

Olds, D.L., and H. Kitzman
    1990    Can home visitation improve the health of women and children at environmental risk? *Pediatrics* 86(1):108-116.
    1993    Review of research on home visiting for pregnant women and parents of young children. *The Future of Children* 3(3):53-92.

Olds, D.L., C.R. Henderson, R. Chamberlin, and R. Tatelbaum
    1986    Preventing child abuse and neglect: A randomized trial of nurse home visitation. *Pediatrics* 78(1):65-78.

Olds, D.L., C.R. Henderson, R. Tatelbaum, and R. Chamberlin
    1988    Improving the life-course development of socially disadvantaged mothers: A randomized trial of nurse home visitation. *American Journal of Public Health* 78(11):1436-1445.

Olds, D.L., C.R. Henderson, and H. Kitzman
    1994    Does prenatal and infancy nurse home visitation have enduring effects on qualities of parental caregiving and child health at 25 to 50 months of life? *Pediatrics* 93(1):89-98.

Olds, D.L., C.R. Henderson, H. Kitzman, and R. Cole
    1995    Effects of prenatal and infancy nurse home visitation on surveillance of child maltreatment. *Pediatrics* 95(3):365-372.

Olds, D.L., J. Eckenrode, C.R. Henderson, Jr., H. Kitzman, J. Powers, R. Cole, K. Sidora, P. Morris, L.M. Pettitt, and D. Luckey
    1997    Long-term effects of home visitation on maternal life course and child abuse and neglect. *Journal of the American Medical Association* 278(8):637-643.

O'Leary, K.D., R.E. Heyman, and P.H. Neidig
    1994    Treatment of Wife Abuse: A Comparison of Gender Specific and Couples Approaches. Paper presented at the 4th International Conference on Family Violence Research, Durham, N.H., July.

Olson, L., C. Anctil, L. Fullerton, J. Brillman, J. Arbuckle, and D. Sklar
    1996    Increasing emergency physician recognition of domestic violence. *Annals of Emergency Medicine* 27(6):741-746.

Osofsky, J.D.
    1995a    The effects of exposure to violence on young children. *American Psychologist* 50:782-788.
    1995b    Children who witness domestic violence: The invisible victims. *Social Policy Reports* 9(3):1-16.
    1997    *Children in a Violent Society.* New York: Guilford Publishers.

Pagelow, M.D.
    1984    *Family Violence.* New York: Praeger.

Palmer, S.E.
    1976    *Children in Long-Term Care: Their Experience and Progress.* Canada: Family and Children's Services of London and Middlesex.

Palmer, S.E., R.A. Brown, and M.E. Barrera
    1992    Group treatment program for abusive husbands: Long-term evaluation. *American Journal of Orthopsychiatry* 62(2):276-283.

Parke, R.D., and C.W. Collmer
    1975    Child abuse: An interdisciplinary analysis. Pp. 1-102 in E.M. Hetherington and M.E. Hetherington, eds., *Review of Child Development Research,* Vol. 5. Chicago, Ill.: University of Chicago Press.

Parker, B., J. McFarlane, and K. Soeken
    1994    Abuse during pregnancy: Effects on maternal complications and birth weight in adult and teenage women. *American Journal of Obstetrics and Gynecology* 84(3):323-328.

Parsons, L.H., D. Zaccaro, B. Wells, and T.G. Stovall
  1995    Methods of and attitudes toward screening obstetrics and gynecology patients for domestic violence. *American Journal of Obstetrics and Gynecology* 173(2):381-387.
Pate, A.M., and E.E. Hamilton
  1992    Formal and informal deterrents to domestic violence: The Dade County Spouse Assault Experiment. *American Sociological Review* 57:691-697.
Pecora, P.J., M.W. Fraser, and D.A. Haapala
  1992    Client outcomes and issues for program design. Pp. 3-32 in K. Wells and D.E. Biegel, eds., *Family Preservation Services: Research and Evaluation.* Newbury Park, Calif.: Sage.
Pelton, L.H.
  1981    *The Social Context of Child Abuse and Neglect.* New York: Human Sciences Press.
  1989    *For Reasons of Poverty.* New York: Praeger.
  1994    The role of material factors in child abuse and neglect. Chap. 4 in G.B. Melton and F.D. Barry, eds., *Protecting Children from Abuse and Neglect.* New York: Guilford Press.
Pennsylvania Attorney General's Task Force
  1988    *Violence Against Elders.* Harrisburg, Pa.: Attorney General's Office.
Peraino, J.M.
  1990    Evaluation of a preschool antivictimization prevention program. *Journal of Interpersonal Violence* 5(4):520-528.
Pfannenstiel, J., and D. Seltzer
  1989    New parents as teachers: Evaluation of an early parent education program. *Early Childhood Research Quarterly* 4(1):1-18.
Pillemer, K.A.
  1986    Risk factors in elder abuse: Results from a case-control study. Pp. 239-263 in K. Pillemer and R. Wolf, eds., *Elder Abuse: Conflict in the Family.* Dover, Mass.: Auburn House.
Pillemer, K.A., and D. Finkelhor
  1988    Prevalence of elder abuse: A random sample survey. *Gerontologist* 28(1):51-57.
Pillemer, K.A., and J. Suitor
  1988    Elder abuse. Pp. 247-270 in V.B. Van Hasselt, R.L. Morrison, A.S. Bellack, and M. Hersen, eds., *Handbook of Family Violence.* New York: Plenum Press.
  1992    Violence and violent feelings: What causes them among family caregivers? *Gerontology* 47(4):S165-S172.
Pittman, N.E., and R.G. Taylor
  1992    MMPI profiles of partners of incestuous sexual offenders and partners of alcoholics. *Family Dynamics of Addiction Quarterly* 2:52-59.
Plichta, S.B.
  1995    Domestic Violence: Building Paths for Women to Travel to Freedom and Safety. Paper presented at the Symposium on Domestic Violence and Women's Health: Broadening the Conversation. The Commonwealth Fund, New York, September.
  1996    Chapter in M. Falik and K.S. Collins, eds., *Women's Health.* Baltimore, Md.: Johns Hopkins University Press.
Poertner, J., and A. Press
  1990    Who best represents the interests of the child in court? *Child Welfare* 69(6):537-549.
Pogge, D.L., and K. Stone
  1990    Conflicts and issues in the treatment of child sexual abuse. *Professional Psychology: Research and Practice* 21:354-361.
Polansky, N.A., M.A. Chalmers, E. Buttenwieser, and D.P. Williams
  1981    *Damaged Parents: An Anatomy of Child Neglect.* Chicago, Ill.: University of Chicago Press.

Polansky, N.A., J.M. Gaudin, and A.C. Kilpatrick
1992    Family radicals. *Children and Youth Services Review* 14:19-26.
Powell, K.E., and D.F. Hawkins
1996    Youth violence prevention: Descriptions and baseline data from 13 evaluation projects. *American Journal of Preventive Medicine* Supplement to 12(5).
Quinn, K., M. Hwalek, and C.S. Goodrich
1993    *Determining Effective Interventions in a Community-Based Elder Abuse System: Final Report.* Washington, D.C.:    Administration on Aging, U.S. Department of Health and Human Services.
Quinn, M.J.
1985    Elder abuse and neglect raise new dilemmas. *Generations* 2:22-25.
Quinn, M.J., and S.K. Tomita
1986    *Elder Abuse and Neglect: Causes, Diagnosis, and Intervention Strategies.* New York: Springer.
Quinsey, V.L., G.T. Harris, M.A. Rice, and M.L. Lalumiere
1993    Assessing treatment efficacy in outcome studies of sex offenders. *Journal of Interpersonal Violence* 8(4):512-523.
Quinsey, V.L., M.E. Rice, and G.T. Harris
1995    Actuarial prediction of sexual recidivism. *Journal of Interpersonal Violence* 10(1):85-105.
Randolph, M.K., and C.A. Gold
1994    Child sexual abuse prevention: Evaluation of a teacher training program. *School Psychology Review* 23(3):485-495.
Reid, J.B., P. Taplan, and R. Lorber
1981    A social interactional approach to the treatment of abusive families. Pp. 83-101 in R.B. Stuart, ed., *Violent Behavior: Social Learning Approaches to Prediction, Management, and Treatment.* New York: Brunner/Mazel.
Reppucci, N.D., and J.J. Haugaard
1988    *The Sexual Abuse of Children: A Comprehensive Guide to Current Knowledge and Intervention Strategies.* San Francisco, Calif.: Jossey-Bass.
Resnick, G.
1985    Enhancing parental competencies for high risk mothers: An evaluation of prevention effects. *Child Abuse and Neglect* 9(4):479-489.
Rice, D.P., W. Max, J. Golding, and H. Pinderhughes
1996    The Cost of Domestic Violence to the Health Care System.    Unpublished manuscript, Institute for Health and Aging, School of Nursing, University of California, San Francisco.
Rizley, R., and D. Cicchetti
1981    *Developmental Perspectives on Child Maltreatment. New Directions for Child Development.* San Francisco, Calif.: Jossey-Bass.
Robertson, J.
1995    Domestic violence and health care: An ongoing dilemma. *Albany Law Review* 58(4):1193-1214.
Robins, L.N., J.E. Helzer, M.M. Weissman, H. Orvascel, E. Gruenberg, J.D. Burke, and D.A. Regier
1984    Lifetime prevalence of specific psychiatric disorders in three sites. *Archives of General Psychiatry* 41(10):949-958.
Rosenberg, M.L., and M.A. Fenley
1992    The federal role in injury control. *American Psychologist* 47(8):1031-1035.
Rosenberg, M.L., and J.A. Mercy
1991    Assaultive violence.  Chapter in M.L. Rosenberg and M.A. Fenley, eds., *Violence in America: A Public Health Approach.* New York: Oxford University Press.

Rosenfeld, B.D.
1992    Court-ordered treatment of spouse abuse. *Clinical Psychology Review* 12:205-226.

Rossi, P.
1992    Assessing family preservation programs. *Children and Youth Services Review* 14:75-95.

Royse, D., and V.R. Wiehe
1989    Assessing effects of foster care on adults raised as foster children: A methodological issue. *Psychological Reports* 64(2):677-678.

Rubenstein, J.S., J.A. Armentrout, S. Levin, and D. Herald
1978    The parent-therapist program: Alternate care for emotionally disturbed children. *American Journal of Orthopsychiatry* 48:654-662.

Runyan, D.K., and C.L. Gould
1985    Foster care for child maltreatment: Impact on delinquent behavior. *Pediatrics* 75(3):562-568.

Runyan, D., C. Gould, D. Frost, et al.
1981    Determinants of foster care for the maltreated child. *American Journal of Public Health* 71:706-711.

Runyan, D.K., M.D. Everson, G.A. Edelsohn, W.H. Hunter, and M.L. Coulter
1988    Impact of legal intervention on sexually abused children. *Pediatrics* 113(4):647-653.

Russell, D.
1984    *Sexual Exploitation: Rape, Child Sexual Abuse, and Work Place Harassment.* Newbury Park, Calif.: Sage.

Rutter, M.
1990    Psychosocial resilience and protective mechanisms. Pp. 181-214 in A. Rolf, A.S. Masten, D. Cicchetti, K.H. Nuechtterlein, and S. Weintraub, eds., *Risk and Protective Factors in the Development of Psychopathology.* New York: Cambridge University Press.

Salovitz, B., and D. Keys
1988    Is child protective services still a service? *Protecting Children* 5:17-23.

Salzinger, S., R.S. Feldman, M. Hammer, and M. Rosario
1993    The effects of physical abuse on children's social relationships. *Child Development* 64(1):169-187.

Sameroff, A.J., and M. Chandler
1975    Reproductive risk and the continuum of caretaking casualty. Pp. 187-244 in F. Horowitz, ed., *Review of Child Development Research,*Vol. 4. Chicago, Ill.: University of Chicago Press.

Saslawsky, D.A., and S.K. Wurtele
1986    Educating children about sexual abuse: Implications for pediatric intervention and possible prevention. *Journal of Pediatric Psychology* 11(2):235-245.

Saunders, D.G.
1992    A typology of men who batter. *American Journal of Orthopsychiatry* 62:264-275.
1995    The tendency to arrest victims of domestic violence: A preliminary analysis of officer characteristics. *Journal of Interpersonal Violence* 10(2):147-158.

Saunders, D.G., and S. Azar
1989    Treatment programs for family violence. Pp. 481-541 in L. Ohlin and M.H. Tonry, eds., *Family Violence, Volume 11, Crime and Justice: An Annual Review of Research.* Chicago, Ill.: University of Chicago Press.

Saunders, D.G., K. Hamberger, and M. Hovey
1993    Indicators of woman abuse based on a chart review at a family practice center. *Archives of Family Medicine* 2:537-543.

Saunders, E.
1988    A comparative study of attitudes toward sexual abuse among social work and judicial system professionals. *Child Abuse and Neglect* 12:83-90.

Scarr, S., and K. McCartney
  1988   Far from home: An experimental evaluation of the Mother-Child Home Program in Bermuda. *Child Development* 59(3):531-543.
Schechter, S.
  1982   Toward an analysis of violence against women in the family. Pp. 209-240 in *Women and Male Violence*. Boston, Mass.: South End Press.
Schei, B., S.O. Samuelsen, and L.S. Bakketeig
  1991   Does spousal physical abuse affect the outcome of pregnancy? *Scandinavian Journal of Sociology and Medicine* 19(1):26-31.
Schinke, S.P., R.F. Schilling, R.P. Barth, L.D. Gilchrist, and J.S. Maxwell
  1986   Stress-management intervention to prevent family violence. *Journal of Family Violence* 1(1):13-26.
Schmidt, J., and E.H. Steury
  1989   Prosecutorial discretion in filing charges in domestic violence cases. *Criminology* 27:487-510.
Schneider, E.M.
  1980   Equal rights to trial for women: Sex bias in the law of self-defense claims by battered women charged with homicide. *Harvard Civil Rights-Civil Liberties Law Review* 1:623-647.
Schuerman, J.R., T.L. Rzepnicki, and J.H. Littell
  1994   *Putting Families First: An Experiment in Family Preservation.* New York: Aldine de Gruyter.
Schwartz, I.M., P. AuClaire, and L.J. Harris
  1991   Family preservation services as an alternative to the out-of-home placement of adolescents. Pp. 33-46 in K. Wells and D.E. Biegel, eds., *Preservation Services: Research and Evaluation.* New York: Sage.
Scogin, F., C. Beall, J. Bynum, G. Stephens, N.P. Grote, L.A. Baumhover, and J.M. Bolland
  1989   Training for abusive caregivers: An unconventional approach to an intervention dilemma. *Journal of Elder Abuse and Neglect* 1(4):73-86.
Sedlak, A.
  1991   *National Incidence and Prevalence of Child Abuse and Neglect: 1988.* Washington, D.C.: National Clearinghouse on Child Abuse and Neglect, U.S. Department of Health and Human Services.
Sedlak, A., and D.D. Broadhurst
  1996   *Third National Incidence Study of Child Abuse and Neglect.* Washington, D.C.: Administration for Children and Families, U.S. Department of Health and Human Services.
Seitz, V., L.K. Rosenbaum, and N. Apfel
  1985   Effects of family support intervention: A ten year follow-up. *Child Development* 5(6):376-391.
Shainess, N.
  1979   Masochism as a process. *American Journal of Psychotherapy* 33(2):174-189.
Sherman, L.W.
  1992a  The influence of criminology on criminal law: Evaluating arrests for misdemeanor domestic violence. *Journal of Criminal Law and Criminology* 83(1):1-45.
  1992b  *Policing Domestic Violence.* New York: The Free Press.
Sherman, L.W., and R.A. Berk
  1984a  The specific deterrent effects of arrest for domestic assault. *American Sociological Review* 49(2):261-272.
  1984b  *The Minneapolis Domestic Violence Experiment.* Washington, D.C.: Police Foundation.

Sherman, L.W., and E.G. Cohn
   1989    The impact of research on legal policy: The Minneapolis domestic violence experiment. *Law & Society Review* 23(1):117-144.
Sherman, L.W., J.D. Schmidt, D.P. Rogan, P.R. Gartin, E.G. Cohn, D.J. Collins, and A.R. Bacich
   1991    From initial deterrence to long-term escalation: Short custody arrest for poverty ghetto domestic violence. *Criminology* 29(4):821-850.
Sherman, L.W., J.D. Schmidt, D.P. Rogan, D.A. Smith, P.R. Gartin, E.G. Cohn, D.J. Collins, and A.R. Bacich
   1992a   The variable effects of arrest on criminal careers: The Milwaukee Domestic Violence Experiment. *Journal of Criminal Law and Criminology* 83(1):137-169.
Sherman, L.W., D.A. Smith, J.D. Schmidt, and D.P. Rogan
   1992b   Crime, punishment, and stake in conformity: Legal and informal control of domestic violence. *American Sociological Review* 57:680-690.
Shyne, A.W., and A.G. Schroeder
   1978    *National Study of Social Services to Children and Their Families.* Washington, D.C.: National Center for Child Advocacy.
Smith, B.E., and S.G. Elstein
   1993    The Prosecution of Child Sexual and Physical Abuse Cases. American Bar Association. Final Report to the National Center on Child Abuse and Neglect, Washington, D.C.
Sosin, M.R., I. Piliavin, and H. Westerfelt
   1991    Toward a longitudinal analysis of homelessness. *Journal of Social Issues* 46:157-174.
Spinetta, J.J., and D. Rigler
   1972    The child abusing parent: A psychological review. *Psychological Bulletin* 77:296-304.
Stark, E., and A.H. Flitcraft
   1988    Violence among intimates: An epidemiological review. Pp. 293-317 in V.B. Van Hasselt, R.L. Morrison, A.S. Bellack, and M. Hersen, eds., *Handbook of Family Violence.* New York: Plenum.
Starr, R.H.
   1988    Physical abuse of children. Pp. 119-155 in V.B. Van Hasselt, R.L. Morrison, A.S. Bellack, and M. Hersen, eds., *Handbook of Family Violence.* New York: Plenum.
Starr, R.H., H. Dubowitz, and B.A. Bush
   1990    The epidemiology of child maltreatment. Pp. 23-53 in R.T. Ammerman and M. Hersen, eds., *Children at Risk: An Evaluation of Factors Contributing to Child Abuse and Neglect.* New York: Plenum.
Steele, B.F., and C.B. Pollock
   1974    A psychiatric study of parents who abuse infants and small children. Pp. 89-133 in R.E. Helfer and C.H. Kempe, eds., *The Battered Child.* Chicago, Ill.: University of Chicago Press.
Steinman, M.
   1988    Evaluating a system-wide response to domestic violence: Some initial findings. *Journal of Contemporary Criminal Justice* 4:172-186.
   1990    Lowering recidivism among men who batter women. *Journal of Police Science and Administration* 17(2):124-132.
Steinmetz, S.K.
   1978    Violence between family members. *Marriage and Family Review* 1(3):3-16.
   1990    Elder abuse by adult offspring: The relationship of actual vs. perceived dependency. *Journal of Health and Human Resources Administration* 12(4):434.
Stern, P.
   1997    *Preparing and Presenting Expert Testimony in Child Abuse Litigation.* Thousand Oaks, Calif.: Sage.

Stets, J.E., and M.A. Straus
  1990    Gender differences in reporting marital violence and its medical and psychological conse-
          quences. In M.A. Straus and R.J. Gelles, eds., *Physical Violence in American Families:
          Risk Factors and Adaptations to Violence in 8,145 Families.* New Brunswick, N.J.:
          Transaction Publishers.
Stone, R.
  1993    Panel finds gaps in violence studies. *Science* 260(5114):1584-1585.
Stoto, M.A.
  1992    Public health assessment in the 1990s. *Annual Review of Public Health* 13:59-78.
Straus, M.A.
  1986    The cost of intrafamily assault and homicide to society. *Academic Medicine* 62:556-561.
  1987    The costs of family violence. *Public Health Reports* 102(6):638-641.
  1993    Measurement Issues in Child Abuse Research. Unpublished manuscript, Family Research
          Laboratory, University of New Hampshire, Durham.
  1994    Ten myths about spanking children. In *Beating the Devil Out of Them: Corporal Punish-
          ment in American Families.* Boston, Mass.: Lexington Books.
Straus, M.A., and R.J. Gelles
  1986    Societal change in family violence from 1975 to 1985 as revealed by two national sur-
          veys. *Journal of Marriage and the Family* 48:465-479.
  1988    How violent are American families? Estimates from the National Family Violence Resur-
          vey and other studies. In G.T. Hotaling, D. Finkelhor, J.T. Kirkpatrick, and M.A. Straus,
          eds., *Family Abuse and Its Consequences: New Directions in Research.* Newbury Park,
          Calif.: Sage.
  1990    *Physical Violence in American Families: Risk Factors and Adaptations to Violence in
          8,145 Families.* New Brunswick, N.J.: Transaction.
Straus, M.A., and C. Smith
  1990    Violence in Hispanic families in the United States: Incidence rates and structural inter-
          pretations. Pp. 341-367 in M.A. Straus and R.J. Gelles, eds., *Physical Violence in Ameri-
          can Families: Risk Factors and Adaptations to Violence in 8,145 Families.* New
          Brunswick, N.J.: Transaction.
Straus, M.A., R.J. Gelles, and S.K. Steinmetz
  1980    *Behind Closed Doors: Violence in the American Family.* New York: Doubleday/An-
          chor.
Sturkie, K.
  1983    Structured group treatment for sexually abused children. *Health and Social Work* 8:299-
          308.
Sugg, N.K., and T. Inui
  1992    Primary care physicians' response to domestic violence: Opening Pandora's box. *Journal
          of the American Medical Association* 267(23):3157-3160.
Sullivan, C.M., and W.S. Davidson
  1991    The provision of advocacy services to women leaving abusive partners: An examination
          of short term effects. *American Journal of Community Psychology* 19(6):953-960.
Sullivan, C.M., J. Basta, C. Tan, and W.S. Davidson II
  1992    After the crisis: A needs assessment of women leaving a domestic violence shelter.
          *Violence and Victims* 7(3):267-275.
Susser, E., E.L. Struening, and S. Conover
  1987    Childhood experiences of homelessness. *American Journal of Psychiatry* 144:1599-1601.
Susser, M.
  1995    Editorial: The tribulations of trials: Intervention in communities. *American Journal of
          Public Health* 85(2):156-172.

Swan, W.W., and J.L. Morgan
1993    Collaborating for Comprehensive Services for Young Children and Their Families. Bal-
        timore, Md.: Paul H. Brookes Publishing Company.
Szykula, S.A., and M.J. Fleischman
1985    Reducing out-of-home placements of abused children: Two controlled field studies. Child
        Abuse and Neglect 9:277-283.
Tan, C., J. Basta, C.M. Sullivan, and W.S. Davidson
1995    The role of social support in the lives of women exiting domestic violence shelters: An
        experimental study. Journal of Interpersonal Violence 10(4):437-451.
Taylor, B.
1995    An Evaluation of the Domestic Violence Prevention Project: A Descriptive Analysis. New
        York: Victim Services, Inc.
Terr, L.
1981    Psychic trauma in children: Observations following the Chowchilla school-bus kidnap-
        ping. American Journal of Psychiatry 138:14-19.
1983    Chowchilla revisited: The effects of psychic trauma four years after school-bus kidnap-
        ping. American Journal of Psychiatry 140:1543-1550.
Thomas, J.
1995    Child protective services responses to child maltreatment. Service Provider Perspectives
        on Family Violence Interventions. Proceedings of a Workshop, Committee on the As-
        sessment of Family Violence Interventions, Washington, D.C.: National Academy Press..
Thompson, R.
1994    Social support and the prevention of child maltreatment. Chapter 3 in G. Melton and F.D.
        Barry, eds., Protecting Children from Abuse and Neglect. New York: Guilford Press.
1995    Preventing Child Maltreatment Through Social Support. A Critical Analysis. Thousand
        Oaks, Calif: Sage.
Tilden, V.P., and P. Shepherd
1987    Increasing the rate of identification of battered women in an emergency department: Use
        of a nursing protocol. Research in Nursing and Health 10:209-215.
Tilden, V.P., T.A. Schmidt, B.J. Limandri, G.T. Chiodo, M.J. Garland, and P.A. Loveless
1994    Factors that influence clinicians' assessment and management of family violence. Ameri-
        can Journal of Public Health 84(4):628-633.
Tjaden, P.G., and N. Theonnes
1992    Predictors of legal intervention in child maltreatment cases. Child Abuse and Neglect
        16:807-821.
Tolman, R.M., and G. Bhosley
1989    A comparison of two types of pregroup preparation for men who batter. Journal of Social
        Service Research 13(2):33-43.
Tolman, R.M., and J.L. Edleson
1995    Intervention for men who batter. A research review. Pp. 163-173 in S.M. Stith and M.A.
        Straus, eds., Understanding Partner Violence: Prevalence, Causes, Consequences, and
        Solutions. Minneapolis, Minn.: National Council on Family Relations.
Tomita, S.K.
1982    Detection and treatment of elderly abuse and neglect: A protocol for health care profes-
        sionals. Physical and Occupational Therapy in Geriatrics 2(2):37-51.
Tracy, E.M.
1991    Defining the target population for family preservation services. Pp. 138-158 in K. Wells
        and D. Biegel eds., Family Preservation Services: Research and Evaluation. Newbury
        Park, Calif.: Sage.
Tracy, E.M., and N. Abell
1994    Social network map: Some further refinements on administration. Social Work Research
        18(1):56-60.

Tracy, E.M., and J.K. Whittaker
  1990    The social network map: Assessing social support in clinical practice. *Families in Society* 7:461-470.
Tutty, L.M.
  1995    The Efficacy of Shelter Follow-Up Programs for Abused Women. Paper presented at the 4th International Family Violence Research Conference, Durham, N.H., July 21-24.
U.S. Advisory Board on Child Abuse and Neglect
  1995    *A Nation's Shame: Fatal Child Abuse and Neglect in the United States.* Washington, D.C.: U.S. Government Printing Office.
U.S. Attorney General
  1984    *Final Report.* Task Force on Family Violence. Washington, D.C.: U.S. Government Printing Office.
U.S. Department of Health and Human Services
  1981    *Services to Victims of Domestic Violence: A Review of Selected Department of Health and Human Services Programs.* Washington, D.C.: Office of the Assistant Secretary for Planning and Evaluation.
  1986    *Compendium of Federal Activities Relating to the Prevention and Treatment of Family Violence.* Washington, D.C.: Office of the Assistant Secretary for Planning and Evaluation.
  1995    *Healthy People 2000: Midcourse Review and 1995 Revisions.* Washington, D.C: U.S. Public Health Service.
U.S. General Accounting Office
  1990    *Prospective Evaluation Methods: The Prospective Evaluation Synthesis.* Program Evaluation and Methodology Division. Washington, D.C.: U.S. General Accounting Office.
  1991a   *Child Abuse Prevention: Status of the Challenge Grant Program.* HRD91-95. Washington, D.C.: U.S. General Accounting Office.
  1991b   *Elder Abuse: Effectiveness of Reporting Laws and Other Factors.* Washington, D.C.: U.S. General Accounting Office.
  1993    *Foster Care. Services to Prevent Out-of-Home Placements Are Limited by Funding Barriers.* Washington, D.C.: U.S. General Accounting Office.
  1996    *Sex Offender Treatment: Research Results Inconclusive About What Works to Reduce Recidivism.* GGD96-137. Washington, D.C.: U.S. General Accounting Office.
U.S. House Select Committee on Aging
  1981    *Elder Abuse: An Examination of a Hidden Problem.* Washington, D.C.: U.S. Government Printing Office.
Van Den Berg, J.E.
  1993    Integration of individualized mental health services into the system of care for children and adolescents. *Administration and Policy in Mental Health* 20(4):247-258.
Verleur, D., R.E. Hughes, and M.D. de Rios
  1986    Enhancement of self-esteem among female adolescent incest victims: A controlled comparison. *Adolescence* 21(84):843-854.
Wagar, J.M., and M.R. Rodway
  1995    An evaluation of a group treatment approach for children who have witnessed wife abuse. *Journal of Family Violence* 10(3):295-307.
Wald, M.S., J.M. Carlsmith, and P.H. Leiderman
  1988    *Protecting Abused and Neglected Children.* Stanford, Calif.: Stanford University.
Walker, L.
  1979    *The Battered Woman.* New York: Harper & Row.
  1994    *Abused Women and Survivor Therapy.* Washington, D.C.: American Psychological Association.

Walton, E.
  1994    Intensive In-Home Family Preservation Services to Enhance Child Protective Investiga-
          tive and Assessment Decisions: The Evaluation of an Experimental Model. Unpublished
          manuscript, U.S. Department of Health and Human Services Administration on Children,
          Youth, and Families, Washington, D.C.
Walton, E., M.W. Fraser, R.E. Lewis, P.J. Pecora, and W.K. Walton
  1993    In-home family-focused reunification: An experimental study. *Child Welfare* 72(5):473-
          487.
Warshaw, C.
  1989    Limitations of the medical model in the care of battered women. *Gender and Society*
          3:506-517.
  1993    Domestic violence: Challenges to medical practice. *Journal of Women's Health* 2(1):73-
          79.
  1996    Domestic violence: Changing theory, changing practice. *Journal of the American Medi-
          cal Women's Association* 51(3):87-91, 100.
  1997    Intimate partner abuse: Developing a framework for change in medical education. *Aca-
          demic Medicine* 72(1 Suppl):S26-S37.
Watson, H., and M. Levine
  1989    Psychotherapy and mandated reporting of child abuse. *American Journal of Orthopsy-
          chiatry* 59(2):246-256.
Wauchope, B.A., and M.A. Straus
  1992    Physical punishment and physical abuse of American children: Incidence rates by age,
          gender, and occupational class. Pp. 133-148 in M.A. Straus and R.J. Gelles, eds., *Physi-
          cal Violence in American Families: Risk Factors and Adaptations to Violence in 8,145
          Families.* New Brunswick, N.J.: Transaction.
Weis, J.G.
  1989    Family violence research methodology and design. In L. Ohlin and M. Tonry, eds.,
          *Family Violence. Volume 11: Crime and Justice: An Annual Review of Research.* Chi-
          cago, Ill.: University of Chicago Press.
Weisberg, R., and M. Wald
  1984    Confidentiality laws and state efforts to protect abused or neglected children: The need
          for statutory reform. *Family Law Quarterly* 18(2):143-212.
Weiss, C.H.
  1972    *Evaluation Research: Methods of Assessing Program Effectiveness.* Englewood Cliffs,
          N.J.: Prentice-Hall.
  1995    Nothing as practical as good theory: Exploring theory-based evaluation for comprehen-
          sive community initiatives for children and families. In J.P. Connell, A.C. Kubisch, L.B.
          Schorr, and C.H. Weiss, eds., *New Approaches to Evaluating Community Initiatives.*
          New York: The Aspen Institute.
Weiss, H., and R. Halpern
  1991    *Community-Based Family Support and Education Programs: Something Old or Some-
          thing New?* New York: Columbia University Press.
Weissbourd, B., and S. Kagan, eds.
  1994    *Putting Families First: America's Family Support Movement and the Challenge of
          Change.* San Francisco, Calif.: Jossey-Bass.
Weisz, V.G.
  1995    *Children and Adolescents in Need.* Thousand Oaks, Calif.: Sage.
Wellman, B.
  1981    Applying network analysis to the study of support. Pp. 171-200 in B.H. Gottlieb, ed.,
          *Social Networks and Social Support.* Beverly Hills, Calif.: Sage.

Wells, K., and D. Biegel
1992     Intensive family preservation services research: Current status and future agenda. *Social Work* 28(1):21-27.
Wesch, D., and J. Lutzker
1991     A comprehensive 5-year evaluation of Project 12 Ways: An ecobehavioral program for treating and preventing child abuse and neglect. *Journal of Family Violence* 6(1):17-35.
Westman, J.C.
1995     A better way to reduce AFDC costs. *Wisconsin Medical Journal* 94(3):132.
Wheeler, C.E., G. Reuter, D. Struckman-Johnson, and Y.Y. Yuan
1992     *Evaluation of State of Connecticut Intensive Family Preservation Services: Phase V Annual Report.* Sacramento, Calif.: Walter R. McDonald and Associates.
Whipple, E.E., and C. Webster-Stratton
1991     The role of parental stress in physically abusive families. *Child Abuse and Neglect* 15(3):279-291.
Whitcomb, D.
1992     *When the Victim Is a Child,* 2nd ed. Washington, D.C.: National Institute of Justice.
Whiteman, M., D. Fanshel, and J.F. Grundy
1987     Cognitive-behavioral interventions aimed at anger of parents at risk of child abuse. *Social Work* 32(6):469-474.
Whittaker, J.K., and S.I. Pfeiffer
1994     Research priorities for residential group care. *Child Welfare* 73(5):583-602.
Widom, C.S.
1988     Sampling biases and implications for child abuse research. *American Journal of Orthopsychiatry* 58(2):260-270.
1989a    Does violence beget violence? A critical examination of the literature. *Psychological Bulletin* 106(1):3-28.
1989b    The cycle of violence. *Science* 244:160-166.
1989c    Child abuse, neglect, and violent criminal behavior. *Criminology* 27:251-271.
1991     The role of placement experiences in mediating the criminal consequences of early childhood victimization. *American Journal of Orthopsychiatry* 61(2):195-209.
1992     Child abuse and alcohol use and abuse. Pp. 291-314 in S.E. Martin, ed., *Alcohol and Interpersonal Violence: Fostering Multidisciplinary Perspectives.* Rockville, Md.: National Institute on Alcohol Abuse and Alcoholism.
Widom, C.S., and M.A. Ames
1994     Criminal consequences of childhood sexual victimization. *Child Abuse and Neglect* 18(4):303-318.
Wilber, K.H.
1991     Alternatives to conservatorship: The role of daily money management services. *Gerontologist* 31(2):150-155.
Williams, O.J., and R.L. Becker
1994     Domestic partner abuse treatment programs and cultural competence: The results of a national survey. *Violence and Victims* 9(3):287-296.
Wilson, W.J.
1996     *When Work Disappears.* New York: Simon and Schuster.
Wiltse, K.
1985     Foster care: An overview. Pp. 563-584 in J. Laird and A. Hartman, eds., *A Handbook of Child Welfare: Context, Knowledge, and Practice.* New York: The Free Press.
Wolf, B.M.
1983     Social Network Form: Information and Scoring Instructions. Unpublished manuscript, Temple University, Philadelphia, Penn.

Wolf, R.S.
   1996    Understanding elder abuse and neglect. *Aging* 367:4-9.
Wolf, R.S., and K.A. Pillemer
   1994    What's new in elder abuse programming? Four bright ideas. *Gerontologist* 34(1):126-
           129.
Wolf, R.S., M.A. Godkin, and K.A. Pillemer
   1984    *Elder Abuse and Neglect: Final Report from Three Model Projects.* Worcester: Univer-
           sity Center on Aging, University of Massachusetts Medical Center.
Wolfe, D.A.
   1987    *Child Abuse: Implications for Child Development and Psychopathology.* Newbury Park,
           Calif.: Sage.
   1991    *Preventing Physical and Emotional Abuse of Children.* New York: Guilford Press.
   1994    The role of intervention and treatment services in the prevention of child abuse and
           neglect. Chapter 6 in G. Melton and F.D. Barry, eds., *Protecting Children from Abuse
           and Neglect.* New York: Guilford Press.
Wolfe, D.A., and C. Wekerle
   1993    Treatment strategies for child abuse and neglect: A critical progress report. *Clinical
           Psychology Review* 15:473-500.
Wolfe, D.A., J. Aragona, K. Kaufman, and J. Sandler
   1980    The importance of adjudication in the treatment of child abusers: Some preliminary find-
           ings. *Child Abuse and Neglect* 4(2):127-135.
Wolfe, D.A., T. MacPherson, R.L. Blount, and V.V. Wolfe
   1986    Evaluation of a brief intervention for educating school children in awareness of physical
           and sexual abuse. *Child Abuse and Neglect* 10(1):85-92.
Wollert, R.
   1988    An evaluation of a communications training program within a self-help group for sexu-
           ally abusive parents. *Community Mental Health Journal* 24(3):229-235.
Wolock, I., and B. Horowitz
   1979    Child maltreatment and material deprivation among AFDC-recipient families. *Social
           Service Review* 53(June):175-194.
   1984    Child maltreatment as a social problem: The neglect of neglect. *American Journal of
           Orthopsychiatry* 54(4):530-543.
Wood, S., K. Barton, and C. Schroeder
   1988    In-home treatment of abusive families: Cost and placement at one year. *Psychotherapy*
           25(3):409-414.
Woods, S.J., and J.C. Campbell
   1993    Posttraumatic stress in battered women: Does the diagnosis fit? *Issues in Mental Health
           Nursing* 14(2):173-186.
Worden, A.P.
   1995    Criminal Justice Innovations in Responding to Family Violence: A Review of Reforms
           and Adaptations. Paper prepared for the Committee on the Assessment of Family Vio-
           lence Interventions, National Research Council, Washington, D.C.
Wulczyn, F.H.
   1992    *Status at Birth and Infant Foster Care Placement in New York City.* Albany: New York
           State Department of Social Services.
Wurtele, S.K.
   1987    School-based sexual abuse prevention programs: A review. *Child Abuse and Neglect*
           11:483-495.

Wurtele, S.K., D.A. Saslawsky, C.L. Miller, S.R. Marrs, and J.C. Britcher
  1986    Teaching personal safety skills for potential prevention of sexual abuse: A comparison of treatments. *Journal of Consulting and Clinical Psychology* 54(5):688-692.
Wurtele, S.K., L.L. Currier, E.I. Gillespie, and C.F. Franklin
  1991    The efficacy of a parent-implemented program for teaching preschoolers personal safety skills. *Behavior Therapy* 22:69-83.
Wyatt, G.E., and S.D. Peters
  1986    Issues in the definition of child sexual abuse in prevalence research. *Child Abuse and Neglect* 10:231-240.
Yllo, K.A.
  1993    Through a feminist lens. Gender, power, and violence. Pp. 47-62 in R.J. Gelles and D.R. Loseke, eds., *Current Controversies on Family Violence*. Newbury Park, Calif.: Sage.
Yuan, Y.Y., W.R. McDonald, C.E. Wheeler, D. Struckman-Johnson, and M. Rivest
  1990    *Evaluation of AB 1562 In-Home Care Demonstration Projects: Volume I, Final Report.* Sacramento, Calif.: Walter R. McDonald and Associates.
Zellman, G.L.
  1990    Report decision-making patterns among mandated child abuse reporters. *Child Abuse and Neglect* 14:325-336.
  1992    The impact of case characteristics on child abuse reporting decisions. *Child Abuse and Neglect* 16(1):57-74.
Zimmerman, R.B.
  1982    Foster care in retrospect. *Tulane Studies in Social Welfare* Vol. 14.
Zorza, J.
  1994    Women battering: High costs and the state of the law. *Clearinghouse Review* Special Issue 1994:383-395.
Zuckerman, B., M. Augustyn, B.M. Groves, and S. Parker
  1995    Silent victims revisited: The special case of domestic violence. *Pediatrics* 96:511-513.
Zuravin, S.J.
  1991    Research definitions of child physical abuse and neglect: Current problems. In R. Starr and D. Wolfe, eds., *The Effects of Child Abuse and Neglect: Issues and Research*. New York: Guilford Press.

# APPENDIX
# A

# Site Visit Resources

The following individuals and organizations provided resource materials and shared their expertise with the committee and staff members during a series of site visits conducted from January to May 1996 in the cities of Boston, Dallas, Miami, New York, and Seattle. We gratefully acknowledge their assistance.

**Boston**

Doreen Spence, Social Worker, Elder Abuse Assessment Team
Lisa Gary, Director, Safe Transitions
Beth Israel Hospital

Captain Robert Dunford, Boston Police Department

Patricia Cullen, Project Director
Michele Pouget-Drum, Project Director
Debra Robbin, Project Director
Kimberly Smith-Cofield, Executive Director
Casa Myrna Vazquez, Inc., Boston

Maggie Costa, Teacher
Sister Marie Morris, Counselor
Cathedral Grammar School, Boston

Betty Singer, Director
Child Protection Team, Children's Hospital, Boston

Carmen Del Rosario, Advocate
Debra Drumm, Advocate
Cyntia Lugo, Advocate
Tina Nappi, Advocate
Karen Patykewich, Advocate
Jennifer  Robertson, Director
Graciela Valencia, Advocate
Project Awake, Children's Hospital, Boston

Betsy Groves, Director
Judy Hunt, Social Worker
Steven Parker, Pediatrician
Barry Zuckerman, Chief of Pediatrics
Child Witness to Violence Project, Boston

Joyce Collier, Therapist
Robb Johnson, Victim Advocate
Victim Recovery Program, Fenway Community Health Center, Boston

Suzin Bartley, Executive Director
The Massachusetts Children's Trust Fund, Boston

Beth Leventhal
Network for Battered Lesbians, Boston

Andy Klein, Chief Probation Officer
Quincy Court Model Domestic Violence Program, Quincy, MA

Curt Rogers
Support Services for Gay Male Victims of Violence, Cambridge

## Dallas

Commissioner Mike Cantrell
Tracy Enna
Commissioner's Court, Dallas

Cindy Dyer
The Honorable Marshall Gandy

Vicki Isaacks, Assistant District Attorney
Jeanette Lafontaine, Victim Advocate
Anita Kinne, Victim Witness Unit, Kids in Court
Frank Crowley Court House, Dallas

Claudia Byrnes, Executive Director
Betsy Myers
Fred Rich
Dallas Children's Advocacy Center

M.R. Price, Assistant Chief of Police
W.R. Rollins, Executive Assistant Chief of Police
Dorothy Scott, Youth and Family Crimes Bureau
Judith Stewart, Youth and Family Crimes Bureau
Sergeant Ches Williams, Youth and Family Crimes Bureau
Dallas Police Department

Veletta Forsyth-Lill
Sherry Lundberg
Diane McGauley, Director
Sharon Obregon
The Family Place, Dallas

Jan Langbein
Genesis Shelter, Dallas

Virginia Patrizi
Legal Services of North Texas, Dallas

Joan Holland, Adult Protective Services
Joellen Goff, Lead Program Director
Diane Kellor, Child Protective Services
Texas Department of Protective and Regulatory Services, Dallas

## Miami

David McGriff, Director
Connie McNellis, Supervisor
Advocate Program, Miami

The Honorable Linda Dakis
The Honorable Joseph Farina
The Honorable Amy Karan

The Honorable Lester Langer
The Honorable Mark King Leban
Dade County Domestic Violence Court, Eleventh Judicial Circuit, Miami

Lauren Lazarus, Assistant Director
Ivon Mesa, Assistant Director
Domestic Violence Court Operations, Miami

Robert Morgan, Director
Mailman Center for Child Development, Miami

Joan Farr, Program Director
Family and Victim Services
Metro-Dade Department of Human Resources, Office of Human Development,
    Miami

Joyce Henry, Director
Inn Transition, North Miami

**New York**

Tracy Schneider, Associate Executive Director
North Central Bronx Hospital, Bronx, NY

Rea Stein, Deputy Borough Director
Administration for Children's Services, Brooklyn, NY

Vanessa Amato, Director
Social Work Services, Coney Island Hospital, Brooklyn, NY

Rhonnie Jaus
Sex Crime and Special Victims Bureau, Kings County District Attorney's
    Office, Brooklyn, NY

Pat Henry, Mayor's Office of the Criminal Justice Coordinator, Brooklyn, NY

Carol Anderson, Domestic Violence/Rape Crisis Advocate, New York

Frances Gautieri, Director of Social Work
Margot Williams, Domestic Violence Coordinator
Bellevue Hospital Center, New York

Susan Xenarios
Crime Victims Treatment Center, New York

Cecile Noel
Health and Hospitals Corporation, New York

Susan Urban, Acting Assistant Deputy Commissioner,
HRA- Crisis Programs, New York

Barbara Blackman, Domestic Violence Unit
John Lawson, Domestic Violence Unit
Lewis Caniglia, Special Operations Officer
24th Precinct, New York Police Department

Susan Morley, Special Victims Liaison Unit
New York Police Department

Susan Wilt, Director of Epidemiology and Surveillance
New York City Department of Health

Stacey Donegan, Emergency Medicine Resident
Steven Lynn, Director, Department of Emergency Medicine
Suzanne Pavel, Clinical Specialist
Roberto Robinson, Administrative Manager
Jane Seskin
Roosevelt Hospital, New York

Judith Urrutia, Social Work Department
Gregg Husk, Director, Department of Emergency Medicine
Doriane Mercado, Clinical Coordinator
Fernando Miranda, Administrative Manager
Barbara O'Neill, Corporate Administrator, Department of Emergency Medicine
Ana Rodriguez, Domestic Violence Advocate
St. Luke's Hospital, New York

Frances Anastasi, Director, Domestic Violence Housing
Lucy Friedman, Executive Director
Maureen Geoglis, Deputy Director of Police Programs
Violet Hawkins, Director, Domestic Violence Division
Chris O'Sullivan, Senior Research Associate
Lisanne Rogers, Volunteer Attorney, Westside Office Legal Project
Lorraine Shimoler, Unit Coordinator, Domestic Violence Prevention Project
Ed Stubbing, Director, Police Programs

Kim Susser, Staff Attorney
Julie Domonkos, Legal Project Director, Westside Community Office
Janet Loflin Lee, Westside Community Office
Jane Barker, Director, Brooklyn Child Advocacy Center
Victim Services, Inc., New York

## Seattle

Tamara Brown, Emergency Assistance, Alternative Response System
Gail Dubin, Chief of Staff, Alternative Response System
Irene Eckfeldt, Social Worker/Case Manager, Alternative Response System
Cathy Peters, Regional Director, South King County
Barbara Phalen, Public Health Nurse/Case Manager, Alternative Response
    System
Alice Probert, Program Manager, Alternative Response System
Ann Shirk, Emergency Assistance, Alternative Response System
Amy Vince-Cruz, Public Health Nurse/Case Manager, Alternative Response
    System
Susan Williams, Social Worker Case Manager, Alternative Response System
Catholic Community Services, Kent, WA

Patrick Gogerty, Executive Director
Marlene Carter, Program Director, Patrick Grogerty Branch
Sharon Cryan, Case Manager, Patrick Grogerty Branch
Deloris Culcleasure, Program Supervisor, Patrick Grogerty Branch
Margaret Kennedy, Associate Director, Patrick Grogerty Branch
Beth Nordstrom, Case Manager, Patrick Grogerty Branch
Carol Opoku, Case Manager, Patrick Grogerty Branch
Stacey Walters, Case Manager, Patrick Grogerty Branch
Beth Larson, Case Manager, Eli Creekmore Branch
Nell Robinson, Case Manager, Eli Creekmore Branch
Debra Ronnholm, Program Director, Eli Creekmore Branch
Stephanie Szot, Case Manager, Eli Creekmore Branch
Childhaven, Seattle

Debbie Allen, Chief, Domestic Violence Unit
Nate Janes, Special Assault Unit
Mark Kampf, Special Assault Unit
Rose Mc Mann, Special Assault Unit
Michelle Mullendorf, Special Assault Unit
Seattle Police Department

Ken Patis, Supervisor
Child Protective Services, Washington State Department of Children and
Families Services, Kent, WA

Patrick Noon
King County Juvenile Court, Seattle

April Gerlock, Coordinator
Domestic Violence Program, American Lake Division, VA Puget Sound Health
Care System, Tacoma, WA

Anne Ganley, Director
Batterer Treatment Program, Department of Veterans' Affairs, Medical Center,
Seattle

# APPENDIX
# B

# Biographical Sketches

**PATRICIA A. KING** (*Chair*) is the Carmack Waterhouse professor of law, medicine, ethics, and public policy at the Georgetown University Law Center. She is a senior research fellow with the Kennedy Institute of Ethics. She has served on several committees of the National Research Council (NRC) and the Institute of Medicine (IOM), including the Commission on Behavioral and Social Sciences and Education (1992-1995), the IOM Committee to Study the Social and Ethical Impact of Biomedicine (1992-1994), the IOM Committee on Assessing Genetic Risks (1991-1993), and the IOM Board on Health and Science Policy (1989-1994). King has served as deputy assistant attorney general, Civil Division, of the U.S. Department of Justice; on the faculty of the University of Michigan at Ann Arbor; and as deputy director of the Office of Civil Rights, U.S. Department of Health, Education, and Welfare. She has a J.D. from Harvard Law School and a B.A. from Wheaton College.

**JACQUELYN C. CAMPBELL** is the Anna D. Wolf endowed professor at the Johns Hopkins University School of Nursing. She was formerly a member of the faculty of Wayne State University and served as a support group facilitator and counselor at several shelters for battered women in Detroit and in New York. Campbell has also been a child and adolescent therapist, a LaMaze instructor, a pediatric nurse, and a high school nurse. She has received awards from the University of Rochester School of Nursing, the Midwest Nursing Research Society, the Michigan Association of Governing Boards of State Universities, the Kellogg National Leadership Fellowship, Wayne State University, the American Academy of Nursing, and Duke University. Campbell was one of six nurse researchers in the country featured in the Sigma Theta Tau International Nurse Researchers "CAMEO" video series. She has a Ph.D. from the University of Rochester School of Nursing and a B.S.N. from the Duke University School of Nursing.

**ROSEMARY CHALK** (*Study Director*) is the deputy director of the Board on Children, Youth, and Families of the National Research Council and the Institute of Medicine. She is directing other studies and project initiatives focused on youth development and child welfare. She has previously directed studies on child abuse, research ethics, and science and human rights for the National Academy of Sciences and the Institute of Medicine. Chalk was the staff director of the Committee on Scientific Freedom and Responsibility of the American Association for the Advancement of Science during its formative years. She has edited an anthology of articles on social responsibility and academic freedom in science, titled *Science, Technology, and Society: Emerging Relationships.* She has a B.A. from the University of Cincinnati.

**DAVID S. CORDRAY** is the chair of the Department of Human Resources and professor of public policy and psychology at Vanderbilt University Peabody College. He has previously been a member of the faculty of Northwestern University and also worked in the U.S. Government Accounting Office in Washington, D.C. He has served as president of the American Evaluation Association and also on the National Academy of Public Administration's Panel on the Status of Evaluation in the Federal Government. Cordray has a B.A. and an M.A. from California State University, Northridge, and a Ph.D. from the Claremont Graduate School at Northwestern University.

**NANCY CROWELL** (*Staff Officer*) is a staff officer in the Commission on Behavioral and Social Sciences and Education in the National Research Council. She has organized a number of workshops for the Board on Children, Youth, and Families, and previously she staffed National Research Council studies on violence against women and risk communication and policy implications of greenhouse warming. Trained as a pediatric audiologist, Crowell worked in a demonstration project for preschool hearing-impaired children and their families at Ball State University. She also worked on several political campaigns and for a political polling and consulting firm prior to joining the National Research Council staff. She has a B.S. from St. Lawrence University and an M.A. from Vanderbilt University.

**KATHERINE DARKE** (*Research Assistant*) is a research assistant in the Commission on Behavioral and Social Sciences and Education of the National Research Council. She has an M.P.P. and a B.A. in government from the College of William and Mary.

**DIANA J. ENGLISH** is the research director of the Children's Services Research Unit in the Children's Administration of the Washington State Department of Social and Health Services. She has served on the faculty of the University of Washington and Western Washington University. She has worked as a casework supervisor and caseworker, counselor, and social worker in the United States and in England. Her research fields include child abuse and neglect, risk assessment, and decision making in child protective services. English has B.A. and M.S.W. degrees from Sacramento State University and a Ph.D. in social welfare from the University of Washington.

**JEFFREY A. FAGAN** is director of the Center for Violence Research and Prevention and visiting professor at the Division of Sociomedical Sciences in the School of Public Health at Columbia University. He has previously served as a member of the faculty of the Rutgers University School of Criminal Justice and the John Jay College of Criminal Justice at the City University of New York. Fagan has worked at the New York City Criminal Justice Agency and directed the Center for Law and Public Policy at the URSA Institute in San Francisco. His research interests have focused on the relationship between race, ethnicity, and poverty. He has a Ph.D. and an M.S. from the State University of New York at Buffalo and a B.E. from New York University.

**RICHARD J. GELLES** is the director of the Family Violence Research Program and professor of sociology and psychology at the University of Rhode Island. He is the author of 19 books, including *The Violent Home* (1974), which was the first systematic empirical investigation of family violence and, most recently, *The Book of David* (1996), which advocates for reform of the child welfare system. In 1996 Gelles served as the American Sociological Association's congressional fellow in the office of the Senate Subcommittee on Youth Violence. Gelles has a Ph.D. from the University of New Hampshire, an M.A. from the University of Rochester, and an A.B. from Bates College.

**JOEL B. GREENHOUSE** is professor of statistics at Carnegie Mellon University and adjunct professor of epidemiology and psychiatry at the University of Pittsburgh. He is a member of the National Research Council's Committee on National Statistics and was a member of the NRC Panel on Statistical Issues for Research in the Combination of Information for the Committee on Applied and Theoretical Statistics. Greenhouse is a fellow of the American Statistical Association, the American Association for the Advancement of Science, and an elected member of the International Statistics Institute. He has a B.S. from the University of Maryland and Ph.D., M.P.H., and M.A. degrees from the University of Michigan.

**SCOTT HARSHBARGER** was elected attorney general of the Commonwealth of Massachusetts in November 1990 and took office in January 1991. He was reelected in 1994. He has focused public attention on issues related to urban violence, health care reform, and family violence. Prior to his election as attorney general, Harshbarger served for eight years as district attorney of Middlesex County, Massachusetts. He also served as the first general counsel to the Massachusetts State Ethics Commission, and in the Attorney General's Office as chief of the Public Protection Bureau. He was also deputy chief counsel for the Massachusetts Defenders Committee. Between periods of public service, Harshbarger worked as a trial attorney in Boston. Harshbarger has a J.D. from Harvard Law School and a B.A. from Harvard University.

**DARNELL F. HAWKINS** is a professor in the Departments of African-American Studies and Sociology and a faculty affiliate of the Criminal Justice Department at the University of Illinois at Chicago. He has previously served on the faculty of the University of North Carolina, and has taught grades three and four in the Detroit public schools. His publications have featured research on homicide among young African Americans and press coverage of homicide. Hawkins has a J.D. from the University of North Carolina, a Ph.D. from the University of Michigan, an M.A.T. from Wayne State University, and a B.A. from Kansas State University.

**CINDY LEDERMAN** is a circuit court judge in the 11th Judicial Circuit in and for Dade County, Florida, assigned to the Juvenile Division. Elected to the county court in 1990, she was a leader of the team that created Dade County's Domestic Violence Court and served as its first administrative judge until her elevation to Circuit Court in 1994. Lederman is a faculty member of the National Judicial College and is the coordinator of the National Judicial College's domestic violence course. In 1995, she was appointed by the U.S. attorney general and the secretary of the U.S. Department of Health and Human Services to the National Advisory Council on Violence Against Women. She is the immediate past president of the National Association of Women Judges. On April 15, 1997, Florida governor Lawton Chiles awarded Lederman the Governor's Peace at Home Award in recognition of her work in the field of domestic violence.

**ELIZABETH McLOUGHLIN** is the director of prevention for the San Francisco Injury Center for Research and Prevention at the University of California, San Francisco, and director of programs for the Trauma Foundation at San Francisco General Hospital. She has a faculty appointment with the Department of Surgery of the University of California at San Francisco and the School of Hygiene and Public Health of the Johns Hopkins University. She has conducted injury research for the University of Otago School of Medicine in Dunedin and

Wellington, New Zealand. Prior to her work in public health, she taught English in two high schools in New York. McLoughlin has an Sc.D. from the John Hopkins School of Hygiene and Public Health, an M.A. from the Teachers College at Columbia University, and M.A. and B.A. degrees from Manhattanville College.

**ELI NEWBERGER** is a pediatrician at Children's Hospital in Boston. In 1970 he organized the hospital's first child protection team and has directed the Interdisciplinary Research Training Program on Family Violence at Boston Children's Hospital since 1979, funded by the National Institute of Mental Health. After two years in the Peace Corps in West Africa, he returned to Boston Children's Hospital and Harvard Medical School to complete his residency in pediatrics. Newberger has served on many national boards and committees, including the U.S. Advisory Board to the National Center on Child Abuse and Neglect in the U.S. Department of Health and Human Services, the Council on Accreditation of Services for Children and Families, and the American Orthopsychiatric Association, the latter as president in 1991. He has earned degrees from Yale University (where he was a Scholar of the House in music theory), an M.D. from Yale Medical School, and an M.S. in epidemiology from the Harvard School of Public Health.

**JOY D. OSOFSKY** is professor of pediatrics and psychology at Louisiana State University Medical Center and adjunct professor of psychology at University of New Orleans. Previously, she was a member of the faculty at Cornell University and Temple University. For the past 25 years she has been involved with preventive intervention research with adolescent mothers and their infants, and, more recently, with children and families exposed to violence. In addition to work in the United States, Osofsky has consulted extensively regarding infant mental health issues in Europe, Asia, and South America. She has edited *Children in a Violent Society* (1997), the *Handbook on Infant Development* (1979, 1987), and co-edited *Hurt, Healing and Hope: Caring for Infants and Toddlers in Violent Environments.* She is past president of the World Association for Infant Mental Health, a member of the board of directors of Zero-to-Three/National Center for Infants, Toddlers, and Families, and editor of the *Infant Mental Health Journal.* She has B.A., M.A., and Ph.D. degrees from Syracuse University.

**HELEN RODRIGUEZ-TRIAS** is a pediatrician and consultant on community-based health programs. She is codirector of the Pacific Institute for Women's Health, based in Los Angeles, an organization for applied research, advocacy, and program development to advance women's health. Rodriguez-Trias has directed pediatric programs in Puerto Rico, New York City, and Newark. She has held the rank of associate professor of clinical pediatrics, teaching medical students at the University of Puerto Rico, Albert Einstein College of Medicine, the Sophie Davis Center for Biomedical Sciences at City College of New York, Columbia College of Physicians and Surgeons, and the University of Medicine and Dentistry of New Jersey. Her emphasis in teaching, research, and activism is on improving the social and economic circumstances that affect children's and women's health. She served on the IOM Committee on Unintended Pregnancy and is a past president of the American Public Health Association.

**SUSAN SCHECHTER** is clinical professor at the University of Iowa School of Social Work. She has served on the adjunct faculty of the School of Health Sciences at Hunter College, as director at the Women's Education Institute in New York, as the program coordinator of the AWAKE program at Children's Hospital in Boston, and as coordinator of the Park Slope Safe Homes Project at Children and Youth Development Services in Brooklyn, New York. Schechter has been a social worker, a psychotherapist, and director of a day care training program. She coauthored *When Love Goes Wrong* and is the author of *Women and Male Violence: The Visions and Struggles of the Battered Women's Movement.* She has an M.S.W. from the University of Illinois and a B.A. from Washington University.

**JACK P. SHONKOFF** (*liaison member*) is dean of the Florence Heller Graduate School and Samuel F. and Rose B. Gingold Professor of Human Development at Brandeis University. Shonkoff is chair of the Board on Children, Youth, and Families of the National Research Council and the Institute of Medicine. Over the past 15 years, he has served on numerous committees of the NRC and IOM, including the Panel on Child Care Policy, the Steering Group for the National Forum on the Future of Children and Families, and the Roundtable on Head Start Research. Shonkoff is the principal investigator of the Early Intervention Collaborative Study, a longitudinal investigation of the development of biologically vulnerable infants and their families. He is a member of the board of directors of Zero-to-Three and a member of the governing council of the Society for Research in Child Development. Shonkoff also serves on the core group of the John D. and Catherine T. MacArthur Research Network on Successful Pathways Through Middle Childhood. He has degrees from Cornell University and the New York University School of Medicine. He has received pediatric training at the Bronx Municipal Hospital Center and the Albert Einstein College of Medicine and completed a fellowship in developmental pediatrics at Harvard Medical School and The Children's Hospital in Boston. He has received multiple professional awards, including a Kellogg national fellowship, a fellowship from the National Center for Clinical Infant Programs, and the 1995 distinguished contribution to child advocacy award from the American Psychological Association.

**MICHAEL E. SMITH** is professor at the University of Wisconsin Law School. He was previously the president of the Vera Institute of Justice, where he had worked since 1977; formerly, he held the positions of director and deputy director in the Institute's New York and London offices. Smith is also a visiting lecturer at Yale Law School. He has worked at the Legal Action Center of the City of New York, for New York Senator Charles Goodell, and as overseas correspondent for *Time, Life,* and *Sports Illustrated.* Smith has a J.D. from Harvard Law School, a B.A. from Oxford University, which he attended as a Rhodes scholar, and a B.A. from Princeton University.

**BILL WALSH** is a 17-year veteran of the Dallas Police Department, currently assigned to the Youth and Family Crimes Division as commander of the Investigations Section. He has responsibility over the Child Abuse Unit, which is responsible for the investigation of all cases of intrafamilial physical and sexual child abuse, including fatal child abuse; the Child Exploitation Unit, which investigates cases involving sexual abuse and exploitation of children by nonfamily members; and the Family Violence Unit, which is responsible for investigating assaultive conduct between family members. Walsh started the Child Exploitation Unit in 1988 and also initiated the Crimes Against Children seminar for law enforcers that is held annually in Dallas. In 1992 he created the Dallas County Child Review Death Team, the first child fatality review team to operate independently of Child Protective Services. He is cofounder and a trustee of the Dallas Children's Advocacy Center, a nonprofit public/private partnership through which the Dallas Police Department and Dallas County Child Protective Services conduct joint investigations into allegations of child abuse and neglect.

**CAROLE L. WARSHAW** is the director of behavioral science at Cook County Hospital, Chicago, Illinois, codirector of the Hospital Crisis Intervention project, and adjunct assistant professor of psychiatry at the University of Illinois College of Medicine. She was chair of the American Medical Association's Committee to Develop Guidelines on Domestic Violence, and is a consultant to the Family Violence Prevention Fund. Warshaw is a member of Chicago Mayor Daley's Task Force on Women's Health and adviser to the Chicago Commission of Violence Against Women. She has an M.D. from Loyola University and a B.A. from Mount Holyoke College.

**CATHY SPATZ WIDOM** (*liaison member*) is professor of criminal justice and psychology at the State University of New York at Albany. She is a former faculty member in psychology and social relations at Harvard University and in criminal justice and psychology at Indiana University. She received the 1989 American Association for the Advancement of Science Behavioral Research Prize and was elected a fellow of the American Psychological Association in 1993. She has published extensively on topics that include child abuse and neglect, juvenile delinquency, female criminality, and violence. Her current research interests focus on the intergenerational transmission of violence and the long-term consequences of early childhood abuse and neglect. She has a Ph.D. from Brandeis University.

**ROSALIE S. WOLF** is executive director of the Institute on Aging at the Memorial Hospital in Worcester, Massachusetts, and assistant professor in the Department of Medicine and Community Medicine and Family Practice at the University of Massachusetts Medical Center. Wolf has focused on the study of elder abuse in domestic settings over the last decade. She has directed elder abuse projects and completed evaluations of seven state projects on the subject. Wolf is the president of the National Committee for the Prevention of Elder Abuse and serves on the management team of the National Center on Elder Abuse in Washington, D.C. In addition, she is coeditor of the *Journal of Elder Abuse & Neglect.* Wolf has a Ph.D. from the Florence Heller Graduate School at Brandeis University and a B.S. from the University of Wisconsin.

# Index

# C

# Other Reports from
# the Board on Children, Youth, and Families

*Improving Schooling for Language-Minority Students: A Research Agenda* (1997)

*New Findings on Welfare and Children's Development: Summary of a Research Briefing* (1997)

*Youth Development and Neighborhood Influences: Challenges and Opportunities: Summary of a Workshop* (1996)

*Paying Attention to Children in a Changing Health Care System: Summaries of Workshops* (with the Board on Health Promotion and Disease Prevention of the Institute of Medicine) (1996)

*Beyond the Blueprint: Directions for Research on Head Start's Families: Report of Three Roundtable Meetings* (1996)

*Child Care for Low-Income Families: Directions for Research: Summary of a Workshop* (1996)

*Service Provider Perspectives on Family Violence Interventions: Proceedings of a Workshop* (1995)

"Immigrant Children and Their Families: Issues for Research and Policy" in *The Future of Children* (1995)

*Integrating Federal Statistics on Children* (with the Committee on National Statistics of the National Research Council) (1995)

*Child Care for Low-Income Families: Summary of Two Workshops* (1995)

*New Findings on Children, Families, and Economic Self-Sufficiency: Summary of a Research Briefing* (1995)

*The Impact of War on Child Health in the Countries of the Former Yugoslavia: A Workshop Summary* (with the Institute of Medicine and the Office of International Affairs of the National Research Council) (1995)

*Cultural Diversity and Early Education: Report of a Workshop* (1994)

*Benefits and Systems of Care for Maternal and Child Health: Workshop Highlights* (with the Board on Health Promotion and Disease Prevention of the Institute of Medicine) (1994)

*Protecting and Improving the Quality of Children Under Health Care Reform: Workshop Highlights* (with the Board on Health Promotion and Disease Prevention of the Institute of Medicine) (1994)

*America's Fathers and Public Policy: Report of a Workshop* (1994)

*Violence and the American Family: Report of a Workshop* (1994)